Barbara O'Neill Natural Herbal Remedies Complete Collection

The Ultimate Guide to Knowing ALL of Dr. Barbara O'Neill's Studies and the Non-Toxic Lifestyle.

A Mind-Opening Book

Roberta Lane

Take your bonus! Scan this QR Code, clic on Link you see and follow the instructions:

PREFACE

In a world where modern medicine and pharmaceuticals dominate, the ancient wisdom of natural remedies often goes overlooked. Yet, there remains a timeless truth in the healing power of nature, a truth that has been harnessed and passed down through generations. This book, "Barbara O'Neill Natural Herbal Remedies," seeks to reconnect us with that wisdom, offering a comprehensive guide to the potent and nurturing world of herbal medicine.

Barbara O'Neill, a renowned naturopath and passionate advocate of natural health, has dedicated her life to understanding and teaching the profound benefits of natural remedies. Her extensive experience and deep knowledge are the backbone of this book, which aims to provide practical, effective, and safe herbal solutions for common ailments.

This book is more than just a compilation of herbal recipes; it is a journey into the heart of natural healing. From the soothing properties of chamomile to the invigorating effects of ginseng, Barbara O'Neill introduces us to a diverse array of herbs, each with unique properties and uses. She meticulously explains the science behind these remedies, ensuring that readers not only know how to use them but also understand why they work.

In these pages, you will find remedies for a wide range of conditions—everything from minor cuts and bruises to more complex health issues like chronic inflammation and stress management. Each remedy is crafted with care, emphasizing the importance of quality ingredients and proper preparation techniques. Barbara's holistic approach integrates these remedies into a lifestyle of wellness, encouraging readers to adopt habits that support overall health and vitality.

The book is organized for ease of use, with clear instructions and helpful tips that make incorporating herbal remedies into your daily routine straightforward and accessible. Whether you are a seasoned herbalist or a curious beginner, you will find this book to be an invaluable resource.

In sharing her knowledge, Barbara O'Neill hopes to empower individuals to take control of their health naturally. By turning to the earth's bounty, we can find gentle yet powerful ways to heal, rejuvenate, and thrive.

May this book inspire you to explore the wonders of natural herbal remedies and discover the profound benefits they offer. Here's to a journey of health, healing, and harmony with nature.

Table of Contents

BOOK 1:

Introduction to Herbal Medicine: History, Principles, and Benefits of Medicinal Herbs

The History of Herbal Medicine

Herbal medicine, also known as botanical medicine or phytotherapy, is one of the oldest forms of medical treatment known to humanity. The history of herbal medicine is a rich tapestry woven from the threads of various cultures, each contributing unique knowledge and practices to the collective understanding of plant-based healing. This introduction explores the evolution of herbal medicine from ancient times to the present day, highlighting its enduring significance and the cultural diversity that shapes its practice.

Ancient Practices and Early Records

The practice of using plants for medicinal purposes is as old as humanity itself. Early humans, driven by necessity and guided by observation, experimentation, and instinct, discovered the healing properties of various plants. This knowledge, passed down through generations, laid the foundation for the complex systems of herbal medicine we recognize today. The following sections delve into the ancient practices and early records of herbal medicine across different cultures.

Paleolithic Era: The Dawn of Herbal Medicine

Archaeological evidence suggests that the use of medicinal plants dates to the Paleolithic era, approximately 60,000 years ago. The Shanidar Cave in Iraq, where Neanderthal remains were discovered alongside pollen from medicinal plants, provides one of the earliest records of herbal medicine. These findings indicate that even early humans possessed an understanding of the therapeutic properties of certain plants.

Sumerians: The First Herbal Practitioners

The Sumerians, who lived in Mesopotamia around 3000 BCE, are among the earliest known practitioners of herbal medicine. They documented their herbal knowledge on clay tablets, creating some of the first written records of medicinal plants. These tablets list hundreds of plants, including myrrh, opium, and thyme, and describe their uses in treating various ailments. The Sumerians' sophisticated approach to herbal medicine laid the groundwork for future civilizations.

Ancient Egypt: A Flourishing Herbal Tradition

In ancient Egypt, herbal medicine was an integral part of medical practice. The Egyptians compiled extensive medical texts that detailed the use of herbs for healing. One of the most famous of these texts is the Ebers Papyrus, dating to around 1550 BCE. This comprehensive medical document contains over 700 remedies, including numerous herbal preparations for ailments ranging from digestive issues to skin conditions.

Egyptian healers, known as "swnw," were skilled in the use of medicinal plants and often combined them with other treatments, such as surgery and spiritual healing. The use of garlic, honey, and castor oil in Egyptian medicine highlights their advanced understanding of herbal remedies.

Traditional Chinese Medicine: Ancient Wisdom

Traditional Chinese Medicine (TCM) has a history spanning over 2,000 years. Ancient Chinese texts, such as the "Shennong Bencao Jing" (The Divine Farmer's Materia Medica), compiled during the Han dynasty, document the use of hundreds of medicinal plants. Shennong, a mythical emperor, is credited with tasting hundreds of herbs to determine their properties and effects.

TCM emphasizes the balance of Yin and Yang and the flow of Qi (vital energy) in maintaining health. Herbs are categorized based on their energetic properties, such as cooling or warming, and their ability to affect different organs and systems in the body. Key herbs like ginseng, ginger, and licorice root have been used for centuries to treat a wide range of conditions.

Ayurveda: The Science of Life

Ayurveda, originating in India more than 3,000 years ago, is one of the world's oldest holistic healing systems. The foundational texts of Ayurveda, the "Charaka Samhita" and "Sushruta Samhita," provide detailed guides to herbal treatments, dietary practices, and lifestyle choices for promoting health and longevity.

Ayurveda categorizes herbs based on their tastes (rasa), effects on the body (virya), and post-digestive effects (vipaka). Herbal formulations in Ayurveda are designed to balance the body's three doshas (Vata, Pitta, and Kapha) and promote overall well-being. Turmeric, ashwagandha, and tulsi are among the many herbs used in Ayurvedic medicine.

Greco-Roman Tradition: Bridging East and West

The Greeks and Romans made significant contributions to herbal medicine, with figures like Hippocrates and Galen advancing medical knowledge. Hippocrates, often called the "Father of Medicine," emphasized the importance of diet and lifestyle in maintaining health and used herbs extensively in his treatments.

Dioscorides, a Greek physician in the Roman army, wrote "De Materia Medica," a seminal work that cataloged over 600 medicinal plants and their uses. This text, compiled in the first century CE, became a cornerstone of herbal medicine in Europe for centuries. Dioscorides' work bridged the gap between ancient Eastern and Western herbal traditions.

Native American Herbalism: A Deep Connection to Nature

Indigenous peoples of the Americas possess a profound understanding of their local environments and utilize a wide variety of plants for medicinal purposes. Native American herbalism is characterized by a deep spiritual connection to nature and a holistic approach to healing.

Different tribes have their own unique herbal practices, often passed down orally through generations. Commonly used plants include echinacea for immune support, willow bark for pain relief, and sage for purification. Native American healers, known as medicine men or women, play a crucial role in preserving and transmitting this knowledge.

The history of herbal medicine is a testament to humanity's enduring relationship with the natural world. From the Paleolithic era to the sophisticated systems of ancient civilizations, the use of medicinal plants has been a constant thread in the tapestry of human history. These early practices and records form the foundation of modern herbal medicine, reminding us of the timeless wisdom embedded in nature. As we continue to explore and understand the complex chemistry of medicinal herbs, we honor the legacy of those who first discovered and documented their healing powers.

Herbal Medicine in Different Cultures

Herbal medicine has been an integral part of human history, with each culture developing its own unique system of healing based on local flora, spiritual beliefs, and medical philosophies. These diverse traditions have contributed to a rich global heritage of herbal knowledge. This section explores the herbal practices of several major cultures, highlighting their distinct approaches and key medicinal plants.

Traditional Chinese Medicine (TCM): Ancient Wisdom from the East

Traditional Chinese Medicine (TCM) has a history spanning over 2,000 years. Rooted in the philosophy of balance and harmony, TCM emphasizes the interplay between Yin and Yang and the flow of Qi (vital energy) through the body. Herbs play a crucial role in TCM, often used in combination to create balanced formulas.

- ✓ **Key Concepts:** In TCM, herbs are classified by their energetic properties (cooling, warming, neutral), flavors (sweet, sour, bitter, salty, pungent), and their effects on specific organs and meridians (energy pathways).
- ✓ **Key Herbs:**

    - **Ginseng (Panax ginseng):** Known for its energy-boosting and adaptogenic properties.
    - **Ginger (Zingiber officinale):** Used for its warming effects and to aid digestion.
    - **Licorice Root (Glycyrrhiza glabra):** Often used as a harmonizing herb in formulas and for its anti-inflammatory properties.
    - **Astragalus (Astragalus membranaceus):** Known for its immune-boosting and energy-enhancing effects.

Ayurveda: The Science of Life from India

Ayurveda, originating in India over 3,000 years ago, is one of the world's oldest holistic healing systems. Ayurveda focuses on maintaining balance in the body through diet, lifestyle, and herbal treatments, tailored to the individual's constitution (dosha).

- **Key Concepts:** Ayurvedic herbs are categorized by their tastes (rasa), potency (virya), and post-digestive effects (vipaka). The primary goal is to balance the three doshas: Vata, Pitta, and Kapha.
- **Key Herbs:**
  - **Turmeric (Curcuma longa):** Renowned for its anti-inflammatory and antioxidant properties.
  - **Ashwagandha (Withania somnifera):** An adaptogen used to reduce stress and improve vitality.
  - **Tulsi (Ocimum sanctum):** Known as holy basil, it is used for its immune-boosting and stress-relieving properties.
  - **Neem (Azadirachta indica):** Used for its antibacterial and detoxifying effects.

Greco-Roman Tradition: Bridging East and West

The Greeks and Romans significantly contributed to herbal medicine, integrating knowledge from Egypt, Persia, and India. Greek physician Hippocrates and Roman physician Galen were pivotal figures in developing the foundations of Western herbal medicine.

- **Key Concepts:** The Greeks and Romans focused on the humoral theory, which posited that health was maintained by balancing the four bodily fluids: blood, phlegm, yellow bile, and black bile.
- **Key Herbs:**
  - **Peppermint (Mentha piperita):** Used for its digestive and cooling properties.
  - **Thyme (Thymus vulgaris):** Valued for its antiseptic and respiratory benefits.
  - **Oregano (Origanum vulgare):** Known for its antimicrobial and anti-inflammatory properties.
  - **St. John's Wort (Hypericum perforatum):** Used for its antidepressant and antiviral effects.

Native American Herbalism: A Deep Connection to Nature

Indigenous peoples of the Americas have a profound understanding of their local environments and utilize a wide variety of plants for medicinal purposes. Native American herbalism is characterized by a holistic approach that integrates physical, spiritual, and environmental health.

- **Key Concepts:** Native American herbal practices emphasize a deep spiritual connection to nature, with healers often serving as both medical practitioners and spiritual guides.
- **Key Herbs:**
  - **Echinacea (Echinacea purpurea):** Used for its immune-boosting properties.
  - **Willow Bark (Salix spp.):** Known as a natural source of salicylic acid, the precursor to aspirin.
  - **Sage (Salvia spp.):** Used for purification and respiratory health.

- Goldenseal (Hydrastis canadensis): Valued for its antimicrobial and digestive properties.

Traditional African Medicine: A Rich Heritage of Healing

Traditional African medicine is a holistic discipline involving indigenous herbalism, spirituality, and community-based practices. African herbalists, or traditional healers, use a wide variety of plants to treat physical, emotional, and spiritual ailments.

- **Key Concepts:** African herbal medicine often involves the use of plant-based remedies in conjunction with rituals and spiritual practices to address the root causes of illness.
- **Key Herbs:**
  - **Rooibos (Aspalathus linearis):** Used for its antioxidant properties and overall health benefits.
  - **Devil's Claw (Harpagophytum procumbens):** Known for its anti-inflammatory and pain-relieving effects.
  - **Baobab (Adansonia digitata):** Used for its high vitamin C content and antioxidant properties.
  - **African Potato (Hypoxis hemerocallidea):** Valued for its immune-boosting and anti-inflammatory properties.

European Herbal Traditions: Medieval and Renaissance Knowledge

During the medieval and Renaissance periods, European herbal medicine flourished, integrating knowledge from ancient texts and local folk traditions. Monasteries played a crucial role in preserving and expanding herbal knowledge.

- **Key Concepts:** European herbalism during these periods focused on the use of native plants and the development of herbals (comprehensive plant guides) that documented the medicinal uses of plants.
- **Key Herbs:**
  - **Lavender (Lavandula angustifolia):** Used for its calming and antiseptic properties.
  - **Chamomile (Matricaria chamomilla):** Known for its soothing effects and digestive benefits.
  - **Nettle (Urtica dioica):** Valued for its anti-inflammatory and nutrient-rich properties.
  - **Elderberry (Sambucus nigra):** Used for its immune-boosting and antiviral effects.

The rich diversity of herbal medicine across different cultures reflects humanity's deep connection to the natural world. Each tradition offers unique insights and practices, contributing to a global tapestry of botanical knowledge. By understanding and appreciating these diverse approaches, we can better harness the healing power of plants in modern medicine.

Evolution Through the Ages

Herbal medicine has evolved significantly over millennia, adapting to cultural, scientific, and technological changes. From ancient practices rooted in observation and tradition to modern integrative approaches supported by scientific research, the journey of herbal medicine through the ages is a testament to humanity's enduring relationship with nature's pharmacy.

Ancient Civilizations: Foundations of Herbal Medicine

The earliest use of medicinal plants can be traced back to ancient civilizations such as the Sumerians, Egyptians, Chinese, and Indians. These cultures documented their herbal knowledge through various means, creating a foundational base for future generations.

- **Sumerians:** Around 3000 BCE, the Sumerians recorded their herbal knowledge on clay tablets, listing hundreds of medicinal plants like myrrh, opium, and thyme.
- **Egyptians:** The Ebers Papyrus (circa 1550 BCE) is one of the most comprehensive medical tex
- s from ancient Egypt, detailing over 700 remedies and reflecting the Egyptians' advanced understanding of herbal medicine.
- **Chinese:** Traditional Chinese Medicine (TCM) has ancient texts such as the "Shennong Bencao Jing" (The Divine Farmer's Materia Medica), which categorized hundreds of herbs based on their properties and effects.
- **Indians:** Ayurveda, with its foundational texts like the "Charaka Samhita" and "Sushruta Samhita," provided detailed guidelines on the use of herbs to balance the body's three doshas (Vata, Pitta, Kapha).

Greco-Roman Influence: Integration and Expansion

The Greco-Roman period marked a significant expansion and integration of herbal knowledge. Greek and Roman scholars synthesized information from various cultures, contributing to a more systematic understanding of medicinal plants.

- **Hippocrates:** Often called the "Father of Medicine," Hippocrates emphasized the importance of diet, lifestyle, and the use of herbs in treating diseases.
- **Dioscorides:** His work "De Materia Medica," written in the first century CE, cataloged over 600 medicinal plants and remained a key reference in Europe for centuries.
- **Galen:** A prominent Roman physician, Galen expanded on the humoral theory and developed complex herbal formulas that influenced medical practice for over a thousand years.

Middle Ages: Preservation and Transmission

During the Middle Ages, much of the herbal knowledge was preserved and transmitted through monastic traditions and Islamic scholars. Monasteries became centers of herbal learning, where monks cultivated medicinal plants and transcribed ancient texts.

- **Monastic Gardens:** Monasteries in Europe maintained extensive herb gardens and were key to preserving herbal knowledge during times of social and political turmoil.

- **Islamic Scholars:** Islamic physicians like Avicenna (Ibn Sina) wrote influential texts such as "The Canon of Medicine," which integrated Greco-Roman, Persian, and Indian herbal knowledge.

Renaissance: Revival and Exploration

The Renaissance period sparked a revival of interest in herbal medicine, driven by exploration, scientific inquiry, and the printing presses invention, which facilitated the widespread dissemination of knowledge.

- **Herbals:** Compendiums like Nicholas Culpeper's "The English Physician" made herbal knowledge more accessible to the general public, documenting the uses and preparation of various plants.
- **Botanical Gardens:** The establishment of botanical gardens in Europe promoted the study and cultivation of medicinal plants, contributing to a more systematic and scientific approach to herbal medicine.

Scientific Revolution: Systematization and Decline

The scientific revolution of the 17th and 18th centuries brought about a more systematic approach to studying medicinal plants, but also marked the beginning of a shift towards synthetic pharmaceuticals.

- **Pharmacopoeias:** The development of official pharmacopoeias standardized the use of medicinal plants and documented their properties, dosages, and preparations.
- **Chemistry and Isolation:** Advances in chemistry led to the isolation of active compounds from plants, such as morphine from opium, paving the way for the development of synthetic drugs.

19th and 20th Centuries: Modernization and Marginalization

As synthetic pharmaceuticals gained prominence, herbal medicine became marginalized in mainstream medical practice. However, interest in natural remedies persisted, particularly in rural and indigenous communities.

- **Eclectic and Thomsonian Movements:** In the United States, movements like the Eclectics and Thomsonians promoted the use of herbal medicine as an alternative to conventional medical practices of the time.
- **Herbal Pharmacies:** Despite the dominance of pharmaceuticals, herbal pharmacies and practitioners continued to operate, maintaining traditional knowledge and practices.

Late 20th Century to Present: Resurgence and Integration

The late 20th and early 21st centuries have seen a resurgence of interest in herbal medicine, driven by a growing emphasis on natural and holistic health practices and increasing scientific validation of traditional remedies.

- **Scientific Research:** Modern research has provided evidence for the efficacy of many traditional herbs, leading to their incorporation into integrative and complementary medicine.
- **Regulation and Standardization:** Efforts to regulate and standardize herbal products have improved their safety and reliability, fostering greater acceptance among healthcare professionals and the public.
- **Global Exchange:** The exchange of herbal knowledge across cultures has enriched the global pharmacopeia, integrating diverse traditions and expanding the repertoire of available remedies.

The evolution of herbal medicine reflects humanity's enduring quest for health and healing through natural means. From ancient practices and early records to modern integrative approaches, the journey of herbal medicine is a testament to the timeless wisdom embedded in the natural world. As scientific research continues to validate and expand our understanding of medicinal plants, herbal medicine remains a vital and dynamic component of global healthcare.

Modern Herbal Medicine

The modern era has witnessed a significant resurgence of interest in herbal medicine, driven by a combination of scientific validation, increasing public interest in natural and holistic health practices, and the integration of traditional knowledge with contemporary medical approaches. This chapter explores the current state of herbal medicine, highlighting its benefits, challenges, and the ongoing efforts to integrate it into modern healthcare systems.

Scientific Validation and Research

One of the key factors contributing to the renewed interest in herbal medicine is the growing body of scientific research supporting the efficacy of many traditional herbs. Advances in technology and analytical methods have allowed researchers to isolate and identify the active compounds in plants, understand their mechanisms of action, and evaluate their therapeutic potential through clinical trials.

- **Evidence-Based Approaches:** Modern herbal medicine increasingly relies on evidence-based practices, where the use of herbs is supported by scientific research and clinical evidence. This approach enhances the credibility and acceptance of herbal treatments within the medical community.
- **Phytochemistry:** The study of the chemical compounds in plants, known as phytochemistry, has revealed a wealth of bioactive substances, including alkaloids, flavonoids, terpenoids, and polyphenols, which contribute to the medicinal properties of herbs.
- **Clinical Trials:** Numerous clinical trials have demonstrated the effectiveness of herbal remedies in treating various conditions, such as echinacea for immune support, St. John's wort for depression, and turmeric for inflammation.

Integration into Healthcare Systems

The integration of herbal medicine into modern healthcare systems varies widely across the world, influenced by cultural, regulatory, and economic factors. In many countries, herbal medicine is practiced alongside conventional medicine, often as part of a broader complementary and alternative medicine (CAM) framework.

- **Complementary and Alternative Medicine (CAM):** Herbal medicine is a key component of CAM, which encompasses a wide range of therapies used alongside or instead of conventional medical treatments. CAM practitioners often take a holistic approach, addressing the physical, emotional, and spiritual aspects of health.
- **Regulatory Frameworks:** The regulation of herbal products and practitioners aims to ensure safety, quality, and efficacy. Regulatory agencies, such as the U.S. Food and Drug Administration (FDA) and the European Medicines Agency (EMA), oversee the production and marketing of herbal supplements.
- **Integration in Clinical Practice:** Some healthcare providers incorporate herbal medicine into their practice, offering patients a more holistic approach to treatment. This integration is particularly common in areas such as integrative oncology, where herbal remedies may be used to support conventional cancer treatments.

Benefits and Popularity

The popularity of herbal medicine continues to grow, driven by a range of factors that appeal to modern consumers seeking natural and holistic health solutions.

- **Natural and Holistic Approach:** Many people are drawn to herbal medicine because it aligns with a natural and holistic approach to health, emphasizing the use of whole plants and a focus on overall well-being rather than just symptom relief.
- **Cultural and Historical Appeal:** The rich cultural and historical heritage of herbal medicine adds to its appeal, offering a connection to traditional healing practices and ancestral wisdom.
- **Accessibility and Affordability:** Herbal remedies are often more accessible and affordable than conventional pharmaceuticals, making them an attractive option for individuals seeking cost-effective health solutions.

Challenges and Considerations

Despite its benefits, the practice of modern herbal medicine faces several challenges and considerations that must be addressed to ensure its safe and effective use.

- **Quality and Standardization:** Variability in the quality and potency of herbal products is a major concern. Ensuring consistent quality through standardization and good manufacturing practices (GMP) is essential for consumer safety.
- **Interactions and Side Effects:** While generally considered safe, some herbs can interact with medications or cause side effects. Educating both practitioners and consumers about these potential risks is crucial.
- **Regulatory and Legal Issues:** The regulatory landscape for herbal medicine varies widely between countries, with some regions having more stringent regulations than

others. Navigating these regulations can be complex for both practitioners and manufacturers.
- **Scientific Rigor:** While many herbs have been studied extensively, others lack sufficient scientific evidence to support their use. Ongoing research and rigorous clinical trials are needed to build a robust evidence base for all herbal treatments.

The Future of Herbal Medicine

The future of herbal medicine looks promising, with ongoing research and innovation driving new discoveries and applications. Several trends and developments are shaping the future landscape of herbal medicine.

- **Personalized Medicine:** Advances in genomics and personalized medicine are paving the way for individualized herbal treatments tailored to a person's genetic profile and specific health needs.
- **Sustainability and Conservation:** As demand for herbal products grows, ensuring sustainable sourcing and conservation of medicinal plants is critical to preserving biodiversity and protecting endangered species.
- **Integration with Conventional Medicine:** Efforts to integrate herbal medicine with conventional medical practices are likely to continue, promoting a more holistic and patient-centered approach to healthcare.
- **Technological Advancements:** Innovations in extraction and formulation technologies are enhancing the efficacy and safety of herbal products, making them more appealing to both consumers and healthcare providers.

Modern herbal medicine represents a dynamic and evolving field that bridges ancient wisdom with contemporary science. As research continues to validate the therapeutic potential of medicinal plants, and as regulatory frameworks and integration efforts advance, herbal medicine is poised to play an increasingly significant role in global healthcare. By embracing both the traditional knowledge and modern innovations, we can harness the full potential of herbal medicine to promote health and well-being in the 21st century.

Basic Principles of Medicinal Herbs

Medicinal herbs have been used for centuries to promote health and treat various ailments, with their efficacy grounded in both traditional wisdom and modern science. Understanding the basic principles of medicinal herbs is essential for effectively harnessing their healing properties. These principles encompass the nature of herbal constituents, how herbs interact with the body, the importance of herbal synergy, and the various forms and methods of preparation. By grasping these foundational concepts, one can appreciate the complexity and potential of herbal medicine, paving the way for safe and effective use in promoting overall health and well-being.

Understanding Herbal Constituents

Herbal constituents are the chemical compounds found in plants that contribute to their medicinal properties. These bioactive compounds can vary widely in their chemical structure and physiological effects, making the study of herbal constituents a complex and fascinating field. Understanding these constituents is crucial for recognizing how herbs exert their therapeutic effects and for ensuring their safe and effective use.

Types of Herbal Constituents

- ✓ **Alkaloids:**
  - o **Description:** Alkaloids are nitrogen-containing compounds that often have potent pharmacological effects.
  - o **Examples:** Morphine from the opium poppy, caffeine from coffee beans, and quinine from cinchona bark.
  - o **Effects:** Alkaloids can have a wide range of effects, including pain relief, stimulation, and anti-malarial properties.
- ✓ **Flavonoids:**
  - o **Description:** Flavonoids are a group of polyphenolic compounds known for their antioxidant properties.
  - o **Examples:** Quercetin found in apples and onions, and catechins found in green tea.
  - o **Effects:** Flavonoids have anti-inflammatory, anti-carcinogenic, and cardiovascular-protective effects.
- ✓ **Terpenoids:**
  - o **Description:** Terpenoids, also known as isoprenoids, are a large and diverse class of organic compounds produced by plants.
  - o **Examples:** Menthol from peppermint, ginkgolides from ginkgo biloba, and limonene from citrus peels.
  - o **Effects:** Terpenoids can have anti-inflammatory, antimicrobial, and anticancer properties.
- ✓ **Glycosides:**
  - o **Description:** Glycosides are compounds in which a sugar is bound to a non-carbohydrate moiety, often contributing to the plant's medicinal properties.
  - o **Examples:** Digitalis glycosides from foxglove, and salicin from willow bark.
  - o **Effects:** Glycosides can have a variety of effects, including cardiac, anti-inflammatory, and analgesic actions.
- ✓ **Tannins:**
  - o **Description:** Tannins are polyphenolic compounds that can precipitate proteins and have astringent properties.
  - o **Examples:** Tannic acid found in tea and oak bark.
  - o **Effects:** Tannins are often used for their astringent, anti-diarrheal, and anti-inflammatory properties.
- ✓ **Saponins:**
  - o **Description:** Saponins are glycosides with a distinctive foaming characteristic.
  - o **Examples:** Ginsenosides from ginseng, and diosgenin from wild yam.
  - o **Effects:** Saponins have expectorant, anti-inflammatory, and immune-boosting properties.
- ✓ **Volatile Oils:**

- o **Description:** Volatile oils, or essential oils, are aromatic compounds that can evaporate easily.
- o **Examples:** Eucalyptus oil, lavender oil, and tea tree oil.
- o **Effects:** Volatile oils can have antimicrobial, anti-inflammatory, and calming effects.
- ✓ **Polysaccharides:**
  - o **Description:** Polysaccharides are complex carbohydrates that can modulate the immune system.
  - o **Examples:** Beta-glucans from mushrooms and aloe vera gel.
  - o **Effects:** Polysaccharides are known for their immunomodulatory, wound-healing, and prebiotic effects.

Interaction with the Body

The therapeutic effects of herbs are largely determined by how their constituents interact with the human body. These interactions can occur through various mechanisms, such as binding to receptors, inhibiting enzymes, or modulating cellular signaling pathways. The bioavailability and metabolism of these constituents also play a crucial role in their efficacy and safety.

Herbal Synergy

One of the fundamental principles of herbal medicine is the concept of synergy, where the combined effect of an herb's constituents is greater than the sum of its individual parts. This synergistic effect can enhance therapeutic efficacy and reduce the likelihood of side effects. Understanding the synergistic interactions between different herbal constituents is key to formulating effective herbal remedies.

Preparation and Dosage Forms

The way herbs are prepared and administered can significantly impact their effectiveness. Common forms of herbal preparations include teas, tinctures, extracts, capsules, and topical applications. Each form has its advantages and specific uses, and the choice of preparation depends on the desired therapeutic effect, the nature of the herbal constituents, and the patient's needs.

Understanding herbal constituents is essential for appreciating the complexity and potential of medicinal herbs. By exploring the various types of bioactive compounds, their interactions with the body, and the principles of herbal synergy and preparation, we can harness the full therapeutic potential of herbs. This knowledge not only enhances the efficacy of herbal treatments but also ensures their safe and informed use in promoting health and well-being.

How Herbs Work in the Body?

Herbs work in the body through a variety of mechanisms, influenced by the bioactive compounds they contain. Understanding these mechanisms is crucial for appreciating how herbal remedies can promote health and treat various conditions. This section explores the different ways herbs interact with the body, including their absorption, metabolism, and specific actions at the cellular and systemic levels.

Absorption and Bioavailability

The journey of an herbal compound in the body begins with its absorption. The bioavailability of an herb refers to the proportion of the active compounds that enter the bloodstream and are available for therapeutic action. Several factors influence absorption and bioavailability, including:

- **Form of Preparation:** Different forms of herbal preparations (e.g., teas, tinctures, capsules) can affect the rate and extent of absorption. For example, tinctures and extracts often have higher bioavailability than dried herbs in capsules.
- **Digestive Health:** The state of the digestive system can impact how well herbs are absorbed. Conditions like leaky gut or impaired digestion can reduce the effectiveness of herbal remedies.
- **Compounds' Chemical Nature:** The solubility of herbal compounds in water or fat can influence their absorption. Water-soluble compounds are generally absorbed more easily in the digestive tract, while fat-soluble compounds may require the presence of dietary fats for optimal absorption.

Metabolism and Distribution

Once absorbed, herbal compounds are metabolized and distributed throughout the body. The liver plays a crucial role in metabolizing these compounds, converting them into active or inactive metabolites. Key points include:

- **First-Pass Metabolism:** Some compounds undergo significant metabolism in the liver before reaching systemic circulation, which can reduce their bioavailability. This process is known as the first-pass effect.
- **Active Metabolites:** Certain herbal compounds are converted into more active forms during metabolism. For instance, the compound curcumin in turmeric is metabolized into several active metabolites that contribute to its therapeutic effects.
- **Distribution:** Herbal compounds are distributed via the bloodstream to various tissues and organs. Their distribution can be influenced by factors such as blood flow, tissue affinity, and the presence of transport proteins.

Cellular and Molecular Mechanisms

Herbal compounds exert their effects at the cellular and molecular levels through various mechanisms, including:

- **Receptor Binding:** Many herbal compounds interact with specific receptors on cell surfaces, initiating a cascade of cellular responses. For example, alkaloids like morphine bind to opioid receptors to produce pain-relieving effects.

- ❖ **Enzyme Inhibition:** Some herbs work by inhibiting enzymes involved in disease processes. For instance, the compound salicin in willow bark inhibits cyclooxygenase enzymes, reducing inflammation and pain.
- ❖ **Antioxidant Activity:** Many herbs contain antioxidants that neutralize free radicals, protecting cells from oxidative stress and damage. Flavonoids and polyphenols are examples of potent antioxidant compounds found in herbs.
- ❖ **Modulation of Signaling Pathways:** Herbal compounds can modulate cellular signaling pathways that regulate processes like inflammation, cell growth, and apoptosis. For example, curcumin modulates the NF-κB pathway, which plays a key role in inflammation and immune response.

Systemic Effects

Beyond their cellular actions, herbs can produce systemic effects that contribute to overall health and well-being. These effects include:

- **Immune Modulation:** Certain herbs, such as echinacea and astragalus, boost the immune system's activity, enhancing the body's ability to fight infections and diseases.
- **Hormonal Balance:** Herbs like black cohosh and vitex can regulate hormonal levels, providing relief from symptoms related to hormonal imbalances, such as menstrual irregularities and menopausal symptoms.
- **Detoxification:** Herbs such as milk thistle and dandelion support liver function and promote detoxification, helping the body eliminate toxins and maintain metabolic health.

Synergistic Effects

One of the unique aspects of herbal medicine is the synergistic effect, where the combined action of multiple compounds in an herb enhances its overall therapeutic efficacy. This synergy can result from:

- ✓ **Compound Interactions:** Different compounds within the same herb or a combination of herbs can work together to produce a stronger effect than any single compound alone.
- ✓ **Modulation of Bioavailability:** Certain compounds can enhance the bioavailability of others. For example, piperine in black pepper increases the absorption of curcumin from turmeric.
- ✓ **Balancing Effects:** Synergistic interactions can also help balance the effects of different compounds, reducing the likelihood of side effects and enhancing the herb's safety profile.

Understanding how herbs work in the body involves a complex interplay of absorption, metabolism, cellular actions, and systemic effects. By comprehending these mechanisms, we can better appreciate the therapeutic potential of herbal remedies and utilize them more effectively to promote health and treat various conditions. This knowledge also underscores the importance of using high-quality, well-prepared herbal products and consulting with knowledgeable practitioners to ensure safe and effective use.

Principles of Herbal Synergy

Herbal synergy is a fundamental concept in herbal medicine that refers to the enhanced therapeutic effects achieved when multiple compounds within a single herb or a combination of herbs work together. This principle is central to understanding how herbal remedies can provide more comprehensive and effective treatment than isolated compounds. The following sections explore the different aspects of herbal synergy, including its mechanisms, benefits, and practical applications.

Mechanisms of Herbal Synergy

1. **Compound Interactions:**
   - **Additive Effects:** When two or more compounds produce a combined effect equal to the sum of their individual effects. For example, different anti-inflammatory compounds in an herb can collectively reduce inflammation more effectively.
   - **Potentiation:** When one compound enhances the effect of another. For instance, piperine in black pepper enhances the bioavailability and efficacy of curcumin in turmeric.
   - **Antagonistic Effects:** In some cases, compounds can counteract potential side effects of others, leading to a more balanced and safer overall effect.

2. **Modulation of Bioavailability:**
   - Certain compounds can improve the absorption and metabolism of other compounds. For example, the presence of fats can enhance the absorption of fat-soluble compounds, and specific enzymes can facilitate the breakdown and utilization of complex molecules.

3. **Multiple Pathway Targeting:**
   - Herbal remedies often affect multiple physiological pathways simultaneously, providing a broader spectrum of action. For instance, an herb may have anti-inflammatory, antioxidant, and antimicrobial properties, addressing various aspects of a health condition.

4. **Balancing Effects:**
   - Synergistic interactions can help balance the effects of different compounds, reducing the likelihood of side effects. For example, the calming effects of certain flavonoids in an herb can mitigate the stimulating effects of alkaloids, creating a more harmonious therapeutic profile.

Benefits of Herbal Synergy

1. **Enhanced Efficacy:**
   - The combined action of multiple compounds can lead to more effective treatment outcomes. This is particularly important in complex conditions where multiple therapeutic actions are needed.

2. **Reduced Dosage Requirements:**
   - Synergistic effects can allow for lower doses of individual compounds while still achieving desired therapeutic effects. This can minimize the risk of adverse reactions and improve the safety profile of herbal remedies.

3. **Holistic Approach:**

- Herbal synergy aligns with the holistic approach of traditional medicine systems, which aim to treat the whole person rather than just specific symptoms. By addressing multiple aspects of health, synergistic herbal remedies support overall well-being.
4. **Broader Therapeutic Range:**
   - Herbs that exhibit synergy can be effective in treating a wider range of conditions. For example, an herb with both anti-inflammatory and immune-boosting properties can be used for conditions involving inflammation and immune dysfunction.

Practical Applications of Herbal Synergy

1. **Formulation of Herbal Blends:**
   - Herbalists often create blends of multiple herbs to harness the synergistic effects of their combined constituents. These blends are tailored to address specific health conditions or to provide general support for the body's systems.
2. **Whole Herb Utilization:**
   - Using whole herbs rather than isolated compounds ensures that all the beneficial constituents are present, allowing for natural synergy. This approach is common in traditional herbal practices and is increasingly supported by modern research.
3. **Combining Herbs with Conventional Treatments:**
   - Herbal synergy can also enhance the effects of conventional treatments. For example, combining certain herbs with pharmaceuticals can improve treatment outcomes and reduce side effects, although this should always be done under the guidance of a healthcare professional.
4. **Personalized Herbal Therapy:**
   - By understanding the synergistic properties of herbs, practitioners can personalize herbal therapy to meet the unique needs of each individual. This involves selecting and combining herbs based on the patient's specific health conditions, constitution, and therapeutic goals.

The principle of herbal synergy highlights the complexity and sophistication of herbal medicine. By understanding and utilizing the synergistic interactions between herbal compounds, practitioners can enhance the efficacy, safety, and holistic benefits of herbal remedies. This approach not only aligns with traditional practices but also offers valuable insights for modern integrative medicine, promoting a more comprehensive and effective approach to health and healing.

Dosage Forms and Methods of Preparation

The effectiveness of herbal remedies greatly depends on how they are prepared and administered. Different dosage forms and methods of preparation can influence the potency, absorption, and therapeutic outcomes of herbal medicines. Understanding these various forms and techniques is essential for optimizing the use of herbs in promoting health and treating ailments.

Common Dosage Forms

1. **Teas and Infusions:**
   - **Preparation:** Teas and infusions are made by steeping herbs in hot water. Infusions are typically used for delicate parts of the plant, such as leaves and flowers.
   - **Usage:** Best for extracting water-soluble constituents like flavonoids and tannins. Commonly used for calming, digestive, and general wellness purposes.
   - **Example:** Chamomile tea for relaxation and digestive support.
2. **Decoctions:**
   - **Preparation:** Decoctions involve boiling tougher parts of the plant, such as roots, bark, and seeds, in water for an extended period.
   - **Usage:** Suitable for extracting water-soluble compounds from harder plant materials. Often used for tonic herbs and those requiring longer extraction times.
   - **Example:** Ginger decoction for its anti-inflammatory and digestive properties.
3. **Tinctures:**
   - **Preparation:** Tinctures are concentrated herbal extracts made by soaking herbs in alcohol or glycerin for several weeks.
   - **Usage:** Highly potent and convenient, tinctures preserve active compounds and have a long shelf life. Used for a wide range of therapeutic purposes.
   - **Example:** Echinacea tincture for immune support.
4. **Extracts:**
   - **Preparation:** Extracts are concentrated forms of herbs, created by removing the active ingredients through solvents like alcohol, water, or glycerin, and then concentrating the solution.
   - **Usage:** Often more potent than tinctures, extracts are used for specific therapeutic effects and can be standardized to ensure consistent potency.
   - **Example:** Standardized milk thistle extract for liver health.
5. **Capsules and Tablets:**
   - **Preparation:** Dried and powdered herbs are encapsulated or compressed into tablets.
   - **Usage:** Convenient for precise dosing and for individuals who prefer not to taste herbs. Useful for long-term supplementation.
   - **Example:** Turmeric capsules for their anti-inflammatory benefits.
6. **Oils and Salves:**
   - **Preparation:** Herbal oils are made by infusing plant material in a carrier oil, while salves are thicker preparations combining herbal oils with beeswax or other thickening agents.
   - **Usage:** Applied topically for skin conditions, muscle pain, and inflammation. Oils are also used for massage and aromatherapy.
   - **Example:** Arnica salve for bruises and sore muscles.
7. **Syrups:**
   - **Preparation:** Syrups are made by mixing herbal extracts or decoctions with honey or sugar to create a sweet, thick liquid.
   - **Usage:** Commonly used for respiratory issues and sore throats due to their soothing properties.
   - **Example:** Elderberry syrup for immune support and cold relief.
8. **Poultices and Compresses:**

- **Preparation:** Poultices are made by applying a paste of fresh or dried herbs directly to the skin, while compresses involve soaking a cloth in an herbal infusion or decoction and applying it to the affected area.
- **Usage:** Used for localized skin issues, inflammation, and injuries.
- **Example:** Comfrey poultice for wound healing and inflammation.

Methods of Preparation

1. **Maceration:**
   - **Description:** Soaking herbs in a cold solvent (usually alcohol, water, or glycerin) for an extended period to extract active constituents.
   - **Application:** Used for making tinctures, glycerites, and cold infusions.
   - **Example:** Macerating valerian root in alcohol to produce a sedative tincture.
2. **Percolation:**
   - **Description:** A more complex extraction method where the solvent is slowly passed through a column of powdered herbs, allowing for efficient extraction of active compounds.
   - **Application:** Used to make potent tinctures and extracts.
   - **Example:** Percolated echinacea tincture for enhanced immune support.
3. **Infusion:**
   - **Description:** Steeping herbs in hot water, similar to making tea, typically used for delicate plant parts.
   - **Application:** Used for daily wellness teas and medicinal infusions.
   - **Example:** Preparing a peppermint infusion for digestive relief.
4. **Decoction:**
   - **Description:** Boiling tough plant parts (roots, bark, seeds) to extract water-soluble constituents.
   - **Application:** Used for tonic herbs and harder plant materials.
   - **Example:** Making a decoction of licorice root for its soothing effects on the respiratory system.
5. **Distillation:**
   - **Description:** Extracting essential oils through steam distillation, where steam passes through plant material, capturing volatile compounds, and then condenses back into a liquid.
   - **Application:** Used to produce essential oils and hydrosols.
   - **Example:** Distilling lavender to obtain its essential oil for aromatherapy and topical use.
6. **Cold Pressing:**
   - **Description:** Extracting oils from seeds and fruits without the use of heat, preserving their natural properties.
   - **Application:** Used for obtaining carrier oils and some essential oils.
   - **Example:** Cold-pressed jojoba oil for skin and hair care.

Considerations for Preparation and Use

1. **Herb Quality:**

- o Use high-quality, organic herbs to ensure the absence of contaminants and to maximize therapeutic effects.
2. **Solvent Choice:**
   - o Choose the appropriate solvent based on the solubility of the herb's active compounds. Alcohol is generally best for alkaloids, while water is suitable for flavonoids and tannins.
3. **Storage:**
   - o Properly store prepared herbal products in dark, cool places to preserve their potency and extend their shelf life.
4. **Dosage and Safety:**
   - o Follow recommended dosages and consult with a healthcare provider, especially when combining herbs with conventional medications or treating serious health conditions.

The various dosage forms and methods of preparation of herbs significantly impact their efficacy and application in herbal medicine. By understanding and selecting the appropriate form and preparation method, practitioners and users can optimize the therapeutic benefits of herbs, ensuring safe and effective treatment for a wide range of health conditions.

BOOK 2:

Benefits and Precautions of Herbal Medicine: Classification, Side Effects and Interactions

Herbal medicine offers a multitude of benefits, drawing on centuries of traditional knowledge and supported by modern scientific research. However, like any form of treatment, it also requires careful consideration and awareness of potential risks. Understanding both the advantages and the necessary precautions is essential for the safe and effective use of herbal remedies. This introduction provides an overview of the primary benefits of herbal medicine, including its natural and holistic approach to health, accessibility, and the potential for fewer side effects compared to synthetic drugs. It also highlights the importance of precautions, such as potential interactions with conventional medications, variability in herb quality, and the need for professional guidance, to ensure safe and responsible use.

General Health Benefits of Herbal Remedies

Herbal remedies have been used for thousands of years across various cultures to promote health and treat a wide range of ailments. Today, they continue to be valued for their natural origins, holistic approach, and potential to support overall well-being. The following sections explore the general health benefits of herbal remedies, highlighting their role in modern healthcare and their diverse applications.

1. Natural and Holistic Healing

- **Whole-Person Approach:** Herbal medicine often addresses the root cause of health issues rather than just alleviating symptoms. This holistic approach considers the physical, emotional, and spiritual aspects of health, promoting overall well-being.
- **Balanced Therapies:** Many herbs provide a balanced mix of nutrients and active compounds that work synergistically, offering comprehensive health benefits without the harsh side effects often associated with synthetic drugs.

2. Support for the Immune System

- **Immune Boosting:** Herbs like echinacea, elderberry, and astragalus are known for their immune-boosting properties, helping the body resist infections and recover more quickly from illnesses.
- **Adaptogens:** Herbs such as ashwagandha, ginseng, and rhodiola help the body adapt to stress and support immune function, promoting resilience and overall vitality.

3. Anti-Inflammatory and Antioxidant Properties

- **Inflammation Reduction:** Many herbs possess anti-inflammatory properties, which can help manage chronic inflammation and associated conditions like arthritis. Turmeric and ginger are notable examples.
- **Oxidative Stress Protection:** Antioxidant-rich herbs like green tea, rosemary, and cinnamon help protect the body from oxidative stress and free radical damage, which are linked to aging and various chronic diseases.

4. Digestive Health

- **Digestive Support:** Herbs like peppermint, chamomile, and fennel are commonly used to support digestive health, alleviate symptoms of indigestion, and promote a healthy gut environment.
- **Liver Health:** Milk thistle and dandelion root are known for their liver-protective effects, aiding in detoxification and overall liver function.

5. Mental Health and Cognitive Function

- **Stress and Anxiety Relief:** Herbs such as valerian, passionflower, and lemon balm are often used to reduce stress and anxiety, promoting relaxation and mental clarity.
- **Cognitive Enhancement:** Ginkgo biloba and bacopa monnieri are known for their potential to enhance memory and cognitive function, supporting brain health and reducing the risk of cognitive decline.

6. Cardiovascular Health

- **Heart Health:** Hawthorn and garlic are herbs that support cardiovascular health by improving blood circulation, reducing blood pressure, and lowering cholesterol levels.
- **Blood Sugar Regulation:** Herbs like cinnamon and fenugreek can help regulate blood sugar levels, making them beneficial for managing diabetes and metabolic syndrome.

7. Skin and Hair Health

- **Skin Healing:** Aloe vera, calendula, and neem are commonly used to promote skin health, treat wounds, and manage skin conditions like eczema and acne.
- **Hair Growth:** Herbs such as rosemary, nettle, and amla are known to support hair growth, strengthen hair follicles, and improve scalp health.

8. Hormonal Balance

- **Women's Health:** Herbs like black cohosh, chaste tree (vitex), and red clover are used to balance hormones and alleviate symptoms of menopause, PMS, and menstrual irregularities.
- **Men's Health:** Saw palmetto and tribulus terrestris are herbs that support prostate health and hormonal balance in men.

The general health benefits of herbal remedies are vast and varied, reflecting their long-standing use in traditional medicine and growing recognition in modern healthcare. By incorporating herbal remedies into daily routines, individuals can support their immune system, reduce inflammation, enhance mental and cognitive function, promote digestive and cardiovascular health, and maintain skin and hair vitality. However, it is important to use herbal remedies responsibly and in consultation with healthcare professionals to ensure their safe and effective integration into health and wellness practices.

Potential Side Effects and Interactions

While herbal remedies offer numerous health benefits, it is essential to recognize that they can also pose risks, particularly if used improperly. Understanding potential side effects and interactions with other medications or health conditions is crucial for ensuring safe and effective use of herbal medicine. This section explores common side effects, possible interactions, and guidelines for minimizing risks.

Common Side Effects

1. **Gastrointestinal Issues:**
   - **Symptoms:** Nausea, vomiting, diarrhea, and abdominal pain.
   - **Examples:** Herbs like senna (used as a laxative) can cause cramping and diarrhea if taken in large doses or for extended periods.
2. **Allergic Reactions:**
   - **Symptoms:** Skin rashes, itching, swelling, and, in severe cases, anaphylaxis.
   - **Examples:** Chamomile and echinacea, which belong to the daisy family, can cause allergic reactions in individuals sensitive to this plant family.
3. **Photosensitivity:**
   - **Symptoms:** Increased sensitivity to sunlight, leading to sunburn or skin rash.
   - **Examples:** St. John's wort can cause photosensitivity, making the skin more prone to sunburn.
4. **Toxicity:**

- **Symptoms:** Depending on the herb, toxicity can affect various organs, leading to liver damage, kidney issues, or other serious health problems.
- **Examples:** Kava, used for anxiety, has been associated with liver toxicity when used excessively or improperly.

Interactions with Medications

1. **Anticoagulants and Antiplatelet Drugs:**
   - **Risk:** Increased risk of bleeding.
   - **Examples:** Garlic, ginkgo biloba, and ginger can enhance the effects of blood-thinning medications like warfarin, increasing the risk of bleeding.
2. **Antidepressants:**
   - **Risk:** Serotonin syndrome or reduced efficacy of medication.
   - **Examples:** St. John's wort can interact with antidepressants such as SSRIs, leading to potentially dangerous increases in serotonin levels or reducing the effectiveness of the medication.
3. **Blood Pressure Medications:**
   - **Risk:** Additive effects or reduced efficacy.
   - **Examples:** Licorice can raise blood pressure and counteract the effects of antihypertensive drugs, while hawthorn may enhance the effects, leading to excessively low blood pressure.
4. **Diabetes Medications:**
   - **Risk:** Altered blood sugar levels.
   - **Examples:** Herbs like ginseng and fenugreek can lower blood sugar, potentially causing hypoglycemia when taken with diabetes medications.
5. **Immunosuppressants:**
   - **Risk:** Reduced efficacy of the medication.
   - **Examples:** Echinacea may stimulate the immune system and counteract the effects of immunosuppressive drugs used in transplant patients.

Guidelines for Safe Use

1. **Consultation with Healthcare Providers:**
   - Always consult with a healthcare professional before starting any herbal remedy, especially if you are taking prescription medications, have underlying health conditions, or are pregnant or breastfeeding.
2. **Quality and Source:**
   - Use high-quality, standardized herbal products from reputable sources to ensure consistency and purity. Avoid products with contaminants or adulterants.
3. **Dosage and Duration:**
   - Follow recommended dosages and avoid prolonged use of herbs without professional guidance. Some herbs are safe for short-term use but can cause adverse effects when used long-term.
4. **Monitoring for Side Effects:**
   - Be vigilant for any adverse reactions when starting a new herbal remedy. Discontinue use and seek medical advice if you experience any unexpected symptoms.

5. **Awareness of Contraindications:**
   - Understand the contraindications of specific herbs, such as those that should not be used during pregnancy, in children, or in individuals with certain medical conditions.
6. **Drug-Herb Interaction Check:**
   - Use resources like drug-herb interaction checkers or consult with a pharmacist or herbalist to identify potential interactions between herbs and medications.

While herbal remedies offer valuable health benefits, it is essential to approach their use with caution and awareness. Understanding potential side effects and interactions with medications is crucial for ensuring their safe and effective use. By consulting healthcare providers, choosing high-quality products, adhering to recommended dosages, and monitoring for adverse effects, individuals can minimize risks and safely incorporate herbal remedies into their health and wellness practices.

Guidelines for Safe Usage

The safe use of herbal remedies requires a thorough understanding of the herbs themselves, their potential interactions, and best practices for their preparation and administration. Following these guidelines can help ensure that herbal treatments are both effective and safe, minimizing the risk of adverse effects and interactions.

Consultation with Healthcare Providers

1. **Seek Professional Advice:**
   - Always consult a healthcare provider, such as a doctor, pharmacist, or qualified herbalist, before starting any herbal remedy, especially if you have existing health conditions, are pregnant, breastfeeding, or taking other medications.
2. **Full Disclosure:**
   - Inform your healthcare provider about all the herbs and supplements you are taking to prevent potential interactions with prescription medications or treatments.

Quality and Source

1. **Choose Reputable Brands:**
   - Purchase herbal products from reputable brands known for high-quality standards. Look for certifications such as Good Manufacturing Practices (GMP) or third-party testing.
2. **Check for Contaminants:**
   - Ensure that herbal products are free from contaminants such as heavy metals, pesticides, and microorganisms. Reputable brands often provide Certificates of Analysis (COA) to verify product purity and potency.
3. **Standardization:**
   - Opt for standardized extracts, which guarantee a consistent concentration of active ingredients, ensuring reliable dosage and efficacy.

Dosage and Administration

1. **Follow Recommended Dosages:**
   - Adhere to the dosage instructions provided by the manufacturer or your healthcare provider. Do not exceed recommended doses, as this can increase the risk of side effects.
2. **Duration of Use:**
   - Use herbs for the recommended duration. Some herbs are suitable for short-term use only, while others may be safe for long-term use under professional supervision.
3. **Correct Preparation:**
   - Use appropriate methods to prepare herbal remedies, such as making teas, tinctures, or decoctions, according to guidelines. Proper preparation ensures the extraction of beneficial compounds while minimizing harmful substances.

Monitoring and Adjustments

1. **Monitor for Side Effects:**
   - Be vigilant for any side effects or allergic reactions when starting a new herbal remedy. Common signs include gastrointestinal upset, skin rashes, and headaches.
2. **Adjust Dosage if Necessary:**
   - If you experience mild side effects, consult your healthcare provider to adjust the dosage or switch to a different preparation. Never self-adjust dosages without professional guidance.
3. **Stop if Severe Reactions Occur:**
   - Discontinue use immediately and seek medical attention if you experience severe reactions such as difficulty breathing, swelling, or intense pain.

Awareness of Contraindications and Interactions

1. **Know Contraindications:**
   - Be aware of any contraindications for the herbs you are using. Some herbs may not be suitable for pregnant women, children, or individuals with certain medical conditions.
2. **Check for Interactions:**
   - Use reliable resources to check for potential interactions between herbs and medications. This is crucial for avoiding adverse effects and ensuring the efficacy of both the herbs and medications.
3. **Avoid Self-Medicating for Serious Conditions:**
   - Do not use herbal remedies as a substitute for conventional medical treatment for serious health conditions. Herbs can complement but should not replace prescribed treatments for serious illnesses.

Education and Resources

1. **Educate Yourself:**

- o Take the time to learn about the herbs you are using, including their benefits, side effects, and proper usage. Reliable sources include books by reputable herbalists, scientific studies, and educational websites.

2. **Use Trusted Resources:**
   - o Refer to trusted resources such as the National Center for Complementary and Integrative Health (NCCIH), the American Herbalists Guild, or the European Scientific Cooperative on Phytotherapy (ESCOP) for accurate and up-to-date information.

3. **Join Herbal Communities:**
   - o Engage with herbal communities and forums to share experiences and gain insights from other users and professionals. However, always verify information from non-professional sources with a qualified healthcare provider.

Herbal remedies can offer significant health benefits when used correctly and safely. By following these guidelines, individuals can minimize risks and maximize the therapeutic potential of herbs. Consultation with healthcare providers, choosing high-quality products, adhering to recommended dosages, monitoring for side effects, and staying informed are all essential practices for the safe and effective use of herbal medicine.

Special Considerations for Different Populations (Pregnant Women, Children, Elderly)

Herbal remedies can be beneficial for various populations, but certain groups require special considerations to ensure their safe and effective use. Pregnant women, children, and the elderly may have unique physiological needs and sensitivities that necessitate tailored approaches to herbal medicine. This section outlines key guidelines and precautions for these specific populations.

Pregnant Women

1. **Consultation with Healthcare Providers:**
   - o Pregnant women should always consult with a healthcare provider before using any herbal remedies. Some herbs can affect pregnancy and fetal development, and professional guidance is essential to avoid potential risks.

2. **Herbs to Avoid:**
   - o Certain herbs can stimulate uterine contractions, potentially leading to miscarriage or preterm labor. Examples include:
     - **Blue Cohosh (Caulophyllum thalictroides):** Known to induce labor.
     - **Pennyroyal (Mentha pulegium):** Can cause uterine contractions and is toxic in high doses.
     - **Mugwort (Artemisia vulgaris):** May stimulate menstruation and should be avoided.

3. **Safe Herbs for Pregnancy:**
   - o Some herbs are generally considered safe and can provide supportive benefits during pregnancy, such as:
     - **Ginger (Zingiber officinale):** Helps alleviate morning sickness and nausea.

- **Peppermint (Mentha piperita):** Useful for relieving digestive discomfort.
- **Red Raspberry Leaf (Rubus idaeus):** Traditionally used to tone the uterus and support labor, typically used in the third trimester.

4. **Dosage and Duration:**
   - Pregnant women should use herbs at the recommended doses and for appropriate durations, avoiding excessive or long-term use without professional supervision.

Children

1. **Pediatric Consultation:**
   - Always consult a pediatrician or qualified healthcare provider before administering herbal remedies to children. Children's bodies process substances differently, and their responses to herbs can vary widely.
2. **Age-Appropriate Dosing:**
   - Dosing for children should be adjusted based on age, weight, and developmental stage. Many herbal reference guides provide pediatric dosing guidelines.
3. **Gentle Herbs for Common Ailments:**
   - Certain herbs are suitable for children and can help with common issues like colic, colds, and digestive discomfort:
     - **Chamomile (Matricaria chamomilla):** Mild sedative and digestive aid.
     - **Fennel (Foeniculum vulgare):** Eases colic and gas.
     - **Elderberry (Sambucus nigra):** Supports immune function and helps with colds and flu.
4. **Herbs to Avoid in Children:**
   - Some herbs are not safe for children and should be avoided:
     - **Aspirin-containing herbs (e.g., willow bark):** Risk of Reye's syndrome.
     - **Goldenseal (Hydrastis canadensis):** Can affect bilirubin levels and is not recommended for infants.
     - **Ephedra (Ephedra sinica):** Can cause severe cardiovascular effects.

Elderly

1. **Healthcare Provider Consultation:**
   - Elderly individuals should consult with their healthcare providers before using herbal remedies, as they may have chronic conditions or be taking multiple medications that could interact with herbs.
2. **Adjusted Dosages:**
   - Dosages may need to be adjusted for the elderly due to changes in metabolism, kidney, and liver function. Lower doses are often recommended to prevent adverse effects.
3. **Herbs for Common Elderly Ailments:**
   - Certain herbs can support health in the elderly, addressing issues such as inflammation, cognitive decline, and cardiovascular health:
     - **Turmeric (Curcuma longa):** Anti-inflammatory properties beneficial for arthritis.
     - **Ginkgo Biloba:** Supports cognitive function and circulation.

- **Hawthorn (Crataegus spp.):** Promotes cardiovascular health and strengthens the heart.
4. **Monitoring for Side Effects:**
   - Elderly individuals should be closely monitored for any adverse reactions or side effects, as they may be more susceptible to these due to age-related physiological changes.
5. **Potential Herb-Drug Interactions:**
   - The risk of herb-drug interactions is higher in the elderly due to polypharmacy (use of multiple medications). Common interactions to be aware of include:
     - **St. John's Wort:** Can interact with a wide range of medications, including antidepressants, anticoagulants, and blood pressure medications.
     - **Ginseng:** May interact with blood thinners and diabetes medications.

Special populations such as pregnant women, children, and the elderly require tailored approaches to the use of herbal remedies. Consulting with healthcare providers, understanding appropriate dosages, and being aware of potential side effects and interactions are crucial for ensuring safe and effective use. By taking these special considerations into account, herbal medicine can be a valuable tool for promoting health and well-being across all stages of life.

Herbal Classification and Properties

Herbal classification and properties form the foundation of understanding how different herbs can be used therapeutically. By categorizing herbs based on their characteristics, actions, and effects on the body, practitioners and users can make informed decisions about their use. This introduction explores the various methods of classifying herbs, including by plant parts used, therapeutic actions, organoleptic properties, and energetic qualities. It also highlights the significance of these classifications in guiding the appropriate selection and application of herbs for promoting health and treating ailments. Understanding the properties of herbs helps ensure their safe and effective integration into health and wellness practices.

Categorization by Plant Parts Used

Herbs can be categorized based on the specific parts of the plant that are used for medicinal purposes. Each part of a plant contains different concentrations and types of bioactive compounds, leading to variations in their therapeutic properties and uses. Understanding the categorization by plant parts helps in selecting the right herb preparation for specific health conditions. The following sections explore the primary plant parts used in herbal medicine and their typical applications.

Leaves

- **Description:** Leaves are often rich in volatile oils, flavonoids, and other phytochemicals that can have a wide range of therapeutic effects.
- **Common Uses:** Leaves are frequently used for their antiseptic, anti-inflammatory, and digestive properties.
- **Examples:**

- **Peppermint (Mentha piperita):** Used for its digestive and cooling effects.
- **Sage (Salvia officinalis):** Known for its antiseptic and astringent properties.

Flowers

- **Description:** Flowers often contain essential oils and flavonoids, making them valuable for their aromatic and therapeutic properties.
- **Common Uses:** Flowers are used for their calming, anti-inflammatory, and antispasmodic effects.
- **Examples:**
  - **Chamomile (Matricaria chamomilla):** Commonly used for its calming and digestive benefits.
  - **Lavender (Lavandula angustifolia):** Known for its relaxing and antiseptic properties.

Roots and Rhizomes

- **Description:** Roots and rhizomes tend to be rich in starches, alkaloids, and other potent compounds, often making them powerful remedies.
- **Common Uses:** These parts are used for their tonic, adaptogenic, and anti-inflammatory properties.
- **Examples:**
  - **Ginger (Zingiber officinale):** Used for its anti-inflammatory and digestive benefits.
  - **Echinacea (Echinacea purpurea):** Known for its immune-boosting properties.

Bark

- **Description:** Bark contains a variety of compounds including tannins, alkaloids, and glycosides, and is often used for its protective and astringent properties.
- **Common Uses:** Bark is commonly used for its astringent, anti-inflammatory, and analgesic effects.
- **Examples:**
  - **Cinnamon (Cinnamomum verum):** Known for its warming and antimicrobial properties.
  - **Willow (Salix spp.):** Used for its pain-relieving and anti-inflammatory effects.

Seeds

- **Description:** Seeds are nutrient-dense and often contain oils, proteins, and various phytochemicals that contribute to their therapeutic effects.
- **Common Uses:** Seeds are used for their nourishing, laxative, and anti-inflammatory properties.
- **Examples:**
  - **Flaxseed (Linum usitatissimum):** Known for its omega-3 fatty acids and laxative properties.
  - **Milk Thistle (Silybum marianum):** Used for its liver-protective effects.

Fruits

- **Description:** Fruits often contain vitamins, minerals, sugars, and antioxidants, making them beneficial for a variety of health purposes.
- **Common Uses:** Fruits are used for their nutritive, laxative, and antioxidant properties.
- **Examples:**
  - **Elderberry (Sambucus nigra):** Known for its immune-boosting and antiviral properties.
  - **Hawthorn (Crataegus spp.):** Used for its cardiovascular benefits.

Berries

- **Description:** Berries are similar to fruits but typically smaller and often higher in certain antioxidants like anthocyanins.
- **Common Uses:** Berries are used for their high antioxidant content and their ability to support the immune system and overall health.
- **Examples:**
  - **Blueberry (Vaccinium spp.):** Known for its high antioxidant content and cognitive support.
  - **Goji Berry (Lycium barbarum):** Used for its immune-boosting and antioxidant properties.

Bulbs

- **Description:** Bulbs store nutrients for the plant and often contain sulfur compounds and other bioactive chemicals.
- **Common Uses:** Bulbs are commonly used for their antimicrobial, digestive, and immune-boosting properties.
- **Examples:**
  - **Garlic (Allium sativum):** Known for its antimicrobial and cardiovascular benefits.
  - **Onion (Allium cepa):** Used for its anti-inflammatory and immune-supportive properties.

Categorizing herbs by plant parts used provides a practical framework for understanding their therapeutic applications. Each part of the plant contains distinct compounds that contribute to its specific health benefits. By recognizing these categories, practitioners and users can make informed decisions about the selection and preparation of herbal remedies, ensuring their effective and safe use in promoting health and treating various ailments.

Classification by Therapeutic Action

Herbal medicine can also be categorized by the therapeutic actions of herbs, which describe the specific health benefits and physiological effects they provide. This method of classification helps practitioners and users select the appropriate herbs for treating specific conditions or achieving desired health outcomes. The following sections outline some of the major therapeutic actions and examples of herbs that fall into each category.

Adaptogens

- **Description:** Adaptogens help the body adapt to stress and promote overall balance and resilience. They support the adrenal glands and improve the body's response to physical, mental, and environmental stressors.
- **Examples:**
  - **Ashwagandha (Withania somnifera):** Reduces stress and anxiety, enhances cognitive function.
  - **Rhodiola (Rhodiola rosea):** Increases energy, stamina, and mental capacity.

Anti-Inflammatories

- **Description:** Anti-inflammatory herbs reduce inflammation in the body, which can help manage conditions like arthritis, allergies, and inflammatory bowel disease.
- **Examples:**
  - **Turmeric (Curcuma longa):** Contains curcumin, which has strong anti-inflammatory properties.
  - **Ginger (Zingiber officinale):** Reduces inflammation and pain.

Antimicrobials

- **Description:** Antimicrobial herbs inhibit the growth of or kill microorganisms such as bacteria, viruses, fungi, and parasites, helping to treat and prevent infections.
- **Examples:**
  - **Garlic (Allium sativum):** Effective against bacteria, viruses, and fungi.
  - **Oregano (Origanum vulgare):** Possesses antibacterial, antiviral, and antifungal properties.

Antioxidants

- **Description:** Antioxidant herbs protect the body from oxidative stress and free radical damage, which are linked to chronic diseases and aging.
- **Examples:**
  - **Green Tea (Camellia sinensis):** Rich in catechins and polyphenols, powerful antioxidants.
  - **Grapeseed Extract (Vitis vinifera):** Contains proanthocyanidins, strong antioxidants.

Nervines

- **Description:** Nervine herbs support the nervous system, helping to calm the mind, reduce anxiety, and improve sleep.
- **Examples:**
  - **Chamomile (Matricaria chamomilla):** Calms the mind and aids in sleep.
  - **Valerian (Valeriana officinalis):** Promotes relaxation and improves sleep quality.

Immunomodulators

- **Description:** Immunomodulating herbs help regulate and support the immune system, enhancing its ability to respond to infections and diseases.
- **Examples:**
    - **Echinacea (Echinacea purpurea):** Boosts immune function and helps fight off infections.
    - **Astragalus (Astragalus membranaceus):** Supports immune system health and increases resistance to illness.

Digestives

- **Description:** Digestive herbs aid in the digestion process, relieve digestive discomfort, and promote a healthy digestive system.
- **Examples:**
    - **Peppermint (Mentha piperita):** Relieves digestive spasms and bloating.
    - **Fennel (Foeniculum vulgare):** Eases gas and bloating, supports healthy digestion.

Cardiotonics

- **Description:** Cardiotonics support heart health by improving cardiovascular function and circulation.
- **Examples:**
    - **Hawthorn (Crataegus spp.):** Strengthens the heart and improves blood flow.
    - **Motherwort (Leonurus cardiaca):** Supports heart function and reduces palpitations.

Hepatics

- **Description:** Hepatic herbs support liver function, aiding in detoxification and promoting overall liver health.
- **Examples:**
    - **Milk Thistle (Silybum marianum):** Protects and regenerates liver cells.
    - **Dandelion Root (Taraxacum officinale):** Supports liver detoxification and bile production.

Diuretics

- **Description:** Diuretic herbs increase urine production, helping to remove excess fluids and toxins from the body.
- **Examples:**
    - **Dandelion Leaf (Taraxacum officinale):** Acts as a mild diuretic.
    - **Nettle (Urtica dioica):** Promotes urine flow and supports kidney function.

Expectorants

- **Description:** Expectorant herbs help clear mucus from the respiratory tract, making it easier to cough up and expel.
- **Examples:**
  - **Licorice Root (Glycyrrhiza glabra):** Soothes the throat and helps expel mucus.
  - **Thyme (Thymus vulgaris):** Acts as an expectorant and antimicrobial for respiratory health.

Analgesics

- **Description:** Analgesic herbs relieve pain without causing a loss of consciousness.
- **Examples:**
  - **Willow Bark (Salix spp.):** Contains salicin, which has pain-relieving properties.
  - **California Poppy (Eschscholzia californica):** Provides mild pain relief and promotes relaxation.

Classifying herbs by their therapeutic actions provides a practical framework for selecting appropriate herbal remedies based on specific health needs and desired outcomes. This method of classification helps users and practitioners understand the distinct benefits and applications of various herbs, facilitating their effective and safe use in promoting health and treating ailments. By recognizing the therapeutic actions of herbs, we can better appreciate their potential and integrate them more effectively into our wellness practices.

Organoleptic Properties (Taste, Color, Smell)

Understanding the organoleptic properties of herbs—such as their taste, color, and smell—is essential in herbal medicine. These sensory attributes not only enhance the therapeutic experience but also provide insights into the herb's potential uses and effects on the body. Here's a detailed look at how these properties are categorized and their significance in herbal practice.

Taste

The taste of an herb can provide clues to its medicinal properties and therapeutic actions. Herbalists often classify herbs based on their primary tastes, which include sweet, bitter, sour, salty, and pungent. Each taste is associated with specific actions and health benefits:

1. **Sweet:**
   - **Properties:** Nourishing, soothing, and often tonifying.
   - **Examples:**
     - **Licorice Root (Glycyrrhiza glabra):** Sweet taste, used to harmonize and soothe the digestive system.
     - **Marshmallow Root (Althaea officinalis):** Provides a soothing effect on mucous membranes.
2. **Bitter:**
   - **Properties:** Stimulates digestion, detoxifies, and promotes bile flow.
   - **Examples:**

- **Dandelion Root (Taraxacum officinale):** Bitter taste, supports liver function and digestion.
- **Gentian Root (Gentiana lutea):** Used to enhance digestive function and appetite.

3. **Sour:**
   - **Properties:** Astringent, helps to tighten tissues and reduce excess moisture.
   - **Examples:**
     - **Hibiscus Flowers (Hibiscus sabdariffa):** Sour taste, rich in vitamin C, and supports cardiovascular health.
     - **Amla (Phyllanthus emblica):** Known for its high vitamin C content and astringent properties.

4. **Salty:**
   - **Properties:** Moistening, softening, and grounding.
   - **Examples:**
     - **Himalayan Salt (Sodium chloride):** Used in various formulations to balance electrolytes.
     - **Kelp (Ascophyllum nodosum):** Rich in minerals, supports thyroid function and detoxification.

5. **Pungent:**
   - **Properties:** Stimulates circulation, clears congestion, and promotes digestion.
   - **Examples:**
     - **Ginger (Zingiber officinale):** Pungent taste, known for its warming and digestive properties.
     - **Turmeric (Curcuma longa):** Pungent flavor, used for its anti-inflammatory and antioxidant effects.

Color

The color of an herb often reflects its chemical composition and potential medicinal properties. Different colors can indicate the presence of specific compounds, influencing the herb's therapeutic uses:

1. **Green:**
   - **Properties:** Typically rich in chlorophyll, antioxidants, and vitamins.
   - **Examples:**
     - **Parsley (Petroselinum crispum):** Fresh green leaves, used for its diuretic and antioxidant properties.
     - **Nettle (Urtica dioica):** Green leaves, known for its mineral-rich content and supportive action on the kidneys.

2. **Yellow:**
   - **Properties:** Often associated with flavonoids and bile-enhancing compounds.
   - **Examples:**
     - **Turmeric (Curcuma longa):** Bright yellow, contains curcumin, known for its anti-inflammatory effects.
     - **Calendula (Calendula officinalis):** Yellow petals, used for skin healing and inflammation.

3. **Red:**

- **Properties:** Rich in anthocyanins and other antioxidants, promoting cardiovascular health.
- **Examples:**
  - **Hawthorn Berries (Crataegus spp.):** Red berries, used to support heart health and circulation.
  - **Rose Hips (Rosa canina):** Red, high in vitamin C and antioxidants.

4. **Blue/Purple:**
   - **Properties:** Contains anthocyanins, known for their antioxidant and anti-inflammatory effects.
   - **Examples:**
     - **Blueberry (Vaccinium spp.):** Blue, rich in antioxidants and vitamins.
     - **Elderberry (Sambucus nigra):** Dark purple berries, used for immune support and antiviral properties.

5. **White:**
   - **Properties:** Often calming and cooling, associated with minerals and cooling properties.
   - **Examples:**
     - **Slippery Elm (Ulmus rubra):** White inner bark, known for its soothing and mucilaginous properties.
     - **White Willow Bark (Salix alba):** White bark, used for its pain-relieving properties due to salicin content.

Smell

The aroma of an herb can provide information about its volatile oils and active constituents, influencing its therapeutic use and therapeutic action. Smells can range from floral and fruity to earthy and pungent:

1. **Floral:**
   - **Properties:** Often calming and uplifting, used for their sedative and mood-enhancing effects.
   - **Examples:**
     - **Lavender (Lavandula angustifolia):** Sweet floral scent, used for its calming and antiseptic properties.
     - **Chamomile (Matricaria chamomilla):** Light, apple-like fragrance, known for its soothing effects on the nervous system.

2. **Citrus:**
   - **Properties:** Refreshing and invigorating, known for their antimicrobial and digestive benefits.
   - **Examples:**
     - **Lemon Balm (Melissa officinalis):** Lemon scent, used for its calming and antiviral properties.
     - **Orange Peel (Citrus sinensis):** Citrus aroma, used to improve digestion and boost mood.

3. **Herbaceous:**
   - **Properties:** Earthy and green, often used for their grounding and detoxifying effects.

- Examples:
    - **Basil (Ocimum basilicum):** Sweet, herbaceous aroma, known for its digestive and antimicrobial properties.
    - **Rosemary (Rosmarinus officinalis):** Woody, herbaceous scent, used for memory enhancement and circulation.
4. **Pungent/Spicy:**
    - **Properties:** Warming and stimulating, used to enhance circulation and digestion.
    - **Examples:**
        - **Ginger (Zingiber officinale):** Spicy, warming scent, known for its digestive and anti-inflammatory benefits.
        - **Cinnamon (Cinnamomum verum):** Sweet, spicy aroma, used for its antimicrobial and warming properties.
5. **Earthy:**
    - **Properties:** Grounding and calming, often used to support detoxification and immune function.
    - **Examples:**
        - **Valerian Root (Valeriana officinalis):** Musky, earthy smell, used for its sedative and muscle-relaxing properties.
        - **Patchouli (Pogostemon cablin):** Deep, earthy aroma, used for its antifungal and calming effects.

The organoleptic properties of herbs—taste, color, and smell—are invaluable tools in herbal medicine. They not only enhance the sensory experience of using herbs but also provide critical information about their actions and uses. By understanding these properties, herbalists and users can better choose and utilize herbs to support health and treat various conditions, ensuring a more informed and holistic approach to herbal medicine.

Energetic Properties (Cooling, Warming, etc.)

The energetic properties of herbs refer to their ability to affect the body's internal balance and temperature. These properties are essential in traditional systems of medicine, such as Traditional Chinese Medicine (TCM) and Ayurveda, which focus on restoring and maintaining harmony within the body. Herbs can be classified based on their energetic qualities, such as cooling, warming, drying, or moistening, which influence their therapeutic applications. Understanding these properties helps in selecting the right herbs for specific conditions and constitutions.

Cooling Herbs

- **Description:** Cooling herbs help to reduce heat and inflammation in the body. They are often used to treat conditions associated with excess heat, such as fever, inflammation, and irritability.
- **Common Uses:** These herbs are beneficial for conditions like fever, hot flashes, skin eruptions, and inflammatory conditions.
- **Examples:**
    - **Peppermint (Mentha piperita):** Cools the body and soothes digestive issues.

- **Chrysanthemum (Chrysanthemum morifolium):** Used in TCM to clear heat and calm the liver.
- **Cucumber (Cucumis sativus):** Hydrating and cooling, often used in skincare and to reduce heat in the body.

Warming Herbs

- **Description:** Warming herbs increase circulation and stimulate body functions. They are often used to treat conditions associated with coldness and stagnation, such as poor circulation, cold extremities, and digestive sluggishness.
- **Common Uses:** These herbs are useful for conditions like cold hands and feet, poor digestion, and respiratory congestion.
- **Examples:**
  - **Ginger (Zingiber officinale):** Warms the body, stimulates digestion, and improves circulation.
  - **Cinnamon (Cinnamomum verum):** Increases warmth, enhances circulation, and has antimicrobial properties.
  - **Black Pepper (Piper nigrum):** Stimulates digestion and circulation, and warms the body.

Drying Herbs

- **Description:** Drying herbs help to reduce excess moisture in the body. They are useful for conditions such as dampness, phlegm, and edema.
- **Common Uses:** These herbs are beneficial for conditions like respiratory congestion, excess mucus, and skin conditions caused by excess moisture.
- **Examples:**
  - **Sage (Salvia officinalis):** Dries up excess moisture, used for sweating and respiratory congestion.
  - **Nettle (Urtica dioica):** Helps with fluid retention and excess mucus.
  - **Thyme (Thymus vulgaris):** Dries and clears respiratory congestion, has antiseptic properties.

Moistening Herbs

- **Description:** Moistening herbs help to hydrate and nourish dry tissues. They are often used to treat conditions associated with dryness, such as dry skin, dry cough, and constipation.
- **Common Uses:** These herbs are beneficial for conditions like dry skin, dry throat, and dry, irritated mucous membranes.
- **Examples:**
  - **Marshmallow Root (Althaea officinalis):** Moistens and soothes dry mucous membranes.
  - **Licorice Root (Glycyrrhiza glabra):** Moistens and nourishes, used for dry cough and digestive irritation.
  - **Flaxseed (Linum usitatissimum):** Provides moisture and lubrication, especially beneficial for the digestive tract.

Balancing Energetic Properties

- **Description:** Some herbs have balancing properties that can adapt to the body's needs, providing both cooling and warming effects depending on the individual's condition.
- **Common Uses:** These herbs are versatile and can be used in various conditions to restore balance.
- **Examples:**
    - **Chamomile (Matricaria chamomilla):** Balances the nervous system, can be both cooling and warming depending on the preparation.
    - **Tulsi (Ocimum sanctum):** Known as holy basil, it adapts to the body's needs and balances stress responses.
    - **Ginseng (Panax ginseng):** Adaptogenic, helps balance energy levels and supports the body's stress response.

The energetic properties of herbs—cooling, warming, drying, and moistening—are critical in understanding how they affect the body's internal balance. These properties guide the selection of herbs for specific conditions and individual constitutions, ensuring a tailored and effective approach to herbal medicine. By recognizing and applying these energetic qualities, practitioners and users can enhance the therapeutic potential of herbs and promote holistic health and well-being.

Key Herbs and Their Traditional Uses

Throughout history, various cultures have relied on specific herbs for their medicinal properties, developing rich traditions around their use. These key herbs have been valued for their ability to treat a wide range of ailments and support overall health. Understanding the traditional uses of these herbs provides valuable insights into their therapeutic potential and applications in modern herbal medicine. This introduction sets the stage for exploring some of the most important herbs and the traditional wisdom behind their use, highlighting their enduring relevance in promoting health and well-being.

Common Herbs for Digestive Health

Digestive health is essential for overall well-being, as it affects the absorption of nutrients and the elimination of waste from the body. Herbal remedies have long been used to support and improve digestive function, alleviate symptoms of digestive discomfort, and promote a healthy gastrointestinal system. The following sections explore some of the most common herbs known for their beneficial effects on digestive health.

Peppermint (Mentha piperita)

- **Traditional Uses:** Peppermint has been used for centuries to soothe digestive issues such as indigestion, gas, and bloating. Its calming effect on the gastrointestinal tract helps relax the muscles of the digestive system, reducing spasms and discomfort.
- **Key Constituents:** Menthol, menthone, and flavonoids.

- **Applications:** Peppermint tea is commonly consumed to relieve digestive discomfort. Peppermint oil is also used in enteric-coated capsules to treat irritable bowel syndrome (IBS).

Ginger (Zingiber officinale)

- **Traditional Uses:** Ginger is widely used to treat nausea, vomiting, and indigestion. Its warming properties stimulate digestion and improve circulation within the gastrointestinal tract.
- **Key Constituents:** Gingerol, shogaol, and zingerone.
- **Applications:** Fresh ginger root can be added to foods or brewed into tea. Ginger supplements are also available for more concentrated doses.

Fennel (Foeniculum vulgare)

- **Traditional Uses:** Fennel seeds have been used to alleviate digestive issues such as bloating, gas, and cramps. Fennel is known for its carminative properties, which help expel gas from the intestines.
- **Key Constituents:** Anethole, fenchone, and estragole.
- **Applications:** Fennel seeds can be chewed after meals, brewed into tea, or used as a spice in cooking to aid digestion.

Chamomile (Matricaria chamomilla)

- **Traditional Uses:** Chamomile is well-known for its soothing effects on the digestive system. It helps relieve indigestion, gas, and colic, and is also used to reduce inflammation in the gastrointestinal tract.
- **Key Constituents:** Apigenin, bisabolol, and chamazulene.
- **Applications:** Chamomile tea is a popular remedy for digestive discomfort and can be consumed regularly for its calming effects.

Dandelion (Taraxacum officinale)

- **Traditional Uses:** Dandelion root is used to stimulate appetite and promote healthy digestion. It acts as a mild laxative and supports liver function, aiding in detoxification.
- **Key Constituents:** Inulin, taraxacin, and sesquiterpene lactones.
- **Applications:** Dandelion root can be consumed as a tea or tincture, and its leaves can be added to salads for their digestive benefits.

Licorice Root (Glycyrrhiza glabra)

- **Traditional Uses:** Licorice root is used to soothe and protect the mucous membranes of the digestive tract. It is particularly helpful for conditions like gastritis and ulcers.
- **Key Constituents:** Glycyrrhizin, flavonoids, and saponins.
- **Applications:** Licorice root can be taken as a tea, extract, or in deglycyrrhizinated form (DGL) to reduce potential side effects like high blood pressure.

Slippery Elm (Ulmus rubra)

- **Traditional Uses:** Slippery elm is known for its mucilaginous properties, which soothe and protect irritated tissues in the digestive tract. It is commonly used to treat conditions like acid reflux and irritable bowel syndrome.
- **Key Constituents:** Mucilage, tannins, and polysaccharides.
- **Applications:** Slippery elm bark can be made into a soothing tea or lozenge, or taken as a powder mixed with water.

Artichoke (Cynara scolymus)

- **Traditional Uses:** Artichoke leaves have been used to stimulate bile production, improve digestion, and reduce symptoms of indigestion such as bloating and gas.
- **Key Constituents:** Cynarin, luteolin, and chlorogenic acid.
- **Applications:** Artichoke extract is available in capsule or tincture form, and the leaves can be brewed into a tea.

Herbal remedies offer a natural and effective way to support digestive health and alleviate common digestive issues. By understanding the traditional uses and applications of these common digestive herbs, individuals can enhance their digestive well-being and overall health. Whether used in teas, tinctures, capsules, or as part of the diet, these herbs provide valuable tools for maintaining a healthy digestive system.

Herbs for Respiratory Support

Respiratory health is crucial for overall well-being, as it ensures the efficient exchange of oxygen and carbon dioxide in the body. Various herbs have been traditionally used to support respiratory function, alleviate symptoms of respiratory conditions, and strengthen the lungs. The following sections explore some of the most common herbs known for their beneficial effects on respiratory health.

Eucalyptus (Eucalyptus globulus)

- **Traditional Uses:** Eucalyptus has been widely used for its decongestant and expectorant properties. It helps clear mucus from the respiratory tract and relieve symptoms of coughs, colds, and sinusitis.
- **Key Constituents:** Eucalyptol (cineole), tannins, and flavonoids.
- **Applications:** Eucalyptus oil can be inhaled through steam inhalation, added to a diffuser, or used in chest rubs to relieve congestion.

Peppermint (Mentha piperita)

- **Traditional Uses:** Peppermint is known for its soothing effects on the respiratory system. Its menthol content helps open airways, reduce congestion, and relieve coughs and colds.
- **Key Constituents:** Menthol, menthone, and flavonoids.

- **Applications:** Peppermint tea, steam inhalation, or peppermint oil in a diffuser can be used to alleviate respiratory discomfort.

Licorice Root (Glycyrrhiza glabra)

- **Traditional Uses:** Licorice root has been used to soothe and protect the mucous membranes of the respiratory tract. It has expectorant, anti-inflammatory, and demulcent properties.
- **Key Constituents:** Glycyrrhizin, flavonoids, and saponins.
- **Applications:** Licorice root tea, extracts, or deglycyrrhizinated licorice (DGL) supplements can be used for respiratory support.

Mullein (Verbascum thapsus)

- **Traditional Uses:** Mullein has traditionally been used to treat respiratory conditions such as bronchitis, asthma, and coughs. It acts as an expectorant, helping to expel mucus from the lungs.
- **Key Constituents:** Mucilage, saponins, and flavonoids.
- **Applications:** Mullein leaves and flowers can be made into tea, tinctures, or extracts for respiratory health.

Thyme (Thymus vulgaris)

- **Traditional Uses:** Thyme is known for its antiseptic and expectorant properties. It helps clear mucus from the respiratory tract and has been used to treat coughs, bronchitis, and sore throats.
- **Key Constituents:** Thymol, carvacrol, and flavonoids.
- **Applications:** Thyme tea, steam inhalation, or thyme oil in a diffuser can be used to support respiratory health.

Ginger (Zingiber officinale)

- **Traditional Uses:** Ginger has been used to relieve respiratory congestion, reduce inflammation, and enhance immune function. Its warming properties help clear mucus and improve circulation in the respiratory tract.
- **Key Constituents:** Gingerol, shogaol, and zingerone.
- **Applications:** Fresh ginger tea, ginger supplements, or adding ginger to foods can help support respiratory health.

Marshmallow Root (Althaea officinalis)

- **Traditional Uses:** Marshmallow root is known for its soothing and demulcent properties. It helps reduce irritation and inflammation in the respiratory tract, making it useful for treating coughs and sore throats.
- **Key Constituents:** Mucilage, flavonoids, and polysaccharides.
- **Applications:** Marshmallow root tea, extracts, or syrups can be used to soothe the respiratory system.

Elecampane (Inula helenium)

- **Traditional Uses:** Elecampane has been used to treat chronic respiratory conditions such as bronchitis and asthma. It acts as an expectorant and has antimicrobial properties.
- **Key Constituents:** Inulin, alantolactone, and isoalantolactone.
- **Applications:** Elecampane root can be made into tea, tinctures, or syrups for respiratory support.

Osha Root (Ligusticum porteri)

- **Traditional Uses:** Osha root has been used by Native American cultures for respiratory infections and congestion. It has antiviral, antibacterial, and expectorant properties.
- **Key Constituents:** Ligustilide, ferulic acid, and phytosterols.
- **Applications:** Osha root can be taken as a tea, tincture, or in capsule form to support respiratory health.

Herbal remedies provide a natural and effective way to support respiratory health and alleviate symptoms of respiratory conditions. By understanding the traditional uses and applications of these common respiratory herbs, individuals can enhance their respiratory well-being and overall health. Whether used in teas, tinctures, steam inhalations, or as part of the diet, these herbs offer valuable tools for maintaining a healthy respiratory system.

Herbal Remedies for Immune System Boosting

A robust immune system is essential for maintaining health and defending the body against infections and diseases. Various herbs have been traditionally used to strengthen and support immune function. These herbs can help enhance the body's natural defenses, reduce the severity of illnesses, and improve overall health. The following sections explore some of the most common herbs known for their immune-boosting properties.

Echinacea (Echinacea purpurea)

- **Traditional Uses:** Echinacea is widely recognized for its immune-stimulating properties. It has been used to prevent and treat colds, flu, and other respiratory infections.
- **Key Constituents:** Alkamides, polysaccharides, and caffeic acid derivatives.
- **Applications:** Echinacea can be taken as a tea, tincture, capsule, or extract to boost immune function, particularly at the onset of symptoms.

Elderberry (Sambucus nigra)

- **Traditional Uses:** Elderberry is known for its antiviral properties and has been traditionally used to reduce the duration and severity of colds and flu.
- **Key Constituents:** Anthocyanins, flavonoids, and vitamins A and C.
- **Applications:** Elderberry syrup, lozenges, or extracts can be used to support immune health and combat viral infections.

Astragalus (Astragalus membranaceus)

- **Traditional Uses:** Astragalus is a key herb in Traditional Chinese Medicine (TCM) for enhancing immune function and increasing vitality. It is used to prevent colds and respiratory infections.
- **Key Constituents:** Polysaccharides, saponins, and flavonoids.
- **Applications:** Astragalus root can be taken as a tea, tincture, or capsule to support long-term immune health and resilience.

Garlic (Allium sativum)

- **Traditional Uses:** Garlic is renowned for its antimicrobial and immune-boosting properties. It has been used to treat infections, support cardiovascular health, and enhance overall immunity.
- **Key Constituents:** Allicin, sulfur compounds, and flavonoids.
- **Applications:** Fresh garlic, garlic supplements, or garlic oil can be incorporated into the diet to support immune function.

Ginger (Zingiber officinale)

- **Traditional Uses:** Ginger is known for its warming and immune-enhancing properties. It helps improve circulation, reduce inflammation, and support the body's defense mechanisms.
- **Key Constituents:** Gingerol, shogaol, and zingerone.
- **Applications:** Fresh ginger tea, ginger supplements, or adding ginger to foods can help boost the immune system.

Turmeric (Curcuma longa)

- **Traditional Uses:** Turmeric has powerful anti-inflammatory and antioxidant properties that support immune health. It has been used to treat infections and reduce inflammation in the body.
- **Key Constituents:** Curcumin, volatile oils, and polysaccharides.
- **Applications:** Turmeric can be taken as a tea, supplement, or added to food to support immune function and overall health.

Reishi Mushroom (Ganoderma lucidum)

- **Traditional Uses:** Reishi mushroom is highly valued in traditional medicine for its immune-modulating properties. It helps enhance immune response and reduce inflammation.
- **Key Constituents:** Polysaccharides, triterpenes, and peptidoglycans.
- **Applications:** Reishi can be consumed as a tea, tincture, or in capsule form to support immune health.

Licorice Root (Glycyrrhiza glabra)

- **Traditional Uses:** Licorice root has been used to support the immune system and treat respiratory infections. It has antiviral and anti-inflammatory properties.
- **Key Constituents:** Glycyrrhizin, flavonoids, and saponins.
- **Applications:** Licorice root tea, extracts, or deglycyrrhizinated licorice (DGL) supplements can be used for immune support.

Andrographis (Andrographis paniculata)

- **Traditional Uses:** Andrographis is known for its immune-stimulating and antiviral properties. It has been used to treat colds, flu, and other infections.
- **Key Constituents:** Andrographolide, diterpenes, and flavonoids.
- **Applications:** Andrographis can be taken as a tea, tincture, or supplement to support immune function.

Herbal remedies offer a natural and effective way to boost the immune system and enhance the body's ability to fight infections. By understanding the traditional uses and applications of these common immune-boosting herbs, individuals can support their immune health and overall well-being. Whether used in teas, tinctures, capsules, or as part of the diet, these herbs provide valuable tools for maintaining a strong and resilient immune system.

Herbs for Mental Health and Cognitive Support

Mental health and cognitive function are critical aspects of overall well-being. Various herbs have been traditionally used to support mental clarity, reduce anxiety, improve mood, and enhance cognitive performance. The following sections explore some of the most common herbs known for their beneficial effects on mental health and cognitive function.

Ginkgo Biloba (Ginkgo biloba)

- **Traditional Uses:** Ginkgo biloba has been used for centuries to enhance cognitive function and improve memory. It is known for increasing blood flow to the brain, which can help with concentration and mental clarity.
- **Key Constituents:** Flavonoids, terpenoids (ginkgolides and bilobalides), and antioxidants.
- **Applications:** Ginkgo can be taken as a tea, extract, or supplement to support cognitive health and improve memory and concentration.

Bacopa Monnieri (Bacopa monnieri)

- **Traditional Uses:** Bacopa, also known as Brahmi, is a staple in Ayurvedic medicine for enhancing cognitive function, reducing anxiety, and improving memory. It is particularly noted for its adaptogenic properties.
- **Key Constituents:** Bacosides, alkaloids, and flavonoids.
- **Applications:** Bacopa can be taken as a tea, tincture, or capsule to support brain health and mental performance.

Ashwagandha (Withania somnifera)

- **Traditional Uses:** Ashwagandha is an adaptogenic herb used in Ayurveda to reduce stress, improve mood, and enhance cognitive function. It helps balance cortisol levels and supports overall mental health.
- **Key Constituents:** Withanolides, alkaloids, and saponins.
- **Applications:** Ashwagandha root can be taken as a tea, tincture, or supplement to support mental resilience and cognitive clarity.

Rhodiola Rosea (Rhodiola rosea)

- **Traditional Uses:** Rhodiola is known for its adaptogenic properties, helping to reduce fatigue, improve mood, and enhance cognitive function. It is particularly useful for managing stress and enhancing mental performance.
- **Key Constituents:** Rosavins, salidrosides, and flavonoids.
- **Applications:** Rhodiola can be taken as a tea, tincture, or supplement to support mental endurance and reduce stress.

Gotu Kola (Centella asiatica)

- **Traditional Uses:** Gotu Kola is an important herb in Ayurveda and Traditional Chinese Medicine for promoting mental clarity, enhancing memory, and reducing anxiety. It supports cognitive function and overall brain health.
- **Key Constituents:** Triterpenoids, asiaticoside, and madecassoside.
- **Applications:** Gotu Kola can be taken as a tea, tincture, or supplement to support cognitive health and reduce anxiety.

St. John's Wort (Hypericum perforatum)

- **Traditional Uses:** St. John's Wort has been traditionally used to treat mild to moderate depression and anxiety. It is known for its mood-stabilizing and antidepressant properties.
- **Key Constituents:** Hypericin, hyperforin, and flavonoids.
- **Applications:** St. John's Wort can be taken as a tea, tincture, or supplement to support emotional well-being and reduce symptoms of depression.

Lemon Balm (Melissa officinalis)

- **Traditional Uses:** Lemon balm is known for its calming and mood-enhancing properties. It helps reduce anxiety, improve sleep, and enhance cognitive function.
- **Key Constituents:** Rosmarinic acid, flavonoids, and essential oils.
- **Applications:** Lemon balm can be taken as a tea, tincture, or supplement to promote relaxation and support mental clarity.

Valerian Root (Valeriana officinalis)

- **Traditional Uses:** Valerian root is commonly used to reduce anxiety, improve sleep quality, and promote relaxation. It is particularly effective for managing stress and nervous tension.

- **Key Constituents:** Valerenic acid, valepotriates, and essential oils.
- **Applications:** Valerian root can be taken as a tea, tincture, or supplement to support relaxation and improve sleep.

Holy Basil (Ocimum sanctum)

- **Traditional Uses:** Holy basil, also known as Tulsi, is an adaptogenic herb used in Ayurveda to reduce stress, enhance mood, and support cognitive function. It helps balance stress hormones and supports overall mental health.
- **Key Constituents:** Eugenol, rosmarinic acid, and ursolic acid.
- **Applications:** Holy basil can be taken as a tea, tincture, or supplement to support stress management and cognitive clarity.

Rosemary (Rosmarinus officinalis)

- **Traditional Uses:** Rosemary has been used traditionally to improve memory, concentration, and overall cognitive function. Its stimulating properties help enhance mental clarity and focus.
- **Key Constituents:** Rosmarinic acid, carnosic acid, and essential oils.
- **Applications:** Rosemary can be used as a culinary herb, essential oil for aromatherapy, or taken as a tea to support cognitive health.

Herbal remedies provide a natural and effective way to support mental health and cognitive function. By understanding the traditional uses and applications of these common herbs, individuals can enhance their mental clarity, reduce anxiety, improve mood, and support overall cognitive health. Whether used in teas, tinctures, supplements, or as part of the diet, these herbs offer valuable tools for maintaining and improving mental well-being.

Topical Herbs for Skin Health

The skin is the largest organ of the body and serves as a protective barrier against external elements. Maintaining healthy skin is crucial for overall health and well-being. Various herbs have been traditionally used topically to support skin health, treat skin conditions, and enhance the skin's appearance. The following sections explore some of the most common herbs known for their beneficial effects on skin health.

Aloe Vera (Aloe barbadensis)

- **Traditional Uses:** Aloe vera is renowned for its soothing, healing, and moisturizing properties. It is commonly used to treat burns, wounds, and skin irritations.
- **Key Constituents:** Polysaccharides, vitamins, minerals, and enzymes.
- **Applications:** Aloe vera gel can be applied directly to the skin to soothe burns, moisturize dry skin, and promote wound healing.

Calendula (Calendula officinalis)

- **Traditional Uses:** Calendula, also known as marigold, is used for its anti-inflammatory, antiseptic, and healing properties. It helps treat minor wounds, rashes, and skin irritations.
- **Key Constituents:** Flavonoids, triterpenoids, and essential oils.
- **Applications:** Calendula can be used in ointments, creams, and infused oils to promote skin healing and reduce inflammation.

Chamomile (Matricaria chamomilla)

- **Traditional Uses:** Chamomile is known for its calming and anti-inflammatory properties. It is used to treat skin conditions such as eczema, dermatitis, and minor wounds.
- **Key Constituents:** Bisabolol, chamazulene, and flavonoids.
- **Applications:** Chamomile-infused oils, creams, and compresses can be applied to the skin to soothe irritation and reduce inflammation.

Lavender (Lavandula angustifolia)

- **Traditional Uses:** Lavender is valued for its antiseptic, anti-inflammatory, and calming properties. It is used to treat burns, wounds, and skin infections.
- **Key Constituents:** Linalool, linalyl acetate, and camphor.
- **Applications:** Lavender essential oil can be diluted and applied to the skin, or used in creams and lotions to promote healing and reduce skin irritation.

Tea Tree (Melaleuca alternifolia)

- **Traditional Uses:** Tea tree oil is known for its potent antiseptic, antifungal, and antibacterial properties. It is used to treat acne, fungal infections, and minor cuts.
- **Key Constituents:** Terpinen-4-ol, cineole, and terpinene.
- **Applications:** Tea tree oil can be diluted and applied to acne spots, fungal infections, and minor wounds to disinfect and promote healing.

Witch Hazel (Hamamelis virginiana)

- **Traditional Uses:** Witch hazel is used for its astringent, anti-inflammatory, and soothing properties. It helps treat acne, minor cuts, and skin irritations.
- **Key Constituents:** Tannins, flavonoids, and volatile oils.
- **Applications:** Witch hazel extract can be applied directly to the skin using a cotton pad to tone, soothe, and reduce inflammation.

Comfrey (Symphytum officinale)

- **Traditional Uses:** Comfrey is known for its cell-regenerating and anti-inflammatory properties. It is used to treat bruises, sprains, and minor wounds.
- **Key Constituents:** Allantoin, rosmarinic acid, and mucilage.
- **Applications:** Comfrey-infused oils, creams, and poultices can be applied to the skin to promote healing and reduce inflammation.

Gotu Kola (Centella asiatica)

- **Traditional Uses:** Gotu kola is used for its skin-healing, anti-inflammatory, and collagen-boosting properties. It helps treat wounds, scars, and skin irritations.
- **Key Constituents:** Asiaticoside, madecassoside, and triterpenoids.
- **Applications:** Gotu kola extracts, creams, and serums can be applied to the skin to enhance healing and improve skin elasticity.

Turmeric (Curcuma longa)

- **Traditional Uses:** Turmeric is known for its anti-inflammatory, antioxidant, and healing properties. It is used to treat acne, wounds, and skin conditions like eczema.
- **Key Constituents:** Curcumin, volatile oils, and polysaccharides.
- **Applications:** Turmeric paste or infused oils can be applied to the skin to reduce inflammation, promote healing, and improve skin health.

Neem (Azadirachta indica)

- **Traditional Uses:** Neem is valued for its antiseptic, antifungal, and anti-inflammatory properties. It is used to treat acne, eczema, and fungal infections.
- **Key Constituents:** Azadirachtin, nimbin, and quercetin.
- **Applications:** Neem oil or neem-based creams and lotions can be applied to the skin to treat infections, reduce inflammation, and improve skin health.

Herbal remedies offer a natural and effective way to support skin health and treat various skin conditions. By understanding the traditional uses and applications of these common topical herbs, individuals can enhance their skin care routines and promote overall skin health. Whether used in gels, oils, creams, or compresses, these herbs provide valuable tools for maintaining healthy, radiant skin.

BOOK 3:

Fundamentals of Non-Toxic Living: Strategies for a Healthier and Cleaner Life

Understanding Toxins

In today's world, toxins are an inescapable part of our environment, infiltrating the air we breathe, the water we drink, and the food we consume. Understanding what toxins are, where they come from, and how they impact our health is crucial for making informed decisions to protect ourselves and our families. This chapter delves into the nature of toxins, their various sources, and the potential health risks associated with exposure. By dispelling common myths and misconceptions, it aims to provide a clear and comprehensive foundation for recognizing and mitigating toxin exposure in our daily lives.

What Are Toxins?

Toxins are harmful substances that can cause damage to living organisms. They come in various forms and can originate from both natural and human-made sources. Understanding the nature and diversity of toxins is essential for recognizing their potential impact on health and taking steps to minimize exposure.

Types of Toxins

1. **Biological Toxins:**

   o **Description:** These are naturally occurring toxins produced by living organisms, including bacteria, fungi, plants, and animals.

   o **Examples:**

      - **Bacterial Toxins:** Botulinum toxin produced by Clostridium botulinum.

      - **Fungal Toxins:** Aflatoxins produced by Aspergillus species.

      - **Plant Toxins:** Ricin from castor beans.

      - **Animal Toxins:** Venom from snakes, spiders, and scorpions.

2. **Chemical Toxins:**

   o **Description:** These are synthetic or naturally occurring chemicals that can be harmful to humans and the environment.

   o **Examples:**

      - **Pesticides:** Chemicals used to kill pests, such as DDT and glyphosate.

      - **Industrial Chemicals:** Asbestos, polychlorinated biphenyls (PCBs), and dioxins.

      - **Heavy Metals:** Lead, mercury, arsenic, and cadmium.

3. **Environmental Toxins:**

   o **Description:** These toxins originate from environmental sources and can accumulate in the air, water, and soil.

- **Examples:**
  - **Air Pollutants:** Particulate matter, carbon monoxide, sulfur dioxide, and nitrogen oxides.
  - **Water Contaminants:** Industrial waste, agricultural runoff, and pharmaceuticals.
  - **Soil Contaminants:** Pesticides, heavy metals, and industrial chemicals.

Sources of Toxins

1. **Industrial Activities:**
   - Manufacturing processes release various chemicals and pollutants into the air, water, and soil.
   - Examples include emissions from factories, chemical spills, and waste disposal.

2. **Agricultural Practices:**
   - The use of pesticides, herbicides, and fertilizers introduces toxins into the environment.
   - Contaminants can enter the food chain through crops and livestock.

3. **Household Products:**
   - Many common household items contain toxic chemicals, such as cleaning agents, personal care products, and synthetic materials.
   - Examples include phthalates in plastics, formaldehyde in furniture, and volatile organic compounds (VOCs) in paints.

4. **Food and Beverages:**
   - Toxins can be present in food due to contamination, additives, and packaging materials.
   - Examples include bisphenol A (BPA) in plastic containers, pesticide residues on fruits and vegetables, and preservatives in processed foods.

5. **Medications and Medical Treatments:**
   - Some pharmaceuticals and medical treatments can introduce toxins into the body.
   - Examples include certain chemotherapy drugs, heavy metal-based medications, and excess use of antibiotics.

Impact of Toxins on Health

1. **Acute Toxicity:**

- Short-term exposure to high levels of toxins can cause immediate health effects, such as poisoning, respiratory distress, and skin irritation.
- Examples include carbon monoxide poisoning, chemical burns, and allergic reactions.

2. **Chronic Toxicity:**

- Long-term exposure to lower levels of toxins can lead to chronic health conditions, including cancer, neurological disorders, and endocrine disruption.
- Examples include lead poisoning, asbestos-related lung disease, and pesticide exposure leading to hormone imbalances.

3. **Bioaccumulation and Biomagnification:**

- Toxins can accumulate in living organisms over time (bioaccumulation) and become more concentrated as they move up the food chain (biomagnification).
- Examples include mercury accumulation in fish and PCBs in marine mammals.

Understanding what toxins are and recognizing their various forms and sources is a crucial first step in protecting health and minimizing exposure. By identifying the types of toxins and their potential impact on the body, individuals can make informed decisions to reduce their toxin burden and create a safer, healthier living environment. This foundational knowledge sets the stage for exploring detoxification strategies and non-toxic living practices in subsequent chapters.

Sources of Toxins in Everyday Life

Toxins are pervasive in our modern environment, often lurking in places we might not expect. Recognizing the common sources of toxins in everyday life is essential for reducing exposure and safeguarding our health. This section explores various sources of toxins that we encounter daily, from the air we breathe to the products we use in our homes.

1. Air Pollution

- **Outdoor Air Pollution:**
  - **Sources:** Vehicle emissions, industrial discharges, power plants, and agricultural activities.
  - **Common Toxins:** Particulate matter (PM), carbon monoxide (CO), nitrogen oxides (NOx), sulfur dioxide (SO2), and volatile organic compounds (VOCs).
  - **Health Effects:** Respiratory problems, cardiovascular diseases, and aggravated asthma.

- **Indoor Air Pollution:**
  - **Sources:** Household cleaning products, tobacco smoke, building materials, and indoor heating appliances.

- Common **Toxins:** Formaldehyde, radon, asbestos, VOCs, and carbon monoxide.
- **Health Effects:** Allergies, asthma, respiratory infections, and indoor air quality syndrome.

2. Water Contamination

- **Drinking Water:**
  - **Sources:** Industrial waste, agricultural runoff, sewage leaks, and contaminated groundwater.
  - **Common Toxins:** Heavy metals (lead, mercury, arsenic), pesticides, nitrates, chlorine, and pharmaceutical residues.
  - **Health Effects:** Gastrointestinal illnesses, neurological disorders, reproductive issues, and cancers.

- **Recreational Water:**
  - **Sources:** Pollution from boats, industrial discharges, and agricultural runoff into lakes, rivers, and oceans.
  - **Common Toxins:** Pathogens (bacteria, viruses), chemical contaminants, and algal toxins.
  - **Health Effects:** Skin infections, gastrointestinal illnesses, and respiratory issues.

3. Food and Beverages

- **Pesticides and Herbicides:**
  - **Sources:** Conventional farming practices that use chemical pesticides and herbicides.
  - **Common Toxins:** Glyphosate, organophosphates, and neonicotinoids.
  - **Health Effects:** Hormonal imbalances, neurological disorders, and cancers.

- **Food Additives and Preservatives:**
  - **Sources:** Processed and packaged foods.
  - **Common Toxins:** Artificial colors, flavors, sweeteners (aspartame), and preservatives (sodium benzoate, BHA, BHT).
  - **Health Effects:** Allergic reactions, hyperactivity, and long-term health risks like cancer.

- **Contaminants in Packaging:**
  - **Sources:** Plastics, cans, and other food packaging materials.

- o **Common Toxins:** Bisphenol A (BPA), phthalates, and styrene.
- o **Health Effects:** Endocrine disruption, developmental issues, and increased cancer risk.

4. Household Products

- **Cleaning Products:**
  - o **Sources:** Common household cleaners, disinfectants, and air fresheners.
  - o **Common Toxins:** Ammonia, bleach, phthalates, and triclosan.
  - o **Health Effects:** Respiratory irritation, skin allergies, and hormone disruption.

- **Personal Care Products:**
  - o **Sources:** Cosmetics, shampoos, lotions, and deodorants.
  - o **Common Toxins:** Parabens, phthalates, formaldehyde-releasing preservatives, and synthetic fragrances.
  - o **Health Effects:** Skin irritation, allergic reactions, and endocrine disruption.

- **Pesticides and Insecticides:**
  - o **Sources:** Household pest control products.
  - o **Common Toxins:** Pyrethroids, organophosphates, and carbamates.
  - o **Health Effects:** Neurological damage, respiratory issues, and hormone disruption.

5. Building Materials and Furnishings

- **Construction Materials:**
  - o **Sources:** Paints, varnishes, adhesives, and insulation materials.
  - o **Common Toxins:** VOCs, formaldehyde, asbestos, and lead.
  - o **Health Effects:** Respiratory problems, skin irritation, and long-term risks like cancer.

- **Furniture and Carpets:**
  - o **Sources:** Upholstered furniture, carpets, and treated wood.
  - o **Common Toxins:** Flame retardants (PBDEs), formaldehyde, and VOCs.
  - o **Health Effects:** Allergic reactions, hormone disruption, and respiratory issues.

6. Electronics and Gadgets

- **Electronic Devices:**

- **Sources:** Computers, smartphones, and household electronics.
- **Common Toxins:** Lead, cadmium, brominated flame retardants, and phthalates.
- **Health Effects:** Neurological damage, reproductive issues, and developmental problems.

Toxins are ubiquitous in our environment, stemming from various everyday sources. By understanding where these toxins come from and how they can affect our health, we can take proactive steps to minimize exposure. This knowledge empowers us to make informed choices about the products we use, the food we eat, and the environments we inhabit, ultimately leading to a healthier, toxin-reduced lifestyle.

The Impact of Toxins on Health

Toxins in our environment can have profound and wide-ranging effects on human health. These effects can be acute or chronic, depending on the type and level of exposure. Understanding the impact of toxins on health is crucial for implementing effective strategies to minimize their harmful effects and promote overall well-being. This section explores the various ways in which toxins affect different systems of the body and the potential health consequences.

1. Respiratory System

- **Acute Effects:**
  - Exposure to high levels of air pollutants and toxic chemicals can cause immediate respiratory issues such as coughing, shortness of breath, and throat irritation.
  - Examples: Inhalation of smoke from fires, industrial emissions, or chemical fumes.

- **Chronic Effects:**
  - Long-term exposure to air pollutants and toxins can lead to chronic respiratory conditions such as asthma, chronic obstructive pulmonary disease (COPD), and lung cancer.
  - Examples: Prolonged exposure to particulate matter, radon, and tobacco smoke.

2. Cardiovascular System

- **Acute Effects:**
  - Sudden exposure to high levels of pollutants can trigger acute cardiovascular events such as heart attacks and strokes.
  - Examples: Short-term spikes in air pollution or exposure to carbon monoxide.

- **Chronic Effects:**

- Long-term exposure to environmental toxins can increase the risk of developing cardiovascular diseases, including hypertension, atherosclerosis, and heart disease.
- Examples: Persistent exposure to heavy metals (lead, mercury) and air pollutants (PM2.5, ozone).

3. Nervous System

- **Acute Effects:**
  - Immediate exposure to neurotoxins can cause symptoms such as headaches, dizziness, confusion, and seizures.
  - Examples: Acute poisoning from pesticides, solvents, or industrial chemicals.

- **Chronic Effects:**
  - Prolonged exposure to neurotoxins can result in long-term neurological disorders, including cognitive decline, memory loss, and developmental delays in children.
  - Examples: Chronic exposure to lead, mercury, and organophosphate pesticides.

4. Endocrine System

- **Acute Effects:**
  - Acute exposure to endocrine disruptors can lead to temporary hormonal imbalances, affecting metabolism, growth, and reproduction.
  - Examples: Short-term exposure to phthalates and bisphenol A (BPA).

- **Chronic Effects:**
  - Long-term exposure to endocrine-disrupting chemicals can lead to significant health issues such as thyroid disorders, reproductive health problems, and increased risk of cancers like breast and prostate cancer.
  - Examples: Persistent exposure to BPA, dioxins, and certain pesticides.

5. Immune System

- **Acute Effects:**
  - Exposure to high levels of certain toxins can cause an immediate weakening of the immune system, making the body more susceptible to infections.
  - Examples: Acute exposure to high doses of radiation or toxic chemicals.

- **Chronic Effects:**

- Long-term exposure to environmental toxins can lead to immune system dysfunction, resulting in increased susceptibility to infections, autoimmune diseases, and allergies.
- Examples: Chronic exposure to heavy metals, PCBs, and pesticides.

6. Reproductive System

- **Acute Effects:**
  - Short-term exposure to reproductive toxins can cause temporary fertility issues and developmental problems in offspring.
  - Examples: Acute exposure to certain solvents, pesticides, and endocrine disruptors.

- **Chronic Effects:**
  - Prolonged exposure to reproductive toxins can result in significant reproductive health problems, including infertility, birth defects, and developmental delays in children.
  - Examples: Persistent exposure to phthalates, lead, and endocrine disruptors.

7. Gastrointestinal System

- **Acute Effects:**
  - Ingestion of toxic substances can cause immediate gastrointestinal symptoms such as nausea, vomiting, diarrhea, and abdominal pain.
  - Examples: Acute food poisoning, ingestion of contaminated water, or toxic chemicals.

- **Chronic Effects:**
  - Long-term exposure to toxins through diet and water can lead to chronic gastrointestinal disorders, including liver disease, gastrointestinal cancers, and inflammatory bowel diseases.
  - Examples: Chronic exposure to aflatoxins, heavy metals, and persistent organic pollutants (POPs).

8. Skin

- **Acute Effects:**
  - Direct contact with certain toxins can cause immediate skin reactions such as rashes, irritation, and burns.
  - Examples: Contact with toxic plants (e.g., poison ivy), chemical spills, and harsh cleaning agents.

- **Chronic Effects:**
    - Long-term exposure to skin irritants and toxic chemicals can lead to chronic skin conditions such as eczema, dermatitis, and skin cancers.
    - Examples: Persistent exposure to industrial chemicals, UV radiation, and certain cosmetics.

Toxins can affect virtually every system in the body, leading to a wide range of acute and chronic health issues. By understanding the impact of toxins on health, we can take proactive measures to reduce exposure and protect ourselves from their harmful effects. This knowledge is essential for developing effective detoxification strategies and adopting non-toxic living practices to promote long-term health and well-being.

Identifying Toxin Exposure

Recognizing and identifying toxin exposure is a crucial step in mitigating its harmful effects and protecting overall health. Toxins can be encountered in various forms and from multiple sources in our everyday environment. By understanding the signs and symptoms of toxin exposure, as well as the methods for detecting and measuring toxins, individuals can take proactive steps to reduce their toxin burden. This section explores how to identify toxin exposure effectively.

Signs and Symptoms of Toxin Exposure

1. **Respiratory Symptoms:**
    - **Common Signs:** Coughing, wheezing, shortness of breath, nasal congestion, throat irritation.
    - **Potential Sources:** Air pollutants, smoke, industrial emissions, household cleaners, mold.

2. **Dermal Symptoms:**
    - **Common Signs:** Rashes, itching, redness, blistering, dry or flaky skin.
    - **Potential Sources:** Contact with toxic plants, chemicals in personal care products, cleaning agents, pesticides.

3. **Gastrointestinal Symptoms:**
    - **Common Signs:** Nausea, vomiting, diarrhea, abdominal pain, bloating.
    - **Potential Sources:** Contaminated food or water, heavy metals, food additives, pesticide residues.

4. **Neurological Symptoms:**
    - **Common Signs:** Headaches, dizziness, confusion, memory loss, tremors, numbness.

- **Potential Sources:** Heavy metals (lead, mercury), solvents, pesticides, industrial chemicals.

5. **Cardiovascular Symptoms:**

   - **Common Signs:** High blood pressure, irregular heartbeat, chest pain.

   - **Potential Sources:** Air pollution, carbon monoxide, heavy metals, endocrine disruptors.

6. **Immune System Symptoms:**

   - **Common Signs:** Frequent infections, allergies, autoimmune disorders.

   - **Potential Sources:** Pesticides, heavy metals, industrial chemicals, environmental pollutants.

7. **Endocrine Symptoms:**

   - **Common Signs:** Hormonal imbalances, weight gain, fatigue, reproductive issues.

   - **Potential Sources:** Endocrine disruptors like BPA, phthalates, pesticides.

Methods for Detecting Toxins

1. **Environmental Testing:**

   - **Air Quality Testing:**

     - **Methods:** Use of air sampling devices to measure pollutants like particulate matter, VOCs, radon.

     - **Applications:** Home air quality monitors, professional air testing services.

   - **Water Quality Testing:**

     - **Methods:** Testing kits and lab analysis to detect contaminants like heavy metals, pesticides, chlorine.

     - **Applications:** Home water testing kits, municipal water reports.

   - **Soil Testing:**

     - **Methods:** Soil sampling and lab analysis to detect contaminants such as pesticides, heavy metals.

     - **Applications:** Home garden soil tests, agricultural soil analysis.

2. **Biomonitoring:**

   - **Blood Tests:**

- **Purpose:** Measure levels of heavy metals (lead, mercury), pesticides, and other toxins in the bloodstream.
- **Applications:** Clinical settings, wellness checks.

- **Urine Tests:**
  - **Purpose:** Detect toxins like heavy metals, BPA, phthalates.
  - **Applications:** Clinical diagnostics, exposure assessment.

- **Hair Analysis:**
  - **Purpose:** Long-term exposure assessment for heavy metals and other persistent toxins.
  - **Applications:** Clinical and forensic settings.

3. **Symptom Tracking and Self-Assessment:**
   - **Purpose:** Monitoring health changes and correlating them with potential exposure sources.
   - **Applications:** Health diaries, symptom tracking apps, consultation with healthcare providers.

4. **Home and Workplace Assessments:**
   - **Purpose:** Identifying and mitigating sources of toxin exposure in living and working environments.
   - **Applications:** Professional home inspections, workplace safety audits, use of non-toxic products and materials.

Reducing Toxin Exposure

1. **Lifestyle Changes:**
   - **Diet:**
     - **Strategies:** Eating organic foods, avoiding processed foods, reducing intake of high-risk foods (e.g., fish high in mercury).
   - **Personal Care:**
     - **Strategies:** Using natural and organic personal care products, avoiding synthetic fragrances and preservatives.
   - **Cleaning:**
     - **Strategies:** Using non-toxic cleaning products, avoiding harsh chemicals.

2. **Environmental Modifications:**

- o **Indoor Air Quality:**

    - **Strategies:** Using air purifiers, increasing ventilation, avoiding indoor smoking.

- o **Water Quality:**

    - **Strategies:** Installing water filters, drinking filtered or bottled water.

- o **Soil Quality:**

    - **Strategies:** Using clean soil for gardening, avoiding pesticide use.

3. **Professional Guidance:**

    - o **Consulting Experts:**

        - **Purpose:** Seeking advice from healthcare providers, environmental health experts, and toxicologists.

        - **Applications:** Developing personalized detox plans, addressing specific health concerns related to toxin exposure.

Identifying toxin exposure involves understanding the signs and symptoms, utilizing various detection methods, and taking proactive steps to reduce exposure. By being aware of the potential sources of toxins and monitoring their presence in our environment and bodies, individuals can take informed actions to protect their health and well-being. This knowledge is essential for creating a cleaner, safer living environment and minimizing the harmful effects of toxins.

Common Myths and Misconceptions About Toxins

Understanding the truth about toxins is essential for making informed decisions about health and safety. However, there are many myths and misconceptions that can lead to unnecessary fear or a false sense of security. This section addresses some of the most common myths and misconceptions about toxins and provides information to help clarify these misunderstandings.

Myth 1: Natural Products Are Always Safe

- **Misconception:** Many people believe that if a product is labeled as "natural," it is completely safe and free of harmful effects.

- **Fact:** Natural does not always mean safe. Some natural substances can be toxic or cause adverse reactions. For example, certain plants like poison ivy or hemlock are highly toxic despite being natural. It's important to research and understand the safety profile of any natural product before use.

Myth 2: Organic Foods Are Completely Free of Toxins

- **Misconception:** Organic foods are often perceived as being completely free of pesticides and other toxins.

- **Fact:** While organic farming practices reduce the use of synthetic pesticides and chemicals, organic foods can still contain natural pesticides or residues from approved organic pesticides. Additionally, organic produce can be contaminated by environmental pollutants. However, organic foods generally have lower levels of pesticide residues compared to conventionally grown foods.

Myth 3: Only Industrial Chemicals Are Harmful

- **Misconception:** Some believe that only chemicals used in industrial processes are harmful, while everyday household chemicals are safe.

- **Fact:** Many household products, such as cleaning agents, personal care products, and air fresheners, contain chemicals that can be harmful with prolonged or excessive exposure. It's important to use these products according to instructions and consider safer, non-toxic alternatives.

Myth 4: Small Amounts of Toxins Are Harmless

- **Misconception:** The belief that exposure to small amounts of toxins is harmless and does not accumulate over time.

- **Fact:** While the body can handle small amounts of many substances, chronic exposure to low levels of certain toxins can accumulate and lead to long-term health issues. For example, continuous exposure to low levels of heavy metals or endocrine disruptors can have significant health impacts over time.

Myth 5: Detox Products Can Instantly Remove Toxins

- **Misconception:** Many detox products on the market claim to instantly cleanse the body of all toxins.

- **Fact:** The body has its own natural detoxification systems, primarily the liver, kidneys, and skin. While certain dietary and lifestyle changes can support these systems, there is no quick fix for detoxification. Over-the-counter detox products often lack scientific backing and may not be effective or necessary.

Myth 6: If You Don't Feel Sick, Toxins Aren't Affecting You

- **Misconception:** The idea that if you don't have immediate symptoms, toxins are not having an impact on your health.

- **Fact:** Some toxins can cause damage without immediate symptoms. Chronic exposure to certain toxins can lead to long-term health effects that may not be apparent until much later. Regular health check-ups and preventive measures are important even in the absence of symptoms.

Myth 7: All Plastics Are Safe

- **Misconception:** The assumption that all plastic products are safe to use, especially those labeled as BPA-free.

- **Fact:** While BPA (Bisphenol A) is a well-known endocrine disruptor, other chemicals used in BPA-free plastics, such as BPS (Bisphenol S), can also be harmful. It is better to minimize the use of plastics for food and beverage storage, opting instead for glass, stainless steel, or other safer alternatives.

Myth 8: You Can't Avoid Toxins

- **Misconception:** The belief that toxins are so pervasive that avoiding them is impossible, leading to a sense of helplessness.

- **Fact:** While it is true that completely avoiding all toxins is unrealistic, there are many practical steps one can take to significantly reduce exposure. Making informed choices about the products you use, the food you eat, and your living environment can greatly minimize your toxin burden.

Myth 9: Filtering Water Removes All Contaminants

- **Misconception:** The belief that using any water filter will remove all contaminants from drinking water.

- **Fact:** Not all water filters are created equal. Different filters are designed to remove different types of contaminants. It's important to choose a filter that is certified to remove specific contaminants present in your water supply. Regular maintenance and replacement of filters are also crucial for effective filtration.

Myth 10: Government Regulations Ensure All Products Are Safe

- **Misconception:** The assumption that government regulations and approvals mean all consumer products are completely safe.

- **Fact:** While regulations aim to ensure safety, they are not foolproof. Some chemicals and products may still pose health risks despite regulatory approval. Staying informed and choosing products with transparent ingredient lists and certifications can help reduce exposure to potentially harmful substances.

Dispelling myths and misconceptions about toxins is crucial for making informed decisions about health and safety. By understanding the facts, individuals can take proactive steps to reduce exposure to harmful substances and create a healthier living environment. Being informed and vigilant about the presence of toxins in everyday life empowers us to make choices that support long-term well-being.

Detoxification Strategies

Detoxification is the process by which the body eliminates toxins and harmful substances to maintain optimal health and well-being. Given the constant exposure to various environmental toxins in our modern world, supporting the body's natural detoxification processes is more important than ever. This chapter introduces a range of detoxification strategies, focusing on dietary choices, lifestyle modifications, and specific practices that can enhance the body's ability to cleanse itself. By understanding and implementing these strategies, individuals can reduce their toxin burden and promote overall health.

The Body's Natural Detoxification Systems

The human body is equipped with sophisticated detoxification systems designed to neutralize and eliminate toxins. These systems involve multiple organs and processes that work together to protect the body from harmful substances. Understanding how these natural detoxification systems function can help individuals support their bodies in effectively managing toxin exposure. This section explores the primary organs and processes involved in the body's natural detoxification systems.

1. Liver

- **Role:** The liver is the central organ in detoxification, responsible for filtering blood coming from the digestive tract before it passes to the rest of the body. It processes and neutralizes toxins, drugs, and metabolic byproducts.

- **Detoxification Phases:**

  - **Phase I:** Involves oxidation, reduction, and hydrolysis reactions to convert toxins into more water-soluble forms. This phase is mediated by enzymes such as cytochrome P450.

  - **Phase II:** Involves conjugation reactions where the liver attaches molecules (e.g., glutathione, sulfate, glycine) to the toxins to make them even more water-soluble and easier to excrete.

- **Support:** Consuming foods rich in antioxidants and compounds that support liver function, such as cruciferous vegetables, turmeric, garlic, and green tea.

2. Kidneys

- **Role:** The kidneys filter blood to remove waste products and excess substances, excreting them in urine. They play a crucial role in maintaining electrolyte balance and regulating blood pressure.

- **Detoxification Process:**

  - Filtration of blood to remove waste products like urea, creatinine, and excess salts.

  - Reabsorption of essential nutrients and water.

  - Secretion of additional wastes and toxins into the urine.

- **Support:** Staying hydrated, reducing salt intake, and consuming foods that support kidney health, such as berries, leafy greens, and hydration-promoting fruits and vegetables.

3. Skin

- **Role:** The skin acts as a barrier to external toxins and also plays a role in excreting waste products through sweat.

- **Detoxification Process:**

  - Sweating helps eliminate water-soluble toxins, heavy metals, and metabolic waste products.

- **Support:** Regular physical activity, sauna use, and maintaining proper skin hygiene to promote healthy sweating and skin function.

4. Lungs

- **Role:** The lungs are responsible for exchanging gases, including the exhalation of carbon dioxide, a waste product of metabolism.

- **Detoxification Process:**

  - Exhalation of carbon dioxide and volatile toxins.

  - Filtering of particulate matter and pathogens through mucus and cilia.

- **Support:** Avoiding smoking, practicing deep breathing exercises, and maintaining indoor air quality to support lung health.

5. Gastrointestinal Tract

- **Role:** The gastrointestinal (GI) tract processes food, absorbs nutrients, and eliminates waste. It plays a key role in preventing toxins from entering the bloodstream.

- **Detoxification Process:**

  - Enzymatic breakdown of food in the stomach and small intestine.

  - Absorption of nutrients and water.

  - Excretion of indigestible substances and toxins through feces.

- **Support:** Eating a high-fiber diet, consuming probiotics and prebiotics, and ensuring regular bowel movements to support a healthy gut.

6. Lymphatic System

- **Role:** The lymphatic system is part of the immune system, responsible for transporting lymph, a fluid containing white blood cells, throughout the body. It helps remove toxins, waste, and other unwanted materials.

- **Detoxification Process:**

  - Collecting and transporting waste products and toxins from tissues to the bloodstream.

  - Filtering lymph through lymph nodes to trap and destroy pathogens and toxins.

- **Support:** Regular exercise, dry brushing, and staying hydrated to promote lymphatic circulation and drainage.

Conclusion

The body's natural detoxification systems are highly efficient and capable of handling a significant toxic load. By understanding how these systems work, individuals can take steps to support and enhance their natural detoxification processes. Proper nutrition, hydration, exercise, and avoiding unnecessary toxin exposure are key strategies to help the body maintain its ability to detoxify and promote overall health.

Dietary Detox: Foods That Cleanse

Incorporating certain foods into your diet can enhance the body's natural detoxification processes, helping to remove toxins and support overall health. These foods provide essential nutrients, antioxidants, and other compounds that aid in detoxification, protect against oxidative stress, and promote healthy organ function. This section explores a variety of foods known for their cleansing properties and explains how they contribute to detoxification.

1. Cruciferous Vegetables

- **Examples:** Broccoli, cauliflower, Brussels sprouts, cabbage, kale.

- **Benefits:** Cruciferous vegetables are rich in sulfur-containing compounds like glucosinolates, which support liver detoxification enzymes. They also contain antioxidants and fiber that help eliminate toxins.

- **Key Compounds:** Glucosinolates, sulforaphane, indole-3-carbinol.

- **How to Use:** Incorporate raw or lightly cooked cruciferous vegetables into salads, stir-fries, and smoothies.

2. Leafy Greens

- **Examples:** Spinach, kale, Swiss chard, collard greens, arugula.

- **Benefits:** Leafy greens are high in chlorophyll, which helps remove heavy metals and other toxins from the bloodstream. They also support liver health and provide essential vitamins and minerals.

- **Key Compounds:** Chlorophyll, fiber, vitamins A, C, and K.

- **How to Use:** Add leafy greens to salads, smoothies, soups, and sautéed dishes.

3. Citrus Fruits

- **Examples:** Lemons, limes, oranges, grapefruits.

- **Benefits:** Citrus fruits are high in vitamin C, which supports the immune system and helps neutralize free radicals. They also stimulate liver enzymes that aid in detoxification.

- **Key Compounds:** Vitamin C, flavonoids, limonoids.

- **How to Use:** Drink warm lemon water in the morning, add citrus slices to water, or use citrus juices in salad dressings and marinades.

4. Berries

- **Examples:** Blueberries, strawberries, raspberries, blackberries.

- **Benefits:** Berries are rich in antioxidants and fiber, which help reduce oxidative stress and support the elimination of toxins through the digestive tract.

- **Key Compounds:** Anthocyanins, vitamin C, fiber.

- **How to Use:** Enjoy berries as a snack, in smoothies, or as a topping for yogurt and oatmeal.

5. Garlic

- **Benefits:** Garlic contains sulfur compounds like allicin that activate liver enzymes responsible for detoxification. It also has antimicrobial properties that support immune health.

- **Key Compounds:** Allicin, sulfur compounds, selenium.

- **How to Use:** Add raw or cooked garlic to soups, stews, sauces, and dressings.

6. Turmeric

- **Benefits:** Turmeric's active compound, curcumin, has potent anti-inflammatory and antioxidant properties that support liver detoxification and protect against cellular damage.

- **Key Compounds:** Curcumin, volatile oils.

- **How to Use:** Incorporate turmeric into curries, soups, smoothies, or take as a supplement.

7. Ginger

- **Benefits:** Ginger aids digestion and has anti-inflammatory properties that support detoxification. It also stimulates circulation and sweating, which can help eliminate toxins.

- **Key Compounds:** Gingerol, shogaol, zingerone.

- **How to Use:** Add fresh or powdered ginger to teas, smoothies, stir-fries, and baked goods.

8. Green Tea

- **Benefits:** Green tea is rich in antioxidants, particularly catechins, which support liver function and help eliminate toxins. It also boosts metabolism and aids in weight management.

- **Key Compounds:** Catechins, EGCG (epigallocatechin gallate), caffeine.
- **How to Use:** Drink green tea daily, either hot or iced, and incorporate it into smoothies or cooking.

9. Beets

- **Benefits:** Beets support liver detoxification and bile production, which aids in the digestion and elimination of fats and toxins. They are also high in antioxidants and fiber.
- **Key Compounds:** Betalains, betaine, fiber.
- **How to Use:** Add raw beets to salads, juice them, or roast them as a side dish.

10. Apples

- **Benefits:** Apples contain pectin, a type of fiber that binds to toxins in the intestines and helps eliminate them. They also support liver health and provide essential vitamins and minerals.
- **Key Compounds:** Pectin, quercetin, vitamin C.
- **How to Use:** Eat apples as a snack, add to salads, or blend into smoothies.

Incorporating detoxifying foods into your diet can enhance the body's natural detoxification processes, helping to remove toxins and support overall health. By regularly consuming a variety of these nutrient-rich foods, you can promote liver function, reduce oxidative stress, and improve digestive health. These dietary choices, combined with a healthy lifestyle, can significantly reduce your toxin burden and contribute to long-term well-being.

Herbal Remedies for Detoxification

Herbal remedies can play a significant role in supporting the body's natural detoxification processes. Various herbs have been traditionally used to cleanse the liver, kidneys, digestive system, and blood, helping to remove toxins and improve overall health. This section explores some of the most effective herbs for detoxification and explains how they can be used to enhance the body's ability to eliminate harmful substances.

1. Milk Thistle (Silybum marianum)

- **Benefits:** Milk thistle is renowned for its liver-protective properties. It contains silymarin, a compound that supports liver cell regeneration, reduces inflammation, and aids in the detoxification of toxins.
- **Key Compounds:** Silymarin, silybin, flavonoids.
- **How to Use:** Milk thistle can be taken as a tea, tincture, or supplement. It is often used in liver detox programs to support liver health and function.

2. Dandelion Root (Taraxacum officinale)

- **Benefits:** Dandelion root acts as a diuretic, increasing urine production and helping to eliminate toxins through the kidneys. It also supports liver health by stimulating bile production.

- **Key Compounds:** Inulin, taraxacin, sesquiterpene lactones.

- **How to Use:** Dandelion root can be consumed as a tea, tincture, or capsule. It is commonly used to support kidney and liver detoxification.

3. Burdock Root (Arctium lappa)

- **Benefits:** Burdock root is known for its blood-purifying properties. It helps remove toxins from the bloodstream, supports liver function, and promotes healthy skin.

- **Key Compounds:** Inulin, polyphenols, tannins.

- **How to Use:** Burdock root can be taken as a tea, tincture, or supplement. It is often used in combination with other detoxifying herbs for comprehensive detoxification support.

4. Cilantro (Coriandrum sativum)

- **Benefits:** Cilantro is effective in binding to heavy metals and aiding their excretion from the body. It supports detoxification of mercury and other heavy metals.

- **Key Compounds:** Linalool, flavonoids, carotenoids.

- **How to Use:** Cilantro can be added to foods, blended into smoothies, or taken as a tincture or supplement. It is particularly useful in heavy metal detox programs.

5. Red Clover (Trifolium pratense)

- **Benefits:** Red clover is a gentle detoxifier that helps purify the blood, support lymphatic function, and improve skin health. It also has mild diuretic properties.

- **Key Compounds:** Isoflavones, coumarins, saponins.

- **How to Use:** Red clover can be consumed as a tea, tincture, or supplement. It is often used in skin detox programs and to support overall detoxification.

6. Nettle (Urtica dioica)

- **Benefits:** Nettle is rich in vitamins and minerals that support detoxification. It acts as a diuretic, promoting the elimination of toxins through urine, and supports kidney health.

- **Key Compounds:** Chlorophyll, vitamins A, C, and K, minerals.

- **How to Use:** Nettle can be consumed as a tea, tincture, or supplement. It is commonly used to support urinary tract health and overall detoxification.

7. Ginger (Zingiber officinale)

- **Benefits:** Ginger aids digestion, improves circulation, and supports detoxification by promoting sweating and the elimination of toxins through the skin.

- **Key Compounds:** Gingerol, shogaol, zingerone.
- **How to Use:** Ginger can be added to foods, brewed into tea, or taken as a supplement. It is often used to enhance digestive detoxification and support immune health.

8. Turmeric (Curcuma longa)

- **Benefits:** Turmeric's active compound, curcumin, has powerful anti-inflammatory and antioxidant properties that support liver detoxification and protect against cellular damage.
- **Key Compounds:** Curcumin, volatile oils.
- **How to Use:** Turmeric can be taken as a tea, added to foods, or taken as a supplement. It is commonly used in liver detox programs and to reduce systemic inflammation.

9. Triphala

- **Benefits:** Triphala is an Ayurvedic herbal formulation consisting of three fruits: Amalaki, Bibhitaki, and Haritaki. It supports digestion, improves bowel movements, and helps detoxify the digestive system.
- **Key Compounds:** Tannins, polyphenols, flavonoids.
- **How to Use:** Triphala can be taken as a powder, capsule, or tea. It is often used to support digestive health and detoxification.

10. Schisandra (Schisandra chinensis)

- **Benefits:** Schisandra supports liver detoxification, enhances mental clarity, and provides adaptogenic benefits to help the body cope with stress.
- **Key Compounds:** Lignans, vitamins C and E, schisandrin.
- **How to Use:** Schisandra can be taken as a tea, tincture, or supplement. It is commonly used in liver detox programs and to support overall vitality.

Conclusion

Herbal remedies offer a natural and effective way to support the body's detoxification processes. By incorporating these detoxifying herbs into your routine, you can enhance liver function, improve kidney health, purify the blood, and promote overall detoxification. These herbs can be used individually or in combination to create a comprehensive detoxification program tailored to your needs. As always, it is advisable to consult with a healthcare provider before starting any new detox regimen, especially if you have underlying health conditions or are taking medications.

Physical Detox Methods (Sweating, Exercise, etc.)

Physical detox methods complement dietary and herbal strategies by promoting the elimination of toxins through natural bodily processes. Sweating, exercise, and other physical activities enhance the body's ability to expel toxins, improve circulation, and support overall health. This section explores various physical detox methods and how they contribute to cleansing the body.

1. Sweating

- **Benefits:** Sweating helps to eliminate toxins through the skin, including heavy metals, pollutants, and metabolic waste products.

- **Methods:**

  - **Saunas:** Using a traditional or infrared sauna increases body temperature, promoting intense sweating and detoxification. Infrared saunas, in particular, penetrate deeper into tissues, enhancing detoxification.

  - **Steam Baths:** Steam baths open up pores and induce sweating, aiding in the elimination of toxins and improving skin health.

  - **Exercise:** Physical activity, especially cardiovascular exercises like running or cycling, promotes sweating and detoxification through the skin.

2. Exercise

- **Benefits:** Regular exercise improves circulation, enhances lymphatic drainage, and supports the detoxification organs such as the liver and kidneys.

- **Types of Exercise:**

  - **Cardiovascular Exercise:** Activities like jogging, cycling, swimming, and brisk walking increase heart rate and promote sweating, aiding in the elimination of toxins.

  - **Strength Training:** Weightlifting and resistance training improve muscle mass and metabolic rate, supporting overall detoxification.

  - **Yoga and Stretching:** Yoga poses and stretches stimulate internal organs, enhance digestion, and promote lymphatic drainage, aiding in detoxification.

3. Hydration

- **Benefits:** Staying well-hydrated supports kidney function, promotes the elimination of toxins through urine, and helps maintain overall cellular health.

- **Methods:**

  - **Water:** Drinking plenty of water throughout the day helps flush out toxins and supports all bodily functions. Aim for at least 8 glasses (64 ounces) per day, or more if exercising or sweating heavily.

  - **Herbal Teas:** Teas made from detoxifying herbs like dandelion, nettle, and ginger support hydration and provide additional detox benefits.

4. Dry Brushing

- **Benefits:** Dry brushing stimulates the lymphatic system, promotes blood circulation, and helps exfoliate dead skin cells, supporting detoxification through the skin.
- **Method:**
  - Use a natural bristle brush to gently brush the skin in long, upward strokes, starting from the feet and moving toward the heart. Perform this routine daily before showering.

5. Epsom Salt Baths

- **Benefits:** Epsom salt (magnesium sulfate) baths help draw out toxins through the skin, relieve muscle tension, and promote relaxation.
- **Method:**
  - Add 1-2 cups of Epsom salt to a warm bath and soak for 20-30 minutes. The magnesium in Epsom salt can also help relax muscles and improve sleep.

6. Deep Breathing Exercises

- **Benefits:** Deep breathing exercises improve oxygenation, enhance lung function, and support the elimination of carbon dioxide and other volatile toxins.
- **Methods:**
  - **Diaphragmatic Breathing:** Breathe deeply into the diaphragm, expanding the abdomen on inhalation and contracting it on exhalation. Practice this for 5-10 minutes daily.
  - **Alternate Nostril Breathing:** Inhale through one nostril while closing the other with a finger, then switch nostrils for the exhale. Repeat for several minutes to enhance respiratory detoxification and relaxation.

7. Lymphatic Drainage Massage

- **Benefits:** Lymphatic drainage massage stimulates the lymphatic system, enhancing the removal of toxins and waste products from the tissues.
- **Method:**
  - A trained therapist uses gentle, rhythmic strokes to promote lymph flow and reduce fluid retention. Self-massage techniques can also be practiced at home.

8. Rebounding

- **Benefits:** Rebounding on a mini trampoline stimulates the lymphatic system, improves circulation, and promotes detoxification through gentle bouncing movements.
- **Method:**
  - Bounce gently on a mini trampoline for 10-20 minutes daily to stimulate lymphatic flow and support detoxification.

9. Skin Exfoliation

- **Benefits:** Exfoliating the skin helps remove dead skin cells, unclog pores, and promote the elimination of toxins through the skin.

- **Methods:**

  - **Scrubs:** Use natural exfoliating scrubs made from ingredients like sugar, salt, or coffee grounds.

  - **Exfoliating Gloves or Brushes:** Use these tools in the shower to gently exfoliate the skin, promoting detoxification.

Physical detox methods such as sweating, exercise, hydration, and other practices play a crucial role in enhancing the body's natural detoxification processes. By incorporating these methods into your routine, you can support the elimination of toxins, improve circulation, and promote overall health. These practices, combined with a healthy diet and herbal remedies, provide a comprehensive approach to detoxification and well-being.

Fasting and Juice Cleanses

Fasting and juice cleanses are popular detoxification methods that can help the body eliminate toxins, improve metabolic health, and enhance overall well-being. Both approaches rely on reducing the intake of solid foods and increasing the consumption of liquids to give the digestive system a break and support the body's natural detox processes. This section explores the benefits, methods, and considerations of fasting and juice cleanses.

Fasting

Benefits of Fasting:

- **Detoxification:** Fasting allows the digestive system to rest and can promote the elimination of stored toxins from fat cells.

- **Cellular Repair:** During fasting, the body initiates autophagy, a process where damaged cells are broken down and recycled.

- **Improved Metabolism:** Fasting can help regulate insulin sensitivity, reduce inflammation, and support metabolic health.

- **Mental Clarity:** Many people experience increased mental clarity and focus during fasting due to stable blood sugar levels and the production of ketones.

Types of Fasting:

1. **Intermittent Fasting:** Alternating periods of eating and fasting, such as the 16/8 method (16 hours fasting, 8 hours eating) or the 5:2 method (eating normally for 5 days, restricting calories for 2 days).

- o **How to Use:** Choose a fasting window that suits your lifestyle and gradually increase the fasting period if necessary. Stay hydrated and focus on nutrient-dense foods during eating periods.

2. **Water Fasting:** Consuming only water for a set period, typically 24-72 hours.

    - o **How to Use:** Prepare by gradually reducing food intake before the fast, stay hydrated, and rest as needed. Consult a healthcare provider before starting, especially for extended fasts.

3. **Extended Fasting:** Fasting for more than 72 hours, which can be more intensive and should be done with medical supervision.

    - o **How to Use:** Similar preparation as water fasting, with added emphasis on monitoring by a healthcare professional to ensure safety and address any potential health issues.

Considerations:

- **Health Conditions:** People with certain health conditions, such as diabetes or eating disorders, should avoid fasting or do so under medical supervision.

- **Hydration:** It's crucial to stay hydrated during fasting periods to support detoxification and prevent dehydration.

- **Electrolytes:** Prolonged fasting may require electrolyte supplementation to maintain balance and prevent deficiencies.

Juice Cleanses

Benefits of Juice Cleanses:

- **Nutrient Intake:** Juices provide a concentrated source of vitamins, minerals, and antioxidants that support detoxification.

- **Digestive Rest:** Similar to fasting, juice cleanses give the digestive system a break, allowing the body to focus on detoxification and healing.

- **Hydration:** Juices contribute to overall hydration, which is essential for flushing out toxins.

Types of Juice Cleanses:

1. **Full Juice Cleanse:** Consuming only freshly pressed fruit and vegetable juices for a set period, typically 1-7 days.

    - o **How to Use:** Prepare by gradually reducing solid food intake, choose a variety of fruits and vegetables to ensure a broad spectrum of nutrients, and consume 4-6 servings of juice per day.

2. **Partial Juice Cleanse:** Combining juices with light, solid meals or snacks, such as salads, smoothies, or soups.

- **How to Use:** Incorporate juices into your regular diet while replacing some meals with juice to reduce calorie intake and support detoxification.

Popular Detox Juices:

- **Green Juice:** Made with leafy greens (kale, spinach), cucumber, celery, lemon, and ginger for a nutrient-dense, detoxifying drink.

- **Carrot-Apple-Ginger Juice:** Combines the sweetness of apples and carrots with the zing of ginger, providing antioxidants and anti-inflammatory compounds.

- **Beetroot Juice:** Includes beets, carrots, and apples, which support liver detoxification and provide essential vitamins and minerals.

Considerations:

- **Quality Ingredients:** Use organic produce to minimize the intake of pesticides and other contaminants.

- **Balance:** Ensure juices are balanced and not overly reliant on high-sugar fruits, which can cause blood sugar spikes.

- **Duration:** Limit juice cleanses to a manageable duration (typically up to 7 days) to avoid potential nutrient deficiencies from prolonged liquid-only diets.

Fasting and juice cleanses are effective methods for supporting the body's natural detoxification processes. By giving the digestive system a break and providing concentrated sources of nutrients, these practices can help eliminate toxins, improve metabolic health, and enhance overall well-being. However, it's important to approach fasting and juice cleanses with caution, especially if you have underlying health conditions or are new to these practices. Consulting with a healthcare provider can ensure that these detoxification methods are safe and effective for your individual needs.

Supporting Liver and Kidney Health

The liver and kidneys are essential organs for detoxification, responsible for filtering and eliminating toxins from the body. Supporting the health and function of these organs is crucial for maintaining overall well-being and enhancing the body's natural detoxification processes. This section explores dietary, lifestyle, and herbal strategies to support liver and kidney health.

Dietary Strategies

1. **Hydration:**

   - **Importance:** Staying well-hydrated is vital for kidney function, as it helps flush out toxins through urine and supports overall cellular health.

   - **Recommendations:** Drink at least 8 glasses (64 ounces) of water daily. Increase intake if exercising or sweating heavily. Herbal teas and water-rich fruits and vegetables can also contribute to hydration.

2. **Nutrient-Dense Foods:**

   o **Liver-Supportive Foods:**

      ▪ **Cruciferous Vegetables:** Broccoli, cauliflower, Brussels sprouts, and kale contain compounds that boost liver detoxification enzymes.

      ▪ **Leafy Greens:** Spinach, kale, and Swiss chard are rich in chlorophyll, which helps detoxify the liver.

      ▪ **Beets:** High in antioxidants and nutrients that support liver function and bile production.

      ▪ **Garlic:** Contains sulfur compounds that activate liver detoxification enzymes.

   o **Kidney-Supportive Foods:**

      ▪ **Berries:** Blueberries, strawberries, and cranberries contain antioxidants that protect the kidneys.

      ▪ **Leafy Greens:** Spinach and kale are also beneficial for kidney health due to their high nutrient content.

      ▪ **Citrus Fruits:** Lemons and oranges provide vitamin C and antioxidants that support kidney function.

      ▪ **Watermelon:** High in water content and helps hydrate the kidneys.

3. **Reduce Processed Foods and Sugars:**

   o **Impact:** Processed foods and high-sugar diets can lead to fatty liver disease and increased kidney workload.

   o **Recommendations:** Limit consumption of processed foods, sugary drinks, and high-fructose corn syrup. Focus on whole, unprocessed foods.

4. **Healthy Fats:**

   o **Importance:** Healthy fats support cell membranes and hormone production, which are essential for liver and kidney health.

   o **Recommendations:** Include sources of healthy fats such as avocados, nuts, seeds, and olive oil in your diet.

Lifestyle Strategies

1. **Regular Exercise:**

   o **Benefits:** Exercise improves circulation, supports cardiovascular health, and enhances the body's detoxification processes.

- **Recommendations:** Aim for at least 30 minutes of moderate exercise most days of the week. Activities like walking, jogging, swimming, and yoga are beneficial.

2. **Limit Alcohol and Caffeine:**

   - **Impact:** Excessive alcohol and caffeine consumption can strain the liver and kidneys.

   - **Recommendations:** Limit alcohol intake to moderate levels and reduce caffeine consumption. Opt for herbal teas or decaffeinated beverages.

3. **Avoid Smoking and Environmental Toxins:**

   - **Impact:** Smoking and exposure to environmental toxins can damage liver and kidney function.

   - **Recommendations:** Avoid smoking and minimize exposure to harmful chemicals. Use natural cleaning products and ensure proper ventilation at home and work.

4. **Maintain a Healthy Weight:**

   - **Importance:** Being overweight or obese can increase the risk of liver and kidney diseases.

   - **Recommendations:** Follow a balanced diet and engage in regular physical activity to maintain a healthy weight.

Herbal Strategies

1. **Milk Thistle (Silybum marianum):**

   - **Benefits:** Contains silymarin, which supports liver cell regeneration, reduces inflammation, and enhances liver detoxification.

   - **How to Use:** Take milk thistle as a tea, tincture, or supplement.

2. **Dandelion Root (Taraxacum officinale):**

   - **Benefits:** Acts as a diuretic, supporting kidney function and increasing urine production. Also stimulates bile production in the liver.

   - **How to Use:** Consume dandelion root as a tea, tincture, or capsule.

3. **Turmeric (Curcuma longa):**

   - **Benefits:** Contains curcumin, which has anti-inflammatory and antioxidant properties that support liver health.

   - **How to Use:** Add turmeric to foods, or take as a tea or supplement.

4. **Burdock Root (Arctium lappa):**

- o **Benefits:** Known for its blood-purifying properties and support for liver and kidney detoxification.
- o **How to Use:** Use burdock root in teas, tinctures, or supplements.

5. **Nettle (Urtica dioica):**
   - o **Benefits:** Rich in vitamins and minerals, supports kidney health and acts as a diuretic to promote urine production.
   - o **How to Use:** Drink nettle tea or take as a tincture or supplement.

6. **Ginger (Zingiber officinale):**
   - o **Benefits:** Aids digestion, improves circulation, and supports liver and kidney health.
   - o **How to Use:** Add ginger to foods, brew into tea, or take as a supplement.

Supporting liver and kidney health is essential for maintaining the body's natural detoxification processes and overall well-being. By incorporating dietary, lifestyle, and herbal strategies, individuals can enhance the function of these vital organs and promote a healthier, toxin-free life. Consistent efforts to support liver and kidney health can lead to improved energy levels, better metabolic health, and a stronger immune system.

BOOK 4:

Non-Toxic Diets and Lifestyles: Organic vs. Conventional Foods

Adopting a non-toxic diet and lifestyle is a proactive approach to enhancing overall health and well-being by minimizing exposure to harmful substances. This involves making informed choices about the foods we eat, the products we use, and the habits we cultivate. By prioritizing natural, whole foods and reducing our reliance on processed items and chemical-laden products, we can significantly lower our toxin burden. This chapter introduces the principles of non-toxic diets and lifestyles, providing practical strategies for creating a healthier, cleaner living environment.

Principles of a Non-Toxic Diet

Adopting a non-toxic diet involves making intentional choices about the foods we consume to minimize exposure to harmful chemicals and maximize nutritional benefits. This approach not only supports detoxification and overall health but also promotes sustainable and ethical food practices. The following principles outline key strategies for creating and maintaining a non-toxic diet.

1. Choose Organic Foods

- **Benefits:** Organic foods are grown without synthetic pesticides, herbicides, and fertilizers, reducing exposure to harmful chemicals.

- **Recommendations:**

  - Prioritize purchasing organic fruits and vegetables, especially those listed on the Environmental Working Group's (EWG) "Dirty Dozen" list, which highlights produce with the highest pesticide residues.

  - Choose organic dairy, meat, and poultry to avoid hormones, antibiotics, and feed additives used in conventional farming.

2. Eat Whole, Unprocessed Foods

- **Benefits:** Whole foods are minimally processed, retaining their natural nutrients and fiber, and free from artificial additives and preservatives.

- **Recommendations:**

  - Focus on a diet rich in fresh fruits and vegetables, whole grains, nuts, seeds, and legumes.

  - Avoid packaged and processed foods that contain artificial colors, flavors, sweeteners, and preservatives.

3. Avoid Genetically Modified Organisms (GMOs)

- **Benefits:** GMOs are often associated with higher pesticide use and potential health risks.

- **Recommendations:**

  - Look for products labeled "Non-GMO" or "Certified Organic," as organic standards prohibit the use of GMOs.

  - Avoid common GMO crops such as corn, soy, canola, and their derivatives unless they are certified organic or non-GMO.

4. Choose Clean Protein Sources

- **Benefits:** Clean protein sources are free from antibiotics, hormones, and harmful feed additives, supporting overall health.

- **Recommendations:**

  - Opt for grass-fed, pasture-raised, and wild-caught animal products.

  - Include plant-based protein sources such as beans, lentils, quinoa, and nuts.

5. Limit Exposure to Environmental Toxins

- **Benefits:** Reducing exposure to environmental toxins helps lower the overall toxin burden on the body.

- **Recommendations:**

    - Wash fruits and vegetables thoroughly to remove pesticide residues. Consider using a vinegar-water solution for washing.

    - Use stainless steel, glass, or BPA-free containers for food storage to avoid leaching chemicals from plastics.

6. Stay Hydrated with Clean Water

- **Benefits:** Drinking clean, filtered water supports hydration and helps flush out toxins from the body.

- **Recommendations:**

    - Use a high-quality water filter to remove contaminants such as chlorine, heavy metals, and other pollutants from tap water.

    - Avoid bottled water stored in plastic containers that may leach harmful chemicals.

7. Incorporate Detoxifying Foods

- **Benefits:** Certain foods support the body's natural detoxification processes and help eliminate toxins.

- **Recommendations:**

    - Include foods like cruciferous vegetables (broccoli, cauliflower), leafy greens (spinach, kale), garlic, ginger, turmeric, and citrus fruits in your diet.

    - Add fiber-rich foods such as flaxseeds, chia seeds, and whole grains to support digestive health and toxin elimination.

8. Reduce Sugar and Refined Carbohydrates

- **Benefits:** Limiting sugar and refined carbohydrates helps prevent blood sugar spikes, supports metabolic health, and reduces inflammation.

- **Recommendations:**

    - Choose whole fruits over fruit juices and sugary snacks.

    - Opt for whole grains like brown rice, quinoa, and oats instead of refined grains like white bread and pasta.

9. Use Natural Sweeteners Sparingly

- **Benefits:** Natural sweeteners have a lower glycemic index and are free from artificial additives.

- **Recommendations:**

  - Use natural sweeteners like honey, maple syrup, stevia, and dates in moderation.

  - Avoid artificial sweeteners such as aspartame, sucralose, and saccharin.

10. Be Mindful of Food Packaging

- **Benefits:** Minimizing exposure to harmful chemicals in packaging materials helps reduce overall toxin intake.

- **Recommendations:**

  - Choose foods packaged in glass, paper, or other non-toxic materials.

  - Avoid canned foods lined with BPA or other harmful chemicals.

Following the principles of a non-toxic diet involves making conscious choices to minimize exposure to harmful chemicals and maximize nutritional intake. By prioritizing organic, whole, and minimally processed foods, staying hydrated with clean water, and being mindful of packaging, individuals can support their body's natural detoxification processes and promote long-term health and well-being.

Organic vs. Conventional Foods

Choosing between organic and conventional foods is a significant consideration for those aiming to reduce toxin exposure and enhance overall health. Understanding the differences between these two types of food production can help individuals make informed decisions about their diet. This section explores the distinctions, benefits, and potential drawbacks of organic and conventional foods.

Definitions

- **Organic Foods:**

  - Produced using methods that do not involve synthetic pesticides, herbicides, fertilizers, genetically modified organisms (GMOs), antibiotics, or growth hormones.

  - Organic farming practices emphasize soil health, ecological balance, and biodiversity, often using natural fertilizers and pest control methods.

- **Conventional Foods:**

  - Produced using modern agricultural practices, which may include the use of synthetic chemicals, GMOs, and other technologies to enhance crop yields and protect against pests and diseases.

- Conventional farming can involve practices that prioritize efficiency and cost-effectiveness, sometimes at the expense of environmental and health considerations.

Differences in Production Methods

1. **Pesticides and Herbicides:**

   - **Organic:** Limited to natural or non-synthetic substances approved by organic certification standards. Organic farmers use crop rotation, biological pest control, and other sustainable practices.

   - **Conventional:** Permits the use of synthetic pesticides and herbicides, which can leave residues on produce and contribute to environmental pollution.

2. **Fertilizers:**

   - **Organic:** Utilizes natural fertilizers such as compost, manure, and green manure. These methods improve soil health and sustainability.

   - **Conventional:** Often relies on synthetic fertilizers to provide nutrients to crops quickly, which can lead to soil degradation and water pollution.

3. **GMOs:**

   - **Organic:** Prohibited in organic farming. Organic foods are free from genetically modified organisms.

   - **Conventional:** GMOs are commonly used to enhance crop yields, resistance to pests, and tolerance to herbicides.

4. **Antibiotics and Hormones:**

   - **Organic:** The use of antibiotics and growth hormones is prohibited in organic livestock production. Organic animals are raised in conditions that allow natural behaviors and are given organic feed.

   - **Conventional:** Antibiotics and growth hormones are often used to promote growth and prevent disease in livestock, which can contribute to antibiotic resistance and hormone residues in food products.

Nutritional Differences

- **Organic Foods:**

  - **Nutrient Density:** Some studies suggest that organic foods can have higher levels of certain nutrients, such as antioxidants, vitamins, and minerals.

  - **Fatty Acids:** Organic meat and dairy products may have a more favorable fatty acid profile, with higher levels of omega-3 fatty acids.

- o **Fewer Contaminants:** Organic produce typically has lower levels of pesticide residues and harmful chemicals.

- **Conventional Foods:**

  - o **Nutrient Content:** Conventional foods provide similar levels of most essential nutrients compared to organic foods. However, the presence of pesticide residues and contaminants may pose health risks.

  - o **Cost-Effectiveness:** Conventional foods are often less expensive due to higher yields and lower production costs.

Environmental Impact

- **Organic Farming:**

  - o **Soil Health:** Organic farming practices improve soil fertility and structure, reduce erosion, and promote biodiversity.

  - o **Water Quality:** Reduced reliance on synthetic chemicals minimizes water pollution and protects aquatic ecosystems.

  - o **Carbon Footprint:** Organic farming can sequester more carbon in the soil, potentially mitigating climate change.

- **Conventional Farming:**

  - o **Efficiency:** Conventional methods can produce higher yields per acre, feeding more people with less land.

  - o **Environmental Degradation:** Intensive use of synthetic chemicals and monoculture practices can lead to soil degradation, water pollution, and loss of biodiversity.

Health Considerations

- **Organic Foods:**

  - o **Reduced Exposure to Pesticides:** Lower levels of synthetic pesticide residues can reduce the risk of health issues associated with chemical exposure, such as endocrine disruption and neurotoxicity.

  - o **Antibiotic Resistance:** Organic farming's prohibition of routine antibiotic use in livestock reduces the risk of antibiotic-resistant bacteria.

- **Conventional Foods:**

  - o **Affordability and Accessibility:** Conventional foods are generally more affordable and widely available, making them an essential option for many consumers.

- **Regulation and Safety:** Conventional foods are subject to regulations and safety standards to minimize health risks, although concerns about long-term exposure to synthetic chemicals remain.

Choosing between organic and conventional foods involves weighing the benefits and potential drawbacks of each. Organic foods offer advantages in terms of reduced chemical exposure, environmental sustainability, and potentially higher nutrient content. However, conventional foods are often more affordable and accessible. By understanding these differences, individuals can make informed decisions that align with their health goals, values, and budget. Integrating organic foods where possible and practical can contribute to a healthier, more sustainable diet.

Avoiding Food Additives and Preservatives

Food additives and preservatives are commonly used in processed foods to enhance flavor, texture, shelf life, and appearance. However, some of these substances can have adverse effects on health, making it important to be mindful of their presence in our diets. This section explores the potential risks associated with food additives and preservatives, common types to watch out for, and strategies for avoiding them to maintain a healthier diet.

Potential Risks of Food Additives and Preservatives

1. **Allergic Reactions:**
   - Some individuals may experience allergic reactions or sensitivities to certain food additives, leading to symptoms such as hives, itching, swelling, and gastrointestinal distress.

2. **Hyperactivity and Behavioral Issues:**
   - Certain artificial colors and preservatives have been linked to hyperactivity and behavioral issues in children, particularly those with attention deficit hyperactivity disorder (ADHD).

3. **Endocrine Disruption:**
   - Some food additives, such as certain artificial sweeteners and preservatives, can disrupt hormone function, potentially leading to metabolic and reproductive issues.

4. **Gastrointestinal Problems:**
   - Additives like artificial sweeteners and emulsifiers can cause digestive issues, including bloating, gas, and diarrhea in some people.

5. **Long-term Health Risks:**
   - Long-term consumption of certain additives and preservatives has been associated with an increased risk of chronic diseases, including cancer, cardiovascular disease, and metabolic disorders.

Common Food Additives and Preservatives to Watch Out For

1. **Artificial Colors:**

    o **Examples:** Red 40, Yellow 5, Blue 1

    o **Risks:** Linked to hyperactivity in children and potential carcinogenic effects.

2. **Artificial Sweeteners:**

    o **Examples:** Aspartame, sucralose, saccharin

    o **Risks:** Associated with metabolic disorders, digestive issues, and potential cancer risks.

3. **Preservatives:**

    o **Examples:** Sodium benzoate, potassium sorbate, BHA (butylated hydroxyanisole), BHT (butylated hydroxytoluene)

    o **Risks:** Linked to allergic reactions, endocrine disruption, and potential carcinogenic effects.

4. **Flavor Enhancers:**

    o **Examples:** Monosodium glutamate (MSG), disodium inosinate, disodium guanylate

    o **Risks:** Can cause headaches, nausea, and other symptoms in sensitive individuals (known as "Chinese Restaurant Syndrome").

5. **Emulsifiers and Stabilizers:**

    o **Examples:** Carrageenan, polysorbates, xanthan gum

    o **Risks:** Associated with gastrointestinal issues and potential inflammatory effects.

6. **Thickeners:**

    o **Examples:** Modified food starch, guar gum, cellulose

    o **Risks:** Generally considered safe, but can cause digestive discomfort in some people.

7. **Antioxidants:**

    o **Examples:** TBHQ (tert-butylhydroquinone), propyl gallate

    o **Risks:** Linked to potential carcinogenic effects and allergic reactions.

Strategies for Avoiding Food Additives and Preservatives

1. **Read Ingredient Labels:**

    o Carefully read the ingredient lists on food packaging to identify and avoid products containing artificial additives and preservatives.

- Look for foods with short ingredient lists and recognizable, natural ingredients.

2. **Choose Whole, Unprocessed Foods:**

   - Focus on consuming fresh fruits, vegetables, whole grains, nuts, seeds, and legumes.
   - These foods are naturally free from additives and preservatives and provide essential nutrients.

3. **Cook at Home:**

   - Prepare meals at home using fresh, whole ingredients to have full control over what goes into your food.
   - Avoid pre-packaged meals, snacks, and convenience foods that often contain additives and preservatives.

4. **Opt for Organic Products:**

   - Organic foods are produced without synthetic additives and preservatives, making them a safer choice for avoiding these substances.
   - Look for certified organic labels when shopping.

5. **Use Natural Preservatives:**

   - If preserving food at home, use natural methods such as freezing, canning, and fermenting.
   - Natural preservatives like vinegar, lemon juice, and salt can be used to extend the shelf life of homemade foods.

6. **Shop at Farmers' Markets:**

   - Buy fresh produce and products directly from local farmers to reduce the likelihood of exposure to additives and preservatives.
   - Farmers' markets often offer seasonal, organic, and minimally processed foods.

7. **Be Cautious with Packaged Foods:**

   - When buying packaged foods, choose brands that prioritize natural ingredients and transparency in labeling.
   - Look for products labeled as "additive-free," "preservative-free," or "all-natural."

8. **Educate Yourself:**

   - Learn about common food additives and preservatives, their potential risks, and how to identify them on labels.

- Stay informed about new research and recommendations regarding food safety and additives.

Avoiding food additives and preservatives is an important aspect of maintaining a non-toxic diet and promoting overall health. By being mindful of ingredient labels, choosing whole and organic foods, and preparing meals at home, individuals can significantly reduce their exposure to potentially harmful substances. These strategies not only support detoxification but also contribute to better nutrition and long-term well-being.

Safe Food Storage and Preparation

Proper food storage and preparation are crucial for maintaining the nutritional quality of food, preventing contamination, and reducing exposure to harmful substances. By following best practices, you can ensure the safety and healthiness of your meals. This section explores safe food storage methods, preparation techniques, and tips for minimizing the risk of toxins and foodborne illnesses.

Safe Food Storage

1. **Use Appropriate Containers:**

   - **Material:** Choose food-grade, BPA-free plastic containers, glass containers, or stainless steel for storage. Avoid using containers that contain BPA, phthalates, or other harmful chemicals that can leach into food.

   - **Lids:** Ensure containers have tight-fitting lids to prevent contamination and maintain freshness.

2. **Refrigeration and Freezing:**

   - **Temperature:** Keep your refrigerator at or below 40°F (4°C) and your freezer at 0°F (-18°C) to slow the growth of bacteria and preserve food quality.

   - **Storage Time:** Follow guidelines for how long different foods can be stored safely in the refrigerator or freezer. Label containers with dates to track storage times.

   - **Organization:** Store raw meat, poultry, and seafood in sealed containers or plastic bags on the bottom shelf to prevent juices from contaminating other foods.

3. **Dry Storage:**

   - **Location:** Store dry goods like grains, cereals, and legumes in a cool, dry, and dark place to prevent spoilage and pest infestations.

   - **Containers:** Use airtight containers to protect dry foods from moisture, air, and pests.

4. **Avoid Cross-Contamination:**

- **Separation:** Keep raw and cooked foods separate to prevent the spread of bacteria. Store raw meat, poultry, and seafood separately from other foods in the refrigerator.

- **Sanitization:** Regularly clean and sanitize your refrigerator, freezer, and storage containers to prevent bacterial growth and contamination.

Safe Food Preparation

1. **Cleanliness:**

   - **Handwashing:** Wash your hands thoroughly with soap and water for at least 20 seconds before and after handling food, especially raw meat, poultry, and seafood.

   - **Surface Cleaning:** Clean and sanitize kitchen surfaces, cutting boards, and utensils before and after preparing food to prevent cross-contamination.

   - **Produce Washing:** Rinse fruits and vegetables under running water to remove dirt, bacteria, and pesticide residues. Use a brush for firm produce like potatoes and apples.

2. **Proper Cooking:**

   - **Temperature:** Cook foods to the appropriate internal temperatures to kill harmful bacteria. Use a food thermometer to check the temperatures:

     - Poultry: 165°F (74°C)

     - Ground meats: 160°F (71°C)

     - Beef, pork, lamb, and veal: 145°F (63°C) with a rest time of 3 minutes

     - Fish: 145°F (63°C)

   - **Avoid Undercooking:** Ensure that meats, poultry, and seafood are cooked thoroughly, and avoid consuming raw or undercooked eggs.

3. **Safe Thawing:**

   - **Refrigerator Thawing:** Thaw frozen foods in the refrigerator, allowing them to defrost slowly and safely.

   - **Cold Water Thawing:** For quicker thawing, place frozen food in a sealed plastic bag and submerge it in cold water, changing the water every 30 minutes.

   - **Microwave Thawing:** Use the defrost setting on your microwave for quick thawing but cook the food immediately after thawing.

4. **Avoiding Cross-Contamination During Preparation:**

   - **Separate Cutting Boards:** Use separate cutting boards for raw meat, poultry, seafood, and vegetables to prevent cross-contamination.

- Utensil Management: Use separate utensils for handling raw and cooked foods. Do not reuse marinades used on raw foods unless boiled first.

5. **Proper Food Handling:**

   - **Marinating:** Marinate foods in the refrigerator, not on the countertop. Discard marinades that have been in contact with raw meat, poultry, or seafood.

   - **Serving:** Use clean plates and utensils for serving cooked foods. Do not place cooked foods on plates that previously held raw foods.

6. **Leftovers:**

   - **Storage:** Refrigerate or freeze leftovers within two hours of cooking to prevent bacterial growth. Use shallow containers for quick cooling.

   - **Reheating:** Reheat leftovers to an internal temperature of 165°F (74°C) to ensure safety. Use a food thermometer to check the temperature.

Tips for Reducing Toxin Exposure

1. **Choose Fresh, Whole Foods:**

   - Focus on fresh, whole foods over processed and packaged items to reduce exposure to additives, preservatives, and packaging chemicals.

2. **Avoid Non-Stick Cookware:**

   - Non-stick cookware can release harmful chemicals like PFOA and PFAS when heated. Use alternatives such as stainless steel, cast iron, or ceramic cookware.

3. **Be Mindful of Charred Foods:**

   - Avoid charring or burning foods during grilling or cooking, as this can produce harmful compounds like acrylamide and heterocyclic amines (HCAs).

4. **Use Natural Cleaning Products:**

   - Opt for natural, non-toxic cleaning products for your kitchen to minimize exposure to harmful chemicals.

Safe food storage and preparation practices are essential for maintaining the nutritional quality of food and preventing contamination. By following these guidelines, you can reduce the risk of foodborne illnesses and exposure to harmful substances. Prioritizing cleanliness, proper cooking, and mindful food handling will contribute to a healthier, safer diet and overall well-being.

Non-Toxic Personal Care Products

Personal care products are a significant part of daily routines, but many conventional products contain chemicals that can be harmful to health. Choosing non-toxic personal care products helps reduce exposure to potentially hazardous substances and supports overall well-being.

This section explores the benefits of non-toxic personal care products, common harmful ingredients to avoid, and tips for selecting safer alternatives.

Benefits of Non-Toxic Personal Care Products

1. **Reduced Chemical Exposure:**

   o Non-toxic products are free from harmful chemicals like parabens, phthalates, and synthetic fragrances, reducing the risk of adverse health effects.

2. **Healthier Skin and Hair:**

   o Natural ingredients in non-toxic products can be gentler on the skin and hair, helping to maintain their natural balance and prevent irritation.

3. **Environmental Sustainability:**

   o Many non-toxic personal care brands prioritize sustainable sourcing, eco-friendly packaging, and ethical practices, reducing the environmental impact.

4. **Lower Risk of Allergic Reactions:**

   o Products made with natural and organic ingredients are less likely to cause allergic reactions and sensitivities compared to those with synthetic chemicals.

Common Harmful Ingredients to Avoid

1. **Parabens:**

   o **Purpose:** Used as preservatives to prevent the growth of bacteria and mold.

   o **Risks:** Linked to endocrine disruption and potential cancer risks.

   o **Alternatives:** Look for products labeled "paraben-free" or those that use natural preservatives like vitamin E or rosemary extract.

2. **Phthalates:**

   o **Purpose:** Used to make plastics flexible and as solvents in fragrances.

   o **Risks:** Associated with endocrine disruption, reproductive issues, and developmental problems.

   o **Alternatives:** Choose products labeled "phthalate-free" and opt for naturally scented or fragrance-free options.

3. **Synthetic Fragrances:**

   o **Purpose:** Added to products for scent.

   o **Risks:** Can contain numerous undisclosed chemicals, potentially causing allergies, skin irritation, and hormone disruption.

- Alternatives: Select products scented with essential oils or those labeled "fragrance-free."

4. **Sodium Lauryl Sulfate (SLS) and Sodium Laureth Sulfate (SLES):**
   - **Purpose:** Used as foaming agents in shampoos, body washes, and toothpaste.
   - **Risks:** Can cause skin and eye irritation and may be contaminated with carcinogenic compounds.
   - **Alternatives:** Look for sulfate-free products that use milder surfactants like coco-glucoside or decyl glucoside.

5. **Formaldehyde and Formaldehyde-Releasing Agents:**
   - **Purpose:** Used as preservatives in cosmetics and personal care products.
   - **Risks:** Known carcinogen and can cause skin irritation and allergic reactions.
   - **Alternatives:** Choose products that do not contain formaldehyde or ingredients like DMDM hydantoin, quaternium-15, and imidazolidinyl urea.

6. **Triclosan:**
   - **Purpose:** Antibacterial agent found in soaps, toothpaste, and deodorants.
   - **Risks:** Linked to endocrine disruption and antibiotic resistance.
   - **Alternatives:** Use products labeled "triclosan-free" and opt for natural antibacterial ingredients like tea tree oil or eucalyptus oil.

7. **Petrolatum and Mineral Oil:**
   - **Purpose:** Used as moisturizing agents in lotions and creams.
   - **Risks:** Can be contaminated with carcinogenic compounds and may clog pores.
   - **Alternatives:** Choose products with natural oils and butters like coconut oil, shea butter, and jojoba oil.

Tips for Selecting Non-Toxic Personal Care Products

1. **Read Labels Carefully:**
   - Check the ingredient list for harmful chemicals and opt for products with natural, recognizable ingredients.
   - Look for certifications such as USDA Organic, EWG Verified, or MADE SAFE to ensure product safety.

2. **Choose Simple Formulations:**
   - Simpler products with fewer ingredients are generally less likely to contain harmful chemicals.

- o Avoid products with long, complex ingredient lists, which can hide potentially toxic substances.

3. **Opt for Fragrance-Free or Naturally Scented Products:**
   - o Synthetic fragrances can contain numerous undisclosed chemicals. Choose fragrance-free products or those scented with essential oils.

4. **Research Brands:**
   - o Support brands that prioritize transparency, sustainability, and the use of non-toxic ingredients.
   - o Check brand websites and third-party reviews for information on their safety and sustainability practices.

5. **DIY Personal Care Products:**
   - o Consider making your own personal care products using simple, natural ingredients like coconut oil, baking soda, and essential oils.
   - o DIY recipes can be tailored to your specific needs and preferences, ensuring the use of safe and effective ingredients.

6. **Patch Test New Products:**
   - o Before using a new product extensively, perform a patch test to check for any adverse reactions or sensitivities.

7. **Use Apps and Resources:**
   - o Utilize apps and websites like EWG's Skin Deep, Think Dirty, and GoodGuide to check the safety ratings of personal care products and ingredients.

Choosing non-toxic personal care products is a crucial step in reducing exposure to harmful chemicals and supporting overall health. By being mindful of the ingredients in your personal care routine and opting for safer, natural alternatives, you can protect yourself and the environment. Educating yourself about common harmful ingredients and making informed choices will contribute to a healthier lifestyle and well-being.

Exercise and Mental Health in a Non-Toxic Lifestyle

Exercise and mental health are critical components of a non-toxic lifestyle. Regular physical activity not only enhances physical health but also has profound benefits for mental well-being. Incorporating exercise into your daily routine and adopting practices to support mental health can significantly reduce stress, improve mood, and promote overall life satisfaction. This section explores the relationship between exercise and mental health and provides strategies for integrating both into a non-toxic lifestyle.

Benefits of Exercise for Mental Health

1. **Stress Reduction:**

- Exercise stimulates the production of endorphins, which are natural mood lifters. It helps reduce levels of the body's stress hormones, such as adrenaline and cortisol.

2. **Improved Mood:**

- Regular physical activity can alleviate symptoms of depression and anxiety by promoting the release of neurotransmitters like serotonin and dopamine.

3. **Enhanced Cognitive Function:**

- Exercise improves blood flow to the brain, supporting cognitive functions such as memory, attention, and executive function. It also promotes neurogenesis, the formation of new brain cells.

4. **Better Sleep:**

- Engaging in regular physical activity can improve sleep quality by helping to regulate the sleep-wake cycle and reduce insomnia.

5. **Increased Energy Levels:**

- Exercise boosts overall energy levels and reduces feelings of fatigue by improving cardiovascular and muscular endurance.

6. **Social Interaction:**

- Participating in group exercises or sports can provide opportunities for social interaction, which is essential for mental well-being.

Types of Exercise for Mental Health

1. **Aerobic Exercise:**

- **Examples:** Running, cycling, swimming, brisk walking.
- **Benefits:** Boosts cardiovascular health, improves mood, reduces anxiety, and enhances cognitive function.

2. **Strength Training:**

- **Examples:** Weightlifting, resistance band exercises, bodyweight exercises.
- **Benefits:** Increases muscle strength, improves body composition, boosts self-esteem, and reduces symptoms of depression.

3. **Yoga and Mind-Body Practices:**

- **Examples:** Yoga, Pilates, Tai Chi, Qigong.
- **Benefits:** Enhances flexibility, reduces stress, promotes relaxation, and improves mental clarity and focus.

4. **Mindfulness and Meditation:**

   o **Examples:** Guided meditation, mindfulness practices, deep breathing exercises.

   o **Benefits:** Reduces stress, improves emotional regulation, enhances self-awareness, and promotes a sense of calm.

5. **Outdoor Activities:**

   o **Examples:** Hiking, gardening, outdoor sports.

   o **Benefits:** Provides exposure to nature, which has been shown to reduce stress and improve mood. Engaging in outdoor activities also increases vitamin D levels.

Integrating Exercise and Mental Health Practices into a Non-Toxic Lifestyle

1. **Create a Routine:**

   o Establish a regular exercise routine that fits your schedule and preferences. Consistency is key to reaping the mental health benefits of physical activity.

2. **Set Realistic Goals:**

   o Set achievable fitness goals to stay motivated and track your progress. Focus on gradual improvements rather than immediate results.

3. **Mix It Up:**

   o Incorporate a variety of exercises to keep your routine interesting and engage different muscle groups. Combining aerobic exercise, strength training, and mind-body practices can provide comprehensive benefits.

4. **Practice Mindfulness:**

   o Integrate mindfulness practices into your daily routine to reduce stress and improve mental clarity. Mindfulness can be practiced through meditation, deep breathing exercises, or simply being present during everyday activities.

5. **Prioritize Self-Care:**

   o Take time for self-care activities that support mental health, such as reading, journaling, or spending time in nature. Balance is essential for maintaining a non-toxic lifestyle.

6. **Stay Hydrated and Eat Well:**

   o Proper hydration and nutrition are vital for physical and mental health. Focus on a balanced diet rich in whole foods, and ensure you drink enough water throughout the day.

7. **Connect with Others:**

- Foster social connections through group exercises, sports, or community activities. Social support is crucial for mental well-being and can enhance the benefits of exercise.

8. **Limit Screen Time:**

   - Reduce exposure to screens and digital devices, especially before bedtime, to improve sleep quality and reduce stress.

9. **Create a Healthy Environment:**

   - Ensure your living and working spaces are free from toxins and conducive to relaxation and focus. Use natural cleaning products, maintain good indoor air quality, and create a clutter-free environment.

10. **Seek Professional Support:**

    - If you struggle with mental health issues, consider seeking support from a mental health professional. Therapy, counseling, and other interventions can provide additional support and guidance.

Incorporating exercise and mental health practices into a non-toxic lifestyle is essential for overall well-being. Regular physical activity, mindfulness practices, and a balanced approach to self-care can significantly enhance mental health, reduce stress, and improve quality of life. By prioritizing these aspects and integrating them into your daily routine, you can create a healthier, more balanced lifestyle that supports both physical and mental health.

Environmental Toxins and How to Avoid Them

Environmental toxins are ubiquitous in our modern world, originating from sources such as industrial pollution, household products, and agricultural practices. These toxins can significantly impact health, contributing to a range of chronic diseases and conditions. Understanding the sources of environmental toxins and implementing strategies to minimize exposure is crucial for maintaining a non-toxic lifestyle. This chapter introduces the various types of environmental toxins, their potential health effects, and practical steps to reduce exposure and protect overall health.

Air Quality: Indoor and Outdoor Pollution

Air quality is a critical factor in maintaining overall health and well-being. Both indoor and outdoor air pollution can have significant impacts on respiratory health, cardiovascular health, and overall quality of life. Understanding the sources of air pollution and implementing strategies to improve air quality can help reduce exposure to harmful pollutants and promote a healthier living environment.

Outdoor Air Pollution

Sources of Outdoor Air Pollution:

1. **Vehicle Emissions:**

o   Cars, trucks, buses, and other motor vehicles emit pollutants such as nitrogen oxides (NOx), carbon monoxide (CO), and particulate matter (PM).

2. **Industrial Emissions:**

   o   Factories, power plants, and other industrial facilities release pollutants including sulfur dioxide (SO_2), volatile organic compounds (VOCs), and heavy metals.

3. **Agricultural Activities:**

   o   Pesticides, fertilizers, and livestock emissions contribute to air pollution through the release of ammonia and methane.

4. **Natural Sources:**

   o   Wildfires, volcanic eruptions, and dust storms can also contribute to outdoor air pollution.

Health Effects of Outdoor Air Pollution:

- Respiratory issues: Asthma, bronchitis, and other chronic respiratory conditions.

- Cardiovascular problems: Increased risk of heart attacks, strokes, and hypertension.

- Reduced lung function: Long-term exposure can lead to decreased lung capacity and function.

- Increased mortality: Higher rates of respiratory and cardiovascular diseases, leading to premature death.

Strategies to Reduce Exposure to Outdoor Air Pollution:

1. **Limit Outdoor Activities:**

   o   Reduce outdoor activities, especially during high pollution days or times of heavy traffic.

2. **Stay Informed:**

   o   Monitor local air quality reports and adjust outdoor plans accordingly.

3. **Use Public Transportation:**

   o   Opt for public transportation, carpooling, or cycling to reduce vehicle emissions.

4. **Support Clean Energy:**

   o   Advocate for and support policies and practices that promote clean energy and reduce industrial emissions.

Indoor Air Pollution

Sources of Indoor Air Pollution:

1. **Household Products:**

   o Cleaning agents, air fresheners, and personal care products can release VOCs and other harmful chemicals.

2. **Building Materials:**

   o Materials such as paint, asbestos, and formaldehyde-containing products can emit pollutants.

3. **Tobacco Smoke:**

   o Smoking indoors releases a variety of harmful pollutants including CO, PM, and carcinogens.

4. **Combustion Appliances:**

   o Gas stoves, heaters, and fireplaces can release pollutants like CO and NO_x.

5. **Biological Contaminants:**

   o Mold, dust mites, and pet dander contribute to indoor air pollution.

Health Effects of Indoor Air Pollution:

- Respiratory issues: Allergies, asthma, and respiratory infections.

- Headaches and fatigue: Short-term exposure to certain indoor pollutants can cause headaches and general fatigue.

- Long-term health risks: Chronic exposure to indoor pollutants can lead to serious health issues such as cancer and heart disease.

Strategies to Improve Indoor Air Quality:

1. **Ventilation:**

   o Ensure proper ventilation by using exhaust fans, opening windows, and using air purifiers to reduce indoor pollutant levels.

2. **Regular Cleaning:**

   o Dust and vacuum regularly to reduce dust mites, pet dander, and other allergens.

3. **Use Natural Products:**

   o Opt for natural, non-toxic cleaning products and personal care items to minimize the release of VOCs and other chemicals.

4. **Smoke-Free Home:**

   o Prohibit smoking indoors to avoid exposure to secondhand smoke.

5. **Monitor Humidity Levels:**

- o Use dehumidifiers to maintain indoor humidity between 30-50% to prevent mold growth.

6. **Regular Maintenance:**

   - o Maintain and clean heating, ventilation, and air conditioning (HVAC) systems to ensure they are functioning properly and not contributing to indoor air pollution.

Air quality, both indoor and outdoor, plays a significant role in overall health and well-being. By understanding the sources and health effects of air pollution and implementing strategies to reduce exposure, individuals can create a healthier living environment. Prioritizing clean air practices and staying informed about air quality can significantly reduce the risk of respiratory and cardiovascular issues, leading to improved quality of life.

Water Quality: Contaminants and Filtration

Ensuring access to clean, safe water is essential for health and well-being. Water quality can be compromised by various contaminants, including chemicals, microorganisms, and heavy metals, which pose significant health risks. Understanding common water contaminants and effective filtration methods can help individuals protect themselves and their families from waterborne illnesses and toxins.

Common Water Contaminants

1. **Microbiological Contaminants:**

   - o **Examples:** Bacteria (E. coli, Salmonella), viruses (norovirus, hepatitis A), protozoa (Giardia, Cryptosporidium).
   - o **Health Risks:** Can cause gastrointestinal illnesses, infections, and other diseases.

2. **Chemical Contaminants:**

   - o **Examples:** Pesticides, herbicides, industrial chemicals (benzene, polychlorinated biphenyls - PCBs).
   - o **Health Risks:** Long-term exposure can lead to cancers, hormonal disruptions, and neurological disorders.

3. **Heavy Metals:**

   - o **Examples:** Lead, mercury, arsenic, cadmium.
   - o **Health Risks:** Can cause developmental issues, neurological damage, and kidney problems.

4. **Radiological Contaminants:**

   - o **Examples:** Radon, uranium.
   - o **Health Risks:** Can increase the risk of cancer and cause organ damage.

5. **Pharmaceuticals and Personal Care Products (PPCPs):**

   o **Examples:** Antibiotics, hormones, painkillers.

   o **Health Risks:** Can lead to antibiotic resistance and hormonal imbalances.

6. **Disinfection Byproducts:**

   o **Examples:** Trihalomethanes (THMs), haloacetic acids (HAAs).

   o **Health Risks:** Associated with an increased risk of cancer and reproductive issues.

Filtration Methods

1. **Activated Carbon Filters:**

   o **How It Works:** Uses activated carbon to adsorb organic contaminants, chlorine, and certain pesticides.

   o **Effective Against:** Chlorine, VOCs, some pesticides, and herbicides.

   o **Limitations:** May not remove heavy metals, fluoride, or microbiological contaminants.

2. **Reverse Osmosis (RO):**

   o **How It Works:** Forces water through a semi-permeable membrane, removing a wide range of contaminants.

   o **Effective Against:** Heavy metals, fluoride, nitrates, and many chemical contaminants.

   o **Limitations:** Wastes a significant amount of water, can be slow, and may remove beneficial minerals.

3. **Ultraviolet (UV) Purification:**

   o **How It Works:** Uses UV light to kill bacteria, viruses, and other microorganisms.

   o **Effective Against:** Microbiological contaminants (bacteria, viruses, protozoa).

   o **Limitations:** Does not remove chemical contaminants, heavy metals, or particulates.

4. **Distillation:**

   o **How It Works:** Heats water to create steam, which is then condensed back into liquid form, leaving contaminants behind.

   o **Effective Against:** Heavy metals, salts, and many chemical contaminants.

   o **Limitations:** Can be slow, energy-intensive, and may not remove VOCs that boil at or below water's boiling point.

5. **Ceramic Filters:**

   o **How It Works:** Uses porous ceramic material to filter out particulates and some pathogens.

   o **Effective Against:** Bacteria, protozoa, and particulates.

   o **Limitations:** May not remove viruses, chemicals, or heavy metals.

6. **Ion Exchange:**

   o **How It Works:** Replaces unwanted ions (e.g., calcium, magnesium) with more desirable ones (e.g., sodium).

   o **Effective Against:** Hard water minerals, some heavy metals.

   o **Limitations:** Does not remove microbiological contaminants or all chemical pollutants.

7. **Gravity-Fed Drip Filters:**

   o **How It Works:** Uses gravity to pass water through a filter medium, such as activated carbon or ceramic.

   o **Effective Against:** Varies based on the filter medium used; commonly removes particulates, chlorine, and some bacteria.

   o **Limitations:** Flow rate can be slow, and effectiveness depends on filter type.

Tips for Ensuring Safe Drinking Water

1. **Test Your Water:**

   o Conduct regular water testing to identify specific contaminants present in your water supply. Use certified labs or home testing kits for accurate results.

2. **Choose the Right Filtration System:**

   o Select a filtration system based on the specific contaminants identified in your water. Consider combining multiple filtration methods for comprehensive protection.

3. **Maintain and Replace Filters:**

   o Regularly maintain and replace filters according to the manufacturer's instructions to ensure continued effectiveness.

4. **Boil Water During Emergencies:**

   o In situations where water quality is compromised, boiling water for at least one minute can kill most pathogens and make it safe to drink.

5. **Use Bottled Water Sparingly:**

- While bottled water can be a temporary solution, it is not a sustainable long-term option due to environmental impact and potential contaminants from plastic bottles.

6. **Protect Your Source:**

   - If you have a private well, ensure it is properly maintained and protected from contamination sources such as septic systems and agricultural runoff.

7. **Stay Informed:**

   - Keep up to date with local water quality reports and advisories. Be proactive in addressing any issues that may arise.

Maintaining high water quality is essential for health and well-being. By understanding common contaminants and utilizing effective filtration methods, individuals can significantly reduce their exposure to harmful substances in drinking water. Regular testing, proper maintenance of filtration systems, and staying informed about local water quality can help ensure access to clean, safe water.

Household Chemicals: Cleaners, Pesticides, and More

Household chemicals, including cleaners, pesticides, and other common products, can introduce toxins into the home environment. Exposure to these chemicals can pose various health risks, ranging from minor irritations to serious long-term health effects. Understanding the potential dangers and adopting safer alternatives can significantly reduce these risks. This section explores the hazards associated with household chemicals and provides strategies for minimizing exposure and maintaining a non-toxic home.

Hazards of Household Chemicals

1. **Cleaners:**

   - **Examples:** Bleach, ammonia, disinfectants, and multi-surface cleaners.

   - **Health Risks:** Respiratory irritation, skin burns, eye damage, and potential long-term effects like asthma and hormone disruption. Mixing certain cleaners (e.g., bleach and ammonia) can produce toxic gases.

2. **Pesticides:**

   - **Examples:** Insecticides, rodenticides, herbicides, and fungicides.

   - **Health Risks:** Neurological damage, endocrine disruption, reproductive issues, and increased cancer risk. Children and pets are particularly vulnerable to pesticide exposure.

3. **Air Fresheners and Scented Products:**

   - **Examples:** Aerosol sprays, plug-ins, scented candles, and diffusers.

- **Health Risks:** Respiratory irritation, allergic reactions, and hormone disruption. Many contain phthalates and VOCs.

4. **Personal Care Products:**
   - **Examples:** Lotions, shampoos, deodorants, and cosmetics.
   - **Health Risks:** Skin irritation, allergies, and potential long-term effects from hormone-disrupting chemicals like parabens and phthalates.

5. **Laundry Products:**
   - **Examples:** Detergents, fabric softeners, stain removers, and dryer sheets.
   - **Health Risks:** Skin irritation, respiratory issues, and allergic reactions. Many contain synthetic fragrances and harsh chemicals.

6. **Paints and Solvents:**
   - **Examples:** Household paints, varnishes, paint thinners, and adhesives.
   - **Health Risks:** Respiratory problems, headaches, dizziness, and long-term risks like liver and kidney damage. VOCs can off-gas for years after application.

Strategies for Minimizing Exposure

1. **Choose Natural and Non-Toxic Cleaners:**
   - **Alternatives:** Use natural cleaning products made from ingredients like vinegar, baking soda, lemon juice, and castile soap.
   - **DIY Recipes:** Make your own cleaning solutions to ensure they are free from harmful chemicals. For example, mix vinegar and water for an all-purpose cleaner, or use baking soda as a scrubbing agent.

2. **Reduce Use of Pesticides:**
   - **Integrated Pest Management (IPM):** Adopt IPM practices to manage pests with minimal chemical use. This includes sealing entry points, maintaining cleanliness, and using traps or natural deterrents.
   - **Natural Alternatives:** Use essential oils, diatomaceous earth, and botanical insecticides like neem oil as safer pest control options.

3. **Avoid Synthetic Fragrances:**
   - **Fragrance-Free Products:** Choose fragrance-free or naturally scented products using essential oils.
   - **Ventilation:** Improve indoor air quality by increasing ventilation and using air purifiers instead of air fresheners.

4. **Opt for Non-Toxic Personal Care Products:**

- o **Natural Ingredients:** Select personal care products made from natural ingredients and free from parabens, phthalates, and synthetic fragrances.

- o **Certification:** Look for products with certifications like USDA Organic, EWG Verified, or MADE SAFE.

5. **Use Eco-Friendly Laundry Products:**

- o **Natural Detergents:** Choose laundry detergents and fabric softeners made from plant-based ingredients and free from synthetic fragrances and harsh chemicals.

- o **Wool Dryer Balls:** Use wool dryer balls instead of dryer sheets to reduce static and soften clothes naturally.

6. **Select Low-VOC or VOC-Free Paints:**

- o **Paint Choices:** Opt for low-VOC or VOC-free paints and finishes to reduce indoor air pollution.

- o **Proper Ventilation:** Ensure proper ventilation during and after painting to minimize exposure to fumes.

7. **Store Chemicals Safely:**

- o **Secure Storage:** Store household chemicals in secure, well-ventilated areas, away from children and pets.

- o **Original Containers:** Keep chemicals in their original containers with labels intact to avoid accidental misuse or mixing.

8. **Regular Maintenance and Cleaning:**

- o **Reduce Dust:** Regularly dust and vacuum to reduce the buildup of allergens and chemical residues.

- o **Mold Prevention:** Address moisture issues and use dehumidifiers to prevent mold growth, which can release harmful spores and mycotoxins.

Reducing exposure to household chemicals is a crucial aspect of maintaining a non-toxic home environment. By choosing natural and non-toxic alternatives, adopting safer practices, and staying informed about the potential hazards of common household products, individuals can significantly decrease their risk of health issues related to chemical exposure. Implementing these strategies promotes a healthier, safer living space for everyone in the household.

Electromagnetic Fields (EMFs) and Radiation

Electromagnetic fields (EMFs) and radiation are pervasive in our modern environment, emanating from various electronic devices and technologies. While the long-term health effects of EMF exposure are still being studied, there is growing concern about potential risks, including neurological disorders, sleep disturbances, and increased cancer risk. Understanding the sources of EMFs and radiation and adopting strategies to minimize exposure can help create a safer living environment. This section explores EMFs, their potential health impacts, and practical steps to reduce exposure.

Sources of EMFs and Radiation

1. **Power Lines and Electrical Wiring:**
   - **Source:** High-voltage power lines, electrical wiring in homes and buildings.
   - **EMF Type:** Extremely Low Frequency (ELF) EMFs.

2. **Electronic Devices:**
   - **Source:** Computers, laptops, tablets, smartphones, and televisions.
   - **EMF Type:** Radiofrequency (RF) EMFs and ELF EMFs.

3. **Wi-Fi Routers and Wireless Devices:**
   - **Source:** Wi-Fi routers, cordless phones, smart home devices, and wireless printers.
   - **EMF Type:** RF EMFs.

4. **Cell Towers and Antennas:**
   - **Source:** Cell towers, broadcast antennas, and satellite dishes.
   - **EMF Type:** RF EMFs.

5. **Household Appliances:**
   - **Source:** Microwaves, refrigerators, washing machines, and other electric appliances.
   - **EMF Type:** ELF EMFs.

6. **Medical Devices:**
   - **Source:** X-ray machines, MRI scanners, and other diagnostic imaging devices.
   - **EMF Type:** Ionizing radiation (X-rays) and non-ionizing radiation (RF and ELF EMFs).

Potential Health Effects of EMFs and Radiation

1. **Neurological Effects:**
   - **Symptoms:** Headaches, dizziness, and cognitive impairments.
   - **Concerns:** Long-term exposure may contribute to neurological disorders such as Alzheimer's disease and dementia.

2. **Sleep Disturbances:**

- **Symptoms:** Insomnia, poor sleep quality, and difficulty falling asleep.
- **Concerns:** EMFs can disrupt the production of melatonin, a hormone that regulates sleep-wake cycles.

3. **Increased Cancer Risk:**

- **Concerns:** Some studies suggest a potential link between long-term EMF exposure and an increased risk of certain cancers, such as leukemia and brain tumors.

4. **Reproductive Effects:**

- **Concerns:** Exposure to high levels of EMFs may impact reproductive health, potentially affecting fertility and fetal development.

5. **Cardiovascular Effects:**

- **Symptoms:** Elevated heart rate, palpitations, and changes in blood pressure.
- **Concerns:** Chronic exposure to EMFs may contribute to cardiovascular health issues.

Strategies to Minimize EMF and Radiation Exposure

1. **Increase Distance from EMF Sources:**

- **Devices:** Keep a safe distance from electronic devices and appliances when not in use. Use speakerphone or headphones for phone calls to keep the device away from your head.
- **Living Spaces:** Arrange furniture to maximize distance from high-EMF sources like Wi-Fi routers and power strips.

2. **Limit Use of Wireless Devices:**

- **Wired Alternatives:** Use wired internet connections instead of Wi-Fi when possible. Opt for wired peripherals like keyboards and mice.
- **Airplane Mode:** Enable airplane mode on smartphones and tablets when not actively using wireless functions.

3. **Turn Off Devices When Not in Use:**

- **Power Down:** Turn off Wi-Fi routers, computers, and other electronics at night or when not in use.
- **Unplug:** Unplug devices and appliances that are not in use to reduce EMF emissions and save energy.

4. **Use EMF Shielding Products:**

- ○ **Shielding Materials:** Consider using EMF shielding products, such as protective cases for smartphones and tablets, or EMF-blocking fabric for curtains and bed canopies.

- ○ **Paints and Films:** Apply EMF shielding paints or window films to reduce EMF penetration from external sources.

5. **Optimize Bedroom Environment:**

- ○ **Sleeping Area:** Keep electronic devices out of the bedroom to minimize nighttime exposure. Use an analog alarm clock instead of a smartphone.

- ○ **Bed Placement:** Position your bed away from walls with electrical wiring and appliances.

6. **Reduce Exposure to Ionizing Radiation:**

- ○ **Medical Imaging:** Limit the use of diagnostic imaging tests like X-rays and CT scans to only when medically necessary. Discuss alternative imaging methods with your healthcare provider.

- ○ **Radon Testing:** Test your home for radon, a naturally occurring radioactive gas that can accumulate indoors and increase lung cancer risk.

7. **Monitor EMF Levels:**

- ○ **EMF Meters:** Use an EMF meter to measure and monitor EMF levels in your home and identify high-exposure areas.

- ○ **Professional Assessment:** Consider hiring a professional to conduct a thorough EMF assessment of your living environment.

Conclusion

While the full extent of health risks associated with EMF exposure is still being researched, taking proactive steps to minimize exposure can help create a safer and healthier living environment. By understanding the sources of EMFs and radiation and implementing practical strategies to reduce exposure, individuals can better protect their health and well-being. Adopting these measures as part of a non-toxic lifestyle supports overall health and promotes a sense of well-being.

Safe Use of Plastics and Alternatives

Plastics are ubiquitous in modern life, but their use comes with potential health risks due to chemicals like bisphenol A (BPA), phthalates, and other additives that can leach into food and beverages. Understanding how to use plastics safely and exploring alternatives can significantly reduce exposure to harmful substances. This section provides guidelines for the safe use of plastics and suggests healthier alternatives.

Risks Associated with Plastics

1. **Chemical Leaching:**

   o **BPA and BPS:** Found in polycarbonate plastics and epoxy resins, these chemicals can leach into food and beverages, particularly when heated, and act as endocrine disruptors.

   o **Phthalates:** Used to soften plastics, phthalates can leach into food and pose risks to the reproductive system and overall health.

2. **Microplastics:**

   o **Sources:** Breakdown of larger plastic items, microbeads in personal care products.

   o **Health Impact:** Ingestion of microplastics can lead to chemical exposure and potential health issues.

Safe Use of Plastics

1. **Identify Safe Plastics:**

   o **Plastic Codes:** Check the recycling codes on plastic products. Avoid plastics with codes 3 (PVC), 6 (PS), and 7 (other, often polycarbonate) which may contain harmful chemicals.

   o **Safer Options:** Opt for plastics labeled 1 (PET), 2 (HDPE), 4 (LDPE), and 5 (PP), which are generally considered safer for food and beverage use.

2. **Avoid Heating Plastics:**

   o **Microwave and Dishwasher:** Do not microwave food in plastic containers or place them in the dishwasher, as heat can cause chemicals to leach out.

   o **Hot Liquids:** Avoid using plastic containers for hot foods and beverages. Use glass or stainless steel instead.

3. **Minimize Plastic Use:**

   o **Food Storage:** Use glass, stainless steel, or silicone containers for storing food and beverages.

   o **Plastic Wrap:** Replace plastic wrap with beeswax wraps, silicone covers, or reusable cloth wraps.

4. **Choose BPA-Free Products:**

   o **Labels:** Look for products labeled "BPA-free." However, be aware that some BPA-free products may contain other harmful chemicals like BPS.

   o **Research:** Check product reviews and recommendations from trusted sources for truly safe alternatives.

5. **Reduce Single-Use Plastics:**

- **Alternatives:** Use reusable bags, water bottles, and straws. Opt for products with minimal or no plastic packaging.
- **Zero Waste Stores:** Shop at stores that offer bulk bins and allow you to bring your own containers.

Healthier Alternatives to Plastics

1. **Glass:**
   - **Benefits:** Non-toxic, does not leach chemicals, durable, and recyclable.
   - **Uses:** Ideal for food storage, drinking bottles, baby bottles, and cooking.

2. **Stainless Steel:**
   - **Benefits:** Durable, non-reactive, and resistant to rust and corrosion. Safe for food and beverages.
   - **Uses:** Water bottles, food containers, cookware, and straws.

3. **Silicone:**
   - **Benefits:** Flexible, durable, and heat resistant. Free from BPA, phthalates, and other harmful chemicals.
   - **Uses:** Baking mats, food storage bags, baby products, and kitchen utensils.

4. **Ceramic and Stoneware:**
   - **Benefits:** Non-toxic and safe for cooking and serving. Often more aesthetically pleasing.
   - **Uses:** Cookware, dinnerware, and storage containers.

5. **Bamboo:**
   - **Benefits:** Renewable resource, biodegradable, and free from harmful chemicals.
   - **Uses:** Cutting boards, utensils, and dishware.

6. **Beeswax Wraps:**
   - **Benefits:** Reusable, biodegradable, and a natural alternative to plastic wrap.
   - **Uses:** Wrapping food items, covering bowls, and storing snacks.

Practical Tips for Transitioning to Safer Alternatives

1. **Gradual Replacement:**
   - **Start Small:** Begin by replacing frequently used plastic items with safer alternatives, such as swapping plastic water bottles for stainless steel ones.

- o **Phase Out:** Gradually phase out plastic food storage containers and replace them with glass or stainless-steel options.

2. **Budget-Friendly Choices:**

   - o **Second-Hand Options:** Look for glass or stainless-steel containers at thrift stores or online marketplaces to save money.

   - o **DIY Solutions:** Make your own beeswax wraps or repurpose glass jars for food storage.

3. **Educate and Advocate:**

   - o **Stay Informed:** Keep up with the latest research on plastic safety and alternatives.

   - o **Spread Awareness:** Encourage friends and family to reduce their plastic use and opt for safer alternatives.

4. **Read Labels and Reviews:**

   - o **Product Research:** Check labels for safety certifications and read reviews from reputable sources to ensure you are choosing truly non-toxic products.

   - o **Trusted Brands:** Support brands known for their commitment to safety and sustainability.

Minimizing the use of plastics and opting for safer alternatives can significantly reduce exposure to harmful chemicals, contributing to better health and a cleaner environment. By being mindful of the plastics, you use and gradually transitioning to non-toxic materials like glass, stainless steel, and silicone, you can create a healthier living space and promote sustainability. These small changes can have a big impact on your overall well-being and the health of the planet.

Reducing Exposure to Heavy Metals

Heavy metals such as lead, mercury, cadmium, and arsenic can have serious health impacts, including neurological damage, kidney disease, and cancer. Reducing exposure to these toxic substances is crucial for maintaining long-term health. This section explores common sources of heavy metals and provides practical strategies for minimizing exposure.

Common Sources of Heavy Metals

1. **Lead:**

   - o **Sources:** Lead-based paint (especially in older homes), contaminated soil, plumbing pipes, batteries, certain cosmetics, and imported toys.

   - o **Health Risks:** Cognitive impairment, developmental delays in children, kidney damage, and hypertension.

2. **Mercury:**

- **Sources:** Contaminated fish and seafood, dental amalgam fillings, some industrial processes, and certain skin-lightening products.
- **Health Risks:** Neurological damage, cognitive deficits, and developmental issues in fetuses and young children.

3. **Cadmium:**

- **Sources:** Cigarette smoke, contaminated food (especially leafy vegetables, grains, and organ meats), industrial emissions, and batteries.
- **Health Risks:** Kidney damage, bone fractures, and an increased risk of cancer.

4. **Arsenic:**

- **Sources:** Contaminated drinking water (particularly from wells), certain pesticides, industrial processes, and rice and rice-based products.
- **Health Risks:** Skin lesions, cardiovascular disease, neurotoxicity, and an increased risk of cancer.

Strategies to Reduce Exposure

1. **Testing and Filtering Water:**

- **Water Testing:** Regularly test your drinking water for heavy metals, especially if you rely on well water.
- **Water Filters:** Use water filters certified to remove heavy metals. Options include reverse osmosis systems and filters with activated alumina.

2. **Dietary Choices:**

- **Fish Consumption:** Limit intake of fish high in mercury, such as shark, swordfish, king mackerel, and tilefish. Opt for lower-mercury fishlike salmon, sardines, and trout.
- **Organic Produce:** Choose organic fruits and vegetables to reduce exposure to cadmium from pesticides. Wash produces thoroughly.
- **Rice Consumption:** Rinse rice thoroughly before cooking, use plenty of water, and consider diversifying your grain intake with alternatives like quinoa, millet, and barley to reduce arsenic exposure.

3. **Home Environment:**

- **Lead Paint:** If you live in an older home, have it inspected for lead paint. Hire professionals to safely remove or encapsulate lead-based paint.
- **Soil Contamination:** Test your garden soil for heavy metals, especially if you live near industrial areas or busy roads. Use raised beds and clean soil for gardening.

- Household Dust: Regularly clean floors, windowsills, and other surfaces to reduce lead-contaminated dust. Use a wet mop and HEPA-filter vacuum.

4. **Consumer Products:**

   - **Safe Toys:** Ensure that children's toys are lead-free. Avoid imported toys that may not meet safety standards.

   - **Cosmetics and Personal Care Products:** Choose cosmetics and personal care products free from heavy metals. Look for reputable brands and certifications.

5. **Avoid Smoking:**

   - **Cigarette Smoke:** Avoid smoking and exposure to secondhand smoke, which contains cadmium and other harmful substances.

6. **Occupational Safety:**

   - **Workplace Safety:** If you work in an industry with potential heavy metal exposure (e.g., construction, battery manufacturing), follow safety guidelines, use protective equipment, and undergo regular health screenings.

7. **Nutritional Support:**

   - **Dietary Antioxidants:** Consume foods rich in antioxidants (e.g., berries, leafy greens, nuts) to support detoxification and reduce oxidative stress from heavy metals.

   - **Chelating Agents:** Certain foods and supplements, like cilantro, chlorella, and garlic, may help bind heavy metals and support their elimination from the body.

Monitoring and Professional Guidance

1. **Regular Health Check-Ups:**

   - Have regular health check-ups and blood tests to monitor for heavy metal exposure, especially if you are at higher risk.

2. **Consult Healthcare Providers:**

   - Seek advice from healthcare providers if you suspect heavy metal exposure. They can provide guidance on testing and detoxification strategies.

3. **Environmental and Occupational Health Resources:**

   - Utilize resources from environmental and occupational health organizations for information on reducing exposure and improving safety practices.

Reducing exposure to heavy metals is essential for protecting health and preventing serious long-term effects. By being aware of common sources and implementing practical strategies to minimize exposure, individuals can significantly lower their risk. Regular monitoring, making informed dietary and consumer choices, and maintaining a clean home environment are key steps in ensuring a healthier, safer lifestyle.

Creating a Non-Toxic Home Environment

A non-toxic home environment is essential for promoting health and well-being. Our homes should be sanctuaries, free from harmful chemicals and pollutants that can adversely affect our health. This chapter introduces practical strategies and tips for reducing toxins in your living space, from choosing safer building materials and cleaning products to improving indoor air quality and managing household waste. By making informed choices and implementing these practices, you can create a healthier, safer home for you and your family.

Choosing Non-Toxic Building Materials

Selecting non-toxic building materials is crucial for creating a healthy home environment. Traditional building materials can release harmful chemicals into the air, contributing to indoor pollution and posing health risks. This section provides guidelines on choosing safer alternatives that minimize exposure to toxins and enhance overall well-being.

Key Considerations for Non-Toxic Building Materials

1. **Volatile Organic Compounds (VOCs):**

   o **Risks:** VOCs are emitted as gases from certain solids and liquids, including paints, coatings, and adhesives. High levels of VOCs can cause respiratory issues, headaches, and long-term health problems.

   o **Solutions:** Choose low-VOC or VOC-free products. Look for certifications like GREENGUARD or Green Seal that indicate low chemical emissions.

2. **Formaldehyde:**

   o **Risks:** Commonly found in pressed wood products, insulation, and adhesives. Formaldehyde is a known carcinogen and can cause respiratory irritation and allergic reactions.

   o **Solutions:** Select formaldehyde-free products, including plywood, particleboard, and medium-density fiberboard (MDF). Use natural adhesives and finishes.

3. **Lead:**

   o **Risks:** Lead-based paints and plumbing fixtures can cause severe neurological and developmental issues, particularly in children.

   o **Solutions:** Use lead-free paints and fixtures. If renovating an older home, have it inspected for lead and hire professionals for safe removal.

4. **Asbestos:**

   o **Risks:** Found in older insulation, roofing, and flooring materials. Asbestos exposure can lead to lung diseases, including cancer.

- **Solutions:** Avoid using materials containing asbestos. For existing asbestos, hire certified professionals for safe removal and disposal.

Non-Toxic Building Material Options

1. **Paints and Finishes:**

   - **Low-VOC and Zero-VOC Paints:** Brands like Benjamin Moore's Natura and Sherwin-Williams' Harmony offer safer alternatives.

   - **Natural Paints:** Made from natural ingredients like clay, chalk, and plant oils, these paints are non-toxic and eco-friendly. Examples include brands like BioShield and ECOS Paints.

2. **Flooring:**

   - **Hardwood:** Opt for sustainably sourced, FSC-certified hardwood. Use water-based, low-VOC sealants and finishes.

   - **Bamboo:** A rapidly renewable resource, bamboo is durable and environmentally friendly. Choose formaldehyde-free options.

   - **Cork:** Naturally anti-microbial and renewable, cork is a healthy flooring choice. Ensure it is sealed with low-VOC finishes.

   - **Natural Linoleum:** Made from linseed oil, cork dust, and wood flour, it is biodegradable and free from harmful chemicals. Brands like Marmoleum offer eco-friendly options.

3. **Cabinetry and Furniture:**

   - **Solid Wood:** Choose solid wood over particleboard or MDF to avoid formaldehyde emissions. Look for FSC-certified wood.

   - **Natural Finishes:** Use natural oils (e.g., tung oil, linseed oil) and waxes for finishing furniture and cabinetry.

4. **Insulation:**

   - **Cellulose Insulation:** Made from recycled paper treated with non-toxic fire retardants, it is a safe and effective insulation option.

   - **Sheep's Wool:** Naturally fire-resistant and non-toxic, sheep's wool provides excellent insulation properties.

   - **Cotton (Denim) Insulation:** Made from recycled cotton fibers, this insulation is free from harmful chemicals and offers good thermal performance.

5. **Adhesives and Sealants:**

   - **Low-VOC Adhesives:** Use adhesives labeled as low-VOC or VOC-free for all construction and renovation projects.

- Natural Alternatives: Consider using natural options like milk protein-based glues or soy-based adhesives.

6. **Wall and Ceiling Materials:**

   - **Plaster:** Natural plaster made from lime or clay is non-toxic and breathable, promoting healthy indoor air quality.

   - **Gypsum Board:** Look for low-VOC gypsum boards that do not contain formaldehyde.

7. **Roofing Materials:**

   - **Metal Roofing:** Durable and recyclable, metal roofing is a sustainable option with no harmful emissions.

   - **Clay and Concrete Tiles:** These materials are non-toxic and long-lasting, providing excellent protection without releasing harmful substances.

Certifications to Look For

1. **GREENGUARD:** Indicates that a product has low chemical emissions and contributes to healthier indoor air quality.

2. **Green Seal:** Certifies products that meet rigorous environmental standards, including low VOC content.

3. **Forest Stewardship Council (FSC):** Ensures that wood products come from responsibly managed forests that provide environmental, social, and economic benefits.

4. **Cradle to Cradle:** Certifies products that are safe for human and environmental health through all lifecycle stages, from production to disposal.

Choosing non-toxic building materials is a crucial step in creating a healthier living environment. By selecting materials that minimize harmful emissions and opting for safer alternatives, you can significantly reduce exposure to toxins in your home. Prioritize products with relevant certifications and consider the long-term benefits of a non-toxic home for your overall health and well-being.

Natural and Green Cleaning Products

Using natural and green cleaning products is a key step in maintaining a non-toxic home environment. Conventional cleaning products often contain harmful chemicals that can contribute to indoor air pollution and pose health risks. Natural and green alternatives offer effective cleaning without the associated health hazards. This section explores the benefits of using natural cleaning products, common toxic ingredients to avoid, and how to make or choose safer cleaning solutions.

Benefits of Natural and Green Cleaning Products

1. **Healthier Indoor Air Quality:**

- Natural cleaning products reduce the emission of volatile organic compounds (VOCs) and other harmful chemicals, improving indoor air quality.

2. **Reduced Health Risks:**

   - Using non-toxic cleaners minimizes exposure to irritants and allergens that can cause respiratory issues, skin irritation, and other health problems.

3. **Environmental Sustainability:**

   - Green cleaning products are often biodegradable and made from renewable resources, reducing environmental impact.

4. **Safe for Children and Pets:**

   - Natural cleaners are safer for homes with children and pets, who are more susceptible to the effects of toxic chemicals.

Common Toxic Ingredients to Avoid

1. **Phthalates:**

   - Found in many fragranced cleaning products.
   - **Risks:** Endocrine disruption, reproductive issues.

2. **Triclosan:**

   - Found in antibacterial cleaners.
   - **Risks:** Hormone disruption, antibiotic resistance.

3. **Ammonia:**

   - Found in glass cleaners and polishing agents.
   - **Risks:** Respiratory irritation, skin burns.

4. **Chlorine Bleach:**

   - Found in disinfectants and whiteners.
   - **Risks:** Respiratory issues, skin irritation, toxic fumes when mixed with other chemicals.

5. **Quaternary Ammonium Compounds (Quats):**

   - Found in disinfectants and fabric softeners.
   - **Risks:** Respiratory and skin irritation, potential allergen.

6. **Sodium Hydroxide (Lye):**

   - Found in oven and drain cleaners.

     o **Risks:** Severe skin and eye irritation, respiratory issues.

Natural Cleaning Ingredients and Their Uses

1. **White Vinegar:**

   o **Uses:** Disinfectant, deodorizer, glass cleaner, and lime scale remover.

   o **How to Use:** Mix equal parts vinegar and water for an all-purpose cleaner. Use undiluted for tougher stains and lime scale.

2. **Baking Soda:**

   o **Uses:** Abrasive cleaner, deodorizer, and stain remover.

   o **How to Use:** Sprinkle on surfaces and scrub with a damp sponge. Mix with water to form a paste for tough stains.

3. **Lemon Juice:**

   o **Uses:** Disinfectant, deodorizer, and stain remover.

   o **How to Use:** Use straight or mixed with vinegar for a powerful cleaner. Combine with baking soda for scrubbing.

4. **Castile Soap:**

   o **Uses:** All-purpose cleaner, dish soap, and laundry detergent.

   o **How to Use:** Dilute with water for various cleaning tasks. Mix with baking soda for a deeper clean.

5. **Essential Oils:**

   o **Uses:** Add fragrance, antibacterial and antifungal properties.

   o **How to Use:** Add a few drops to vinegar or baking soda-based cleaners. Popular choices include tea tree, lavender, and eucalyptus oils.

6. **Hydrogen Peroxide:**

   o **Uses:** Disinfectant and stain remover.

   o **How to Use:** Use a 3% solution for cleaning surfaces and whitening grout. Test on a small area first.

DIY Natural Cleaning Recipes

1. **All-Purpose Cleaner:**

   o **Ingredients:** 1 cup white vinegar, 1 cup water, 10-15 drops essential oil.

   o **Instructions:** Mix ingredients in a spray bottle. Use on countertops, floors, and other surfaces.

2. **Glass Cleaner:**

   o **Ingredients:** 1 cup water, 1 cup vinegar, 1 tablespoon cornstarch.

   o **Instructions:** Mix in a spray bottle. Shake well before each use. Wipe with a microfiber cloth.

3. **Bathroom Scrub:**

   o **Ingredients:** 1/2 cup baking soda, 1/4 cup liquid castile soap, 10 drops tea tree oil.

   o **Instructions:** Mix ingredients to form a paste. Apply to surfaces with a sponge or brush, scrub, and rinse.

4. **Floor Cleaner:**

   o **Ingredients:** 1/2 cup white vinegar, 1 gallon warm water, a few drops of essential oil (optional).

   o **Instructions:** Mix ingredients in a bucket. Mop floors as usual.

5. **Toilet Bowl Cleaner:**

   o **Ingredients:** 1/2 cup baking soda, 1/4 cup white vinegar, 10 drops tea tree oil.

   o **Instructions:** Sprinkle baking soda into the bowl, add vinegar and tea tree oil. Scrub and let sit for 10 minutes before flushing.

Choosing Commercial Green Cleaning Products

1. **Certifications to Look For:**

   o **EPA Safer Choice:** Indicates the product meets stringent safety criteria.

   o **Green Seal:** Ensures the product is environmentally responsible and safe for use.

   o **EcoLogo:** Certifies products that reduce environmental impact and are safer for human health.

2. **Read Labels:**

   o Look for ingredient transparency and avoid products with vague terms like "fragrance" or "surfactant."

3. **Research Brands:**

   o Choose brands known for their commitment to sustainability and non-toxic ingredients. Some reputable brands include Seventh Generation, Ecover, and Mrs. Meyer's.

4. **Consumer Reviews:**

- Check reviews and ratings from other consumers to gauge the effectiveness and safety of the products.

Switching to natural and green cleaning products is a vital step in creating a healthier, non-toxic home environment. By using common household ingredients and understanding how to choose safer commercial products, you can effectively clean your home while minimizing exposure to harmful chemicals. This shift not only benefits your health but also supports environmental sustainability.

Non-Toxic Furnishings and Decorations

Choosing non-toxic furnishings and decorations for your home is an essential aspect of creating a healthy living environment. Traditional furniture and decor items can release harmful chemicals into the air, contributing to indoor pollution and posing health risks. This section provides guidelines on selecting safer alternatives that enhance your home's aesthetics while promoting well-being.

Key Considerations for Non-Toxic Furnishings and Decorations

1. **Avoiding VOCs:**
   - **Sources:** Paints, finishes, adhesives, and synthetic materials.
   - **Solutions:** Opt for low-VOC or VOC-free products. Look for certifications such as GREENGUARD or Green Seal that indicate low emissions.

2. **Natural Materials:**
   - **Benefits:** Natural materials like wood, cotton, wool, and bamboo are less likely to contain harmful chemicals.
   - **Examples:** Solid wood furniture, organic cotton textiles, wool rugs, and bamboo accessories.

3. **Flame Retardants:**
   - **Sources:** Upholstered furniture, mattresses, and textiles.
   - **Risks:** Chemicals like PBDEs (polybrominated diphenyl ethers) can disrupt hormones and have been linked to cancer.
   - **Solutions:** Choose products labeled as free from flame retardants or use naturally flame-resistant materials like wool.

4. **Formaldehyde:**
   - **Sources:** Pressed wood products, some glues, and finishes.
   - **Risks:** A known carcinogen that can cause respiratory issues and skin irritation.
   - **Solutions:** Select formaldehyde-free furniture and use natural finishes.

5. **Pesticides and Heavy Metals:**

- **Sources:** Imported textiles, some rugs, and furniture.
- **Risks:** Exposure can lead to various health issues, including neurological damage.
- **Solutions:** Choose organic and eco-friendly textiles and ensure products comply with safety standards.

Non-Toxic Furniture Options

1. **Solid Wood Furniture:**
   - **Benefits:** Durable, timeless, and free from harmful chemicals found in pressed wood.
   - **Certification:** Look for FSC (Forest Stewardship Council) certified wood to ensure sustainable sourcing.
   - **Finishes:** Use natural oils or water-based, low-VOC finishes.

2. **Eco-Friendly Upholstery:**
   - **Materials:** Choose natural fabrics like organic cotton, linen, hemp, and wool.
   - **Cushions:** Opt for natural latex or wool instead of polyurethane foam, which can off-gas harmful chemicals.
   - **Brands:** Seek out furniture brands that prioritize sustainability and non-toxic materials.

3. **Reclaimed and Vintage Furniture:**
   - **Benefits:** Reusing furniture reduces waste and often avoids the use of modern synthetic materials.
   - **Considerations:** Ensure that older furniture has not been treated with harmful chemicals or lead-based paints.

Non-Toxic Decorations

1. **Natural Textiles:**
   - **Curtains and Drapes:** Use organic cotton, linen, or hemp for window treatments.
   - **Rugs and Carpets:** Choose wool, jute, sisal, or organic cotton rugs. Avoid synthetic materials that can off-gas VOCs.

2. **Eco-Friendly Paints and Finishes:**
   - **Low-VOC or Zero-VOC Paints:** Brands like Benjamin Moore's Natura and Sherwin-Williams' Harmony offer safer options.

- Natural Paints: Made from ingredients like clay, chalk, and plant oils. Examples include BioShield and ECOS Paints.

3. **Houseplants:**
   - **Benefits:** Improve indoor air quality by absorbing toxins and releasing oxygen.
   - **Selection:** Choose easy-care varieties like spider plants, snake plants, and peace lilies.

4. **Non-Toxic Candles:**
   - **Materials:** Opt for candles made from beeswax, soy, or coconut wax. Avoid paraffin candles, which can release harmful chemicals.
   - **Fragrance:** Use candles scented with essential oils rather than synthetic fragrances.

5. **Natural Flooring:**
   - **Wood Flooring:** Select FSC-certified hardwood with natural finishes.
   - **Bamboo:** A sustainable and durable option.
   - **Cork:** Naturally hypoallergenic and anti-microbial.
   - **Natural Stone and Tiles:** Free from synthetic chemicals and easy to clean.

6. **Artwork and Decor:**
   - **Materials:** Choose artwork made from natural or recycled materials.
   - **Framing:** Use frames made from untreated wood or recycled materials.
   - **Handmade Items:** Support local artisans who use natural materials and eco-friendly practices.

Practical Tips for Creating a Non-Toxic Home

1. **Research and Certifications:**
   - Look for certifications such as GREENGUARD, FSC, and GOTS (Global Organic Textile Standard) when purchasing furnishings and decor.
   - Research brands and products to ensure they adhere to non-toxic and sustainable practices.

2. **Ventilation:**
   - Ensure good ventilation during and after the installation of new furnishings to reduce the concentration of any off-gassed chemicals.
   - Use air purifiers to help maintain indoor air quality.

3. **Cleaning and Maintenance:**

   o Regularly clean with non-toxic cleaning products to reduce dust and allergens.

   o Maintain furniture and decor to extend their lifespan and reduce the need for replacements.

4. **DIY Projects:**

   o When refinishing or repurposing furniture, use natural paints, finishes, and adhesives.

   o Consider making your own decor items using natural or recycled materials.

Choosing non-toxic furnishings and decorations is essential for creating a healthy, sustainable living environment. By selecting products made from natural materials, avoiding harmful chemicals, and prioritizing eco-friendly practices, you can significantly reduce exposure to toxins in your home. These choices not only benefit your health but also contribute to a more sustainable and environmentally friendly lifestyle.

Safe Pest Control Methods

Maintaining a pest-free home is essential for health and comfort, but conventional pest control methods often involve harmful chemicals that can pose risks to human health and the environment. Safe, non-toxic pest control methods can effectively manage pests without these risks. This section explores safe pest control strategies and techniques to help create a healthier home environment.

Integrated Pest Management (IPM)

Integrated Pest Management (IPM) is an effective and environmentally sensitive approach to pest control that combines multiple methods to manage pests economically and with minimal risk. The key principles of IPM include:

1. **Prevention:**

   o **Sanitation:** Keep your home clean to reduce food and water sources for pests. Regularly clean kitchen surfaces, store food in sealed containers, and promptly fix leaky pipes.

   o **Exclusion:** Seal cracks and gaps in walls, windows, doors, and foundations to prevent pests from entering your home. Use door sweeps, window screens, and caulk to close entry points.

2. **Monitoring:**

   o **Regular Inspections:** Conduct regular inspections of your home to identify signs of pest activity early. Look for droppings, nests, and damage to food or property.

   o **Pest Identification:** Accurately identify the pests to determine the most effective control methods.

3. **Control:**

   o **Cultural Controls:** Modify habits and environmental conditions to reduce pest populations. This can include crop rotation in gardens, proper waste management, and using pest-resistant plant varieties.

   o **Mechanical Controls:** Use physical methods to remove or exclude pests, such as traps, barriers, and hand-picking.

   o **Biological Controls:** Introduce natural predators or beneficial insects to control pest populations. For example, ladybugs can help control aphids in the garden.

Natural and Non-Toxic Pest Control Methods

1. **Natural Repellents:**

   o **Essential Oils:** Use essential oils such as peppermint, eucalyptus, tea tree, and lavender to repel pests like ants, mosquitoes, and spiders. Mix a few drops with water and spray around entry points and affected areas.

   o **Herbs and Spices:** Place dried herbs and spices like bay leaves, cloves, and cinnamon sticks in pantry shelves and cupboards to deter pests.

2. **Homemade Pest Control Sprays:**

   o **Vinegar and Water:** A solution of equal parts vinegar and water can repel ants and spiders. Spray around entry points and areas of pest activity.

   o **Soap and Water:** A mixture of dish soap and water can be sprayed directly on insects like aphids, mites, and whiteflies to kill them on contact.

3. **Physical Barriers and Traps:**

   o **Sticky Traps:** Use sticky traps to catch flying insects like fruit flies and gnats. Place them near windows, plants, and other areas of pest activity.

   o **Diatomaceous Earth:** Sprinkle food-grade diatomaceous earth around the perimeter of your home, in cracks and crevices, and other pest entry points. This natural powder is abrasive to insects and can help control ants, bed bugs, and other crawling pests.

   o **Copper Tape:** Use copper tape around garden beds, plant pots, and other areas to repel slugs and snails.

4. **Biological Controls:**

   o **Beneficial Insects:** Introduce beneficial insects like ladybugs, lacewings, and predatory mites to your garden to control pests naturally.

   o **Nematodes:** Use beneficial nematodes to control soil-dwelling pests like grubs, termites, and root-knot nematodes.

5. **Baits and Traps:**

   - **Boric Acid:** Use boric acid baits to control ants and cockroaches. Mix boric acid with sugar or peanut butter and place it in bait stations or small containers near pest activity.

   - **DIY Traps:** Create homemade traps for pests like fruit flies and gnats using apple cider vinegar and a few drops of dish soap in a small bowl. The vinegar attracts the pests, and the soap breaks the surface tension, causing them to drown.

Safe Use of Commercial Pest Control Products

1. **Eco-Friendly Products:**

   - **Natural Insecticides:** Choose insecticides made from natural ingredients like neem oil, pyrethrin, and insecticidal soap. These products are less harmful to humans and the environment.

   - **Rodent Control:** Use humane traps to catch and release rodents. Avoid rodenticides, which can be toxic to pets and wildlife.

2. **Read Labels Carefully:**

   - **Active Ingredients:** Check the labels for active ingredients and choose products with low toxicity to humans and pets.

   - **Application Instructions:** Follow the manufacturer's instructions for proper application and safety precautions.

Professional Pest Control Services

1. **Green Pest Control:**

   - **Eco-Friendly Companies:** Choose pest control companies that use eco-friendly and non-toxic methods. Ask about their IPM practices and the types of products they use.

   - **Integrated Approach:** Ensure the company uses an integrated approach that includes prevention, monitoring, and control.

2. **Regular Maintenance:**

   - **Ongoing Services:** Consider regular maintenance services from a professional pest control company to prevent infestations and address pest problems early.

Safe pest control methods are essential for maintaining a healthy home environment without exposing yourself, your family, and your pets to harmful chemicals. By adopting integrated pest management principles and using natural and non-toxic solutions, you can effectively manage pest problems while promoting a healthier, safer living space. These strategies not only protect your health but also support environmental sustainability.

Improving Indoor Air Quality

Maintaining high indoor air quality is essential for overall health and well-being, as poor air quality can lead to respiratory issues, allergies, and other health problems. Various factors, including dust, chemicals, mold, and outdoor pollutants, can compromise indoor air quality. This section explores practical strategies for improving indoor air quality and creating a healthier living environment.

Key Strategies for Improving Indoor Air Quality

1. **Ventilation:**

   o **Natural Ventilation:** Regularly open windows and doors to allow fresh air to circulate and reduce indoor pollutants.

   o **Mechanical Ventilation:** Use exhaust fans in kitchens and bathrooms to remove moisture, odors, and pollutants. Consider installing a whole-house ventilation system for consistent air exchange.

2. **Air Purification:**

   o **Air Purifiers:** Invest in high-quality air purifiers with HEPA (High-Efficiency Particulate Air) filters to capture dust, pollen, pet dander, and other airborne particles. Some models also include activated carbon filters to remove odors and volatile organic compounds (VOCs).

   o **HVAC Filters:** Use high-efficiency filters in your heating, ventilation, and air conditioning (HVAC) system and replace them regularly to ensure optimal performance.

3. **Reducing Indoor Pollutants:**

   o **No Smoking Indoors:** Prohibit smoking inside your home to prevent exposure to harmful tobacco smoke.

   o **Minimize VOCs:** Choose low-VOC or VOC-free paints, finishes, and cleaning products. Avoid synthetic fragrances and air fresheners that can release VOCs.

   o **Control Humidity:** Maintain indoor humidity levels between 30-50% to prevent mold growth and dust mite proliferation. Use dehumidifiers in damp areas and ensure proper ventilation in bathrooms and kitchens.

4. **Houseplants:**

   o **Natural Air Purifiers:** Certain houseplants can help improve indoor air quality by absorbing pollutants and releasing oxygen. Effective options include spider plants, snake plants, peace lilies, and Boston ferns.

5. **Regular Cleaning:**

   o **Dust and Vacuum:** Regularly dust surfaces and vacuum floors using a vacuum cleaner with a HEPA filter to reduce dust, pet dander, and other allergens.

- **Mop Floors:** Use a damp mop or microfiber cloth to clean hard floors and remove fine particles that vacuuming may miss.
- **Wash Bedding:** Wash bedding, curtains, and soft furnishings regularly to remove dust mites and allergens.

6. **Avoiding Toxic Materials:**

- **Furniture and Furnishings:** Choose furniture and decor made from natural materials and free from harmful chemicals. Look for certifications such as GREENGUARD or OEKO-TEX.
- **Building Materials:** Select low-VOC or VOC-free building materials and finishes when renovating or building your home.

7. **Controlling Allergens:**

- **Pet Care:** Bathe and groom pets regularly to reduce dander. Keep pets out of bedrooms and off furniture to minimize allergens.
- **Pest Control:** Use non-toxic pest control methods to prevent infestations and reduce exposure to pesticides.

8. **Reducing Combustion Pollutants:**

- **Proper Ventilation:** Ensure proper ventilation when using gas stoves, fireplaces, and other combustion appliances. Install exhaust fans and regularly check for leaks.
- **Alternative Heating:** Consider using electric or radiant heaters instead of wood-burning stoves or fireplaces, which can produce indoor air pollutants.

Monitoring Indoor Air Quality

1. **Air Quality Monitors:**

- Use indoor air quality monitors to track levels of pollutants such as VOCs, particulate matter, carbon dioxide (CO_2), and humidity. These devices can help you identify problem areas and take corrective action.

2. **Radon Testing:**

- Test your home for radon, a naturally occurring radioactive gas that can accumulate indoors and pose serious health risks. Radon test kits are available for home use, or you can hire a professional for testing.

3. **Carbon Monoxide Detectors:**

- Install carbon monoxide (CO) detectors near sleeping areas and fuel-burning appliances to detect dangerous levels of this colorless, odorless gas.

Practical Tips for Maintaining Air Quality

1. **Seasonal Maintenance:**

   o Perform seasonal maintenance on your HVAC system, including cleaning ducts and vents to prevent the buildup of dust and allergens.

   o Inspect and clean gutters, downspouts, and roof areas to prevent water damage and mold growth.

2. **Mindful Cooking:**

   o Use range hoods or exhaust fans while cooking to remove smoke, grease, and cooking odors from the kitchen.

3. **Eco-Friendly Cleaning Products:**

   o Use natural and eco-friendly cleaning products that do not release harmful chemicals into the air. Look for products with third-party certifications for safety and environmental impact.

4. **Shoes Off Policy:**

   o Implement a "shoes off" policy in your home to prevent bringing in dirt, pollen, and other outdoor pollutants.

5. **Reduce Indoor Clutter:**

   o Minimize clutter to reduce dust accumulation and make cleaning easier. Regularly declutter and organize your living spaces.

Improving indoor air quality is essential for maintaining a healthy home environment. By implementing these strategies, you can significantly reduce exposure to indoor pollutants and allergens, creating a safer and more comfortable living space. Regular monitoring, proper ventilation, and the use of natural and non-toxic products are key to ensuring high indoor air quality and overall well-being.

Sustainable and Non-Toxic Gardening Practices

Creating a sustainable and non-toxic garden not only enhances the beauty and productivity of your outdoor space but also contributes to environmental health and personal well-being. By adopting eco-friendly practices and avoiding harmful chemicals, you can cultivate a thriving garden that supports biodiversity and reduces your ecological footprint. This section explores sustainable and non-toxic gardening methods, including soil health, pest management, water conservation, and plant selection.

Key Principles of Sustainable and Non-Toxic Gardening

1. **Soil Health:**

   o **Composting:** Create a compost pile to recycle kitchen scraps and garden waste into nutrient-rich compost. This improves soil structure, fertility, and microbial activity.

- **Organic Mulching:** Use organic mulch, such as straw, leaves, or wood chips, to conserve moisture, suppress weeds, and enhance soil health as it decomposes.
- **Cover Crops:** Plant cover crops like clover, rye, or legumes to prevent soil erosion, improve soil fertility, and increase organic matter.

2. **Pest and Disease Management:**

- **Integrated Pest Management (IPM):** Implement IPM practices, including cultural, mechanical, biological, and chemical controls, to manage pests with minimal environmental impact.
- **Natural Predators:** Encourage beneficial insects like ladybugs, lacewings, and predatory beetles that prey on garden pests.
- **Companion Planting:** Use companion planting techniques to naturally repel pests and promote plant health. For example, plant marigolds to deter nematodes or basil to repel aphids and mosquitoes.
- **Non-Toxic Sprays:** Use homemade or commercially available non-toxic sprays, such as neem oil, insecticidal soap, or garlic spray, to manage pests and diseases.

3. **Water Conservation:**

- **Drip Irrigation:** Install drip irrigation systems to deliver water directly to plant roots, reducing water waste and promoting efficient usage.
- **Rainwater Harvesting:** Collect and store rainwater in barrels to use for garden irrigation, reducing reliance on municipal water supplies.
- **Mulching:** Apply mulch around plants to retain soil moisture and reduce the need for frequent watering.

4. **Plant Selection:**

- **Native Plants:** Choose native plants that are adapted to your local climate and soil conditions. They typically require less water, fertilizer, and pest control.
- **Drought-Tolerant Plants:** Incorporate drought-tolerant plants into your garden to reduce water consumption and maintain a vibrant landscape during dry periods.
- **Diverse Planting:** Cultivate a diverse range of plants to support biodiversity, attract pollinators, and create a resilient garden ecosystem.

5. **Organic Fertilizers:**

- **Compost and Manure:** Use compost and well-rotted manure to provide essential nutrients to your plants naturally.
- **Natural Fertilizers:** Apply natural fertilizers like fish emulsion, seaweed extract, and bone meal to enhance soil fertility without synthetic chemicals.

Practical Tips for Sustainable and Non-Toxic Gardening

1. **Start with Healthy Soil:**
   - Conduct a soil test to determine nutrient levels and pH. Amend the soil with organic matter and natural fertilizers based on test results to create a healthy growing environment.

2. **Practice Crop Rotation:**
   - Rotate crops annually to prevent soil depletion, reduce pest and disease buildup, and maintain soil health.

3. **Use Non-Toxic Materials:**
   - Avoid using treated wood, synthetic fertilizers, and chemical pesticides in your garden. Opt for non-toxic, biodegradable materials whenever possible.

4. **Create Wildlife Habitats:**
   - Provide habitats for birds, beneficial insects, and other wildlife by planting native shrubs, wildflowers, and creating water sources like birdbaths or small ponds.

5. **Manual Weed Control:**
   - Use hand weeding, hoeing, and mulching to control weeds naturally. Avoid herbicides that can harm beneficial plants and soil organisms.

6. **Seasonal Planting:**
   - Plant seasonally appropriate crops to reduce the need for excessive watering and pest control. Use a planting calendar to time your garden activities effectively.

7. **Reduce Plastic Use:**
   - Minimize the use of plastic pots, trays, and garden tools. Opt for biodegradable pots, recycled materials, and durable tools that have a longer lifespan.

DIY Non-Toxic Pest Control Recipes

1. **Neem Oil Spray:**
   - **Ingredients:** 2 teaspoons neem oil, 1 teaspoon mild liquid soap, 1 quart water.
   - **Instructions:** Mix all ingredients in a spray bottle and apply to plants to control aphids, mites, and other pests.

2. **Garlic Spray:**
   - **Ingredients:** 1 bulb of garlic, 1 quart water.
   - **Instructions:** Blend garlic with water, strain, and spray on plants to repel insects like aphids and caterpillars.

3. **Insecticidal Soap:**

   - **Ingredients:** 1 tablespoon mild liquid soap, 1 quart water.

   - **Instructions:** Mix soap and water in a spray bottle and apply directly to insects on plants.

4. **Baking Soda Fungicide:**

   - **Ingredients:** 1 tablespoon baking soda, 1 teaspoon mild liquid soap, 1 gallon water.

   - **Instructions:** Mix all ingredients and spray on plants to control fungal diseases like powdery mildew.

Adopting sustainable and non-toxic gardening practices is essential for creating a healthy, vibrant garden that benefits both you and the environment. By focusing on soil health, natural pest control, water conservation, and plant selection, you can cultivate a garden that thrives without the use of harmful chemicals. These practices not only enhance the beauty and productivity of your garden but also support biodiversity and promote a sustainable lifestyle.

BOOK 5:

Herbs for the Immune System: Naturally Boosting the Body's Defenses

Echinacea: The Immunity Ally

Echinacea, a revered herb in traditional and modern herbal medicine, has long been celebrated for its powerful immune-boosting properties. Native to North America, Echinacea has been used for centuries by indigenous peoples and later adopted by European settlers for its medicinal benefits. Known for its vibrant purple flowers and cone-shaped seed heads, Echinacea is not only a beautiful addition to gardens but also a potent ally in supporting the body's natural defenses.

The herb's reputation as an "immunity ally" is well-deserved, thanks to its ability to enhance the body's immune response, combat infections, and reduce the severity and duration of illnesses such as the common cold and flu. In this chapter, we will explore the history and traditional uses of Echinacea, the scientific basis for its immune-enhancing effects, and practical ways to incorporate this powerful herb into your daily routine to maintain optimal health. Whether you are new to herbal remedies or a seasoned practitioner, Echinacea offers valuable benefits that can help you stay healthy and resilient year-round.

History and Traditional Uses of Echinacea

Echinacea, also known as the purple coneflower, has a rich history deeply rooted in the medicinal practices of Native American tribes. For centuries, these indigenous peoples recognized and utilized the healing properties of Echinacea, making it a cornerstone of their traditional medicine.

Native American Use

The earliest recorded use of Echinacea dates back to the Great Plains tribes, such as the Cheyenne, Sioux, and Pawnee. These tribes employed Echinacea for a variety of ailments, thanks to its purported ability to boost immunity and treat infections. They used different parts of the plant, including the roots, flowers, and leaves, in various preparations:

- **Wound Healing:** The Cheyenne and other tribes applied Echinacea root poultices to wounds, burns, and insect bites to reduce inflammation and promote healing.

- **Respiratory Infections:** Echinacea was used to treat colds, coughs, sore throats, and other respiratory conditions. It was often chewed raw or brewed into teas.

- **Snake Bites and Venomous Stings:** The Plains tribes used Echinacea to counteract the effects of snake bites and stings from venomous insects, relying on its believed detoxifying properties.

- **Pain Relief:** Echinacea was also employed as an analgesic to alleviate pain from toothaches, sore throats, and other common ailments.

Introduction to European Settlers

When European settlers arrived in North America, they quickly adopted Echinacea into their own medicinal practices, learning from Native American traditions. By the 19th century,

Echinacea had become a popular remedy among settlers and was widely used in the eclectic medicine movement, which emphasized botanical treatments.

- **Eclectic Medicine:** Eclectic physicians in the United States promoted the use of Echinacea for various conditions, including infections, inflammation, and as a general immune booster. It was particularly valued for its ability to treat ailments that were difficult to manage with the limited pharmaceutical options available at the time.

Modern Use and Scientific Validation

In the early 20th century, Echinacea's popularity waned in the United States due to the rise of synthetic pharmaceuticals. However, it gained traction in Europe, particularly in Germany, where it became a staple in herbal medicine.

- **Renewed Interest:** In recent decades, there has been a resurgence of interest in Echinacea, driven by a growing preference for natural and holistic health solutions. Modern scientific research has begun to validate many of the traditional uses of Echinacea, highlighting its immune-boosting and anti-inflammatory properties.

- **Scientific Studies:** Numerous studies have shown that Echinacea can stimulate the immune system by increasing the activity of white blood cells, enhancing the body's ability to fight off infections. It has been found to reduce the duration and severity of colds and flu when taken at the onset of symptoms.

Practical Applications Today

Today, Echinacea is widely available in various forms, including teas, tinctures, capsules, and extracts. It is commonly used to:

- **Support Immune Function:** Regular use of Echinacea can help strengthen the immune system, making it less susceptible to infections.

- **Treat Acute Illnesses:** Echinacea is often taken at the first sign of a cold or flu to reduce symptoms and shorten the duration of the illness.

- **General Wellness:** Many people incorporate Echinacea into their wellness routines to maintain overall health and resilience against common ailments.

The history and traditional uses of Echinacea demonstrate its long-standing reputation as a powerful medicinal herb. From its origins with Native American tribes to its modern applications, Echinacea has proven to be a valuable ally in promoting health and wellness. As we continue to explore and understand its benefits, Echinacea remains a cornerstone of natural herbal remedies, offering a safe and effective way to support the body's defenses.

Active Compounds and Mechanisms of Action

Echinacea's reputation as a powerful immune-boosting herb is supported by its rich array of active compounds, each contributing to its medicinal properties. Understanding these compounds and their mechanisms of action can provide insight into how Echinacea enhances the immune system and helps the body combat infections.

Active Compounds in Echinacea

1. **Alkylamides:**

   - **Description:** Alkylamides are fatty acid-derived compounds that are considered the primary active constituents in Echinacea. They are responsible for the characteristic tingling sensation on the tongue when consuming Echinacea extracts.

   - **Functions:** Alkylamides have immunomodulatory effects, helping to modulate the immune response by interacting with cannabinoid receptors (CB2) on immune cells. This interaction can enhance the activity of macrophages and other white blood cells, improving the body's ability to detect and respond to pathogens.

2. **Polysaccharides:**

   - **Description:** Polysaccharides are complex carbohydrates found in the cell walls of plants. In Echinacea, these include arabinogalactan and inulin.

   - **Functions:** Polysaccharides stimulate the immune system by activating macrophages, natural killer cells, and other components of the innate immune system. They also promote the production of cytokines, signaling molecules that regulate the immune response.

3. **Caffeic Acid Derivatives:**

   - **Description:** This group includes compounds such as echinacoside, cichoric acid, and chlorogenic acid.

   - **Functions:** Caffeic acid derivatives have antioxidant, anti-inflammatory, and antimicrobial properties. They help protect cells from oxidative stress and enhance the body's ability to fight infections by inhibiting the growth of bacteria and viruses.

4. **Glycoproteins:**

   - **Description:** Glycoproteins are proteins with carbohydrate groups attached to them, which play a role in cell signaling and immune response.

   - **Functions:** Glycoproteins in Echinacea enhance immune function by stimulating the activity of immune cells, promoting the production of cytokines, and supporting the overall immune response.

5. **Flavonoids:**

   - **Description:** Flavonoids are a group of plant metabolites that provide antioxidant benefits.

   - **Functions:** In Echinacea, flavonoids contribute to reducing inflammation and protecting cells from oxidative damage. They also support the immune system by modulating the activity of various immune cells.

Mechanisms of Action

1. **Immune System Modulation:**

   - Echinacea's active compounds interact with the immune system in several ways to enhance its function. Alkylamides, for example, modulate the immune response by binding to CB2 receptors on immune cells, which can enhance the activity and effectiveness of macrophages, natural killer cells, and other white blood cells. This modulation helps the body to recognize and respond more effectively to pathogens.

2. **Stimulation of Cytokine Production:**

   - Polysaccharides and glycoproteins in Echinacea stimulate the production of cytokines such as interleukins and tumor necrosis factor-alpha (TNF-α). Cytokines are crucial for immune signaling, coordinating the response of various immune cells to infection and inflammation. By increasing cytokine production, Echinacea helps to amplify the immune response, enabling the body to combat infections more effectively.

3. **Antimicrobial Properties:**

   - Caffeic acid derivatives and other compounds in Echinacea exhibit antimicrobial properties, inhibiting the growth of bacteria, viruses, and fungi. This direct antimicrobial action helps to prevent and manage infections by reducing the load of pathogenic organisms in the body.

4. **Antioxidant and Anti-Inflammatory Effects:**

   - The flavonoids and caffeic acid derivatives in Echinacea provide significant antioxidant and anti-inflammatory benefits. By neutralizing free radicals and reducing oxidative stress, these compounds help protect immune cells from damage. Additionally, their anti-inflammatory effects can mitigate excessive immune responses, preventing chronic inflammation and associated health issues.

5. **Activation of Innate Immune Cells:**

   - Polysaccharides in Echinacea activate innate immune cells, including macrophages and natural killer cells. These cells are essential for the body's first line of defense against infections, as they can rapidly respond to and eliminate pathogens. By boosting the activity of these cells, Echinacea enhances the body's ability to fend off infections at an early stage.

The active compounds in Echinacea work synergistically to enhance immune function through various mechanisms. Alkylamides, polysaccharides, caffeic acid derivatives, glycoproteins, and flavonoids each contribute to modulating the immune response, stimulating cytokine production, providing antimicrobial effects, and offering antioxidant and anti-inflammatory benefits. These combined actions make Echinacea a potent ally in supporting the body's natural defenses and maintaining overall health. Understanding these mechanisms helps to appreciate the profound impact Echinacea can have on the immune system and underscores its value as a natural remedy for boosting immunity.

Benefits of Echinacea for Immune Health

Echinacea is widely recognized for its ability to enhance immune health and support the body in fighting off infections. This powerful herb offers several key benefits that make it a valuable addition to any natural health regimen. Here, we delve into the primary benefits of Echinacea for immune health and how it can help you maintain overall well-being.

1. Boosts Immune Function

Enhanced White Blood Cell Activity:

- Echinacea stimulates the activity of white blood cells, particularly macrophages, natural killer cells, and T-cells. These cells play crucial roles in identifying, attacking, and eliminating pathogens like bacteria, viruses, and fungi.

Increased Production of Cytokines:

- The herb promotes the production of cytokines, which are signaling molecules that regulate the immune response. By enhancing cytokine production, Echinacea helps coordinate a more efficient and effective immune response.

Activation of Innate and Adaptive Immunity:

- Echinacea supports both innate and adaptive immune responses. Innate immunity provides the first line of defense against infections, while adaptive immunity develops a targeted response to specific pathogens. Echinacea helps optimize the function of both systems, providing comprehensive immune support.

2. Reduces the Severity and Duration of Colds and Flu

Early Intervention:

- When taken at the first sign of illness, Echinacea can reduce the severity and duration of colds and flu. Studies have shown that individuals who use Echinacea at the onset of symptoms experience milder symptoms and recover more quickly compared to those who do not use the herb.

Symptom Relief:

- Echinacea helps alleviate common cold and flu symptoms such as sore throat, cough, congestion, and fatigue. Its anti-inflammatory and immune-modulating properties contribute to this symptom relief, making the illness more manageable and less disruptive.

3. Antimicrobial and Antiviral Properties

Fights Bacterial Infections:

- Echinacea has demonstrated antibacterial activity against a range of pathogenic bacteria, including Streptococcus pyogenes and Staphylococcus aureus. This antimicrobial action helps prevent and manage bacterial infections that can complicate respiratory illnesses.

Inhibits Viral Replication:

- Research indicates that Echinacea can inhibit the replication of certain viruses, including influenza and herpes viruses. By interfering with viral replication, Echinacea helps reduce the viral load and supports the body's efforts to eliminate the infection.

4. Anti-Inflammatory Effects

Reduces Inflammation:

- Chronic inflammation can weaken the immune system and contribute to various health issues. Echinacea's anti-inflammatory properties help mitigate excessive inflammation, promoting a balanced immune response and reducing the risk of chronic inflammatory conditions.

Supports Respiratory Health:

- Echinacea's ability to reduce inflammation is particularly beneficial for respiratory health. It can help alleviate inflammation in the respiratory tract, making it easier to breathe and reducing the discomfort associated with respiratory infections.

5. Antioxidant Protection

Neutralizes Free Radicals:

- Echinacea contains powerful antioxidants, including flavonoids and caffeic acid derivatives, that neutralize free radicals. By reducing oxidative stress, these antioxidants protect immune cells from damage, ensuring they function optimally.

Supports Cellular Health:

- The antioxidant activity of Echinacea helps protect cells throughout the body, not just immune cells. This broad-spectrum protection supports overall health and well-being, making the body more resilient to infections and diseases.

6. Adaptogenic Benefits

Stress Reduction:

- Chronic stress can suppress the immune system and make the body more susceptible to infections. Echinacea exhibits adaptogenic properties, helping the body manage stress more effectively and supporting a balanced immune response.

Enhanced Resilience:

- As an adaptogen, Echinacea helps enhance the body's overall resilience to physical, emotional, and environmental stressors. This increased resilience supports immune health and overall vitality.

Echinacea offers a range of benefits for immune health, making it a valuable tool for preventing and managing infections. Its ability to boost immune function, reduce the severity and duration of colds and flu, provide antimicrobial and antiviral effects, reduce inflammation, offer antioxidant protection, and act as an adaptogen makes it a comprehensive and effective herbal remedy. By incorporating Echinacea into your wellness routine, you can support your immune system and maintain better overall health.

Echinacea Varieties: Purpurea, Angustifolia, and Pallida

Echinacea, commonly known as coneflower, comprises several species, each with unique properties and benefits. The most commonly used varieties in herbal medicine are Echinacea purpurea, Echinacea angustifolia, and Echinacea pallida. Understanding the differences between these varieties can help you select the most appropriate one for your needs.

Echinacea Purpurea

Description:

- **Appearance:** Echinacea purpurea is known for its vibrant purple petals and large, cone-shaped seed head. It is the most widely cultivated and recognized species.

- **Habitat:** Native to the central and southeastern United States, E. purpurea thrives in prairies and open woodlands. It is commonly grown in gardens and used ornamentally.

Active Compounds:

- **Polysaccharides:** High in polysaccharides, which are known for their immune-stimulating properties.

- **Caffeic Acid Derivatives:** Contains significant amounts of cichoric acid and other caffeic acid derivatives, contributing to its antioxidant and antimicrobial effects.

- **Alkylamides:** Present in moderate concentrations, contributing to its overall immunomodulatory effects.

Uses and Benefits:

- **Immune Support:** E. purpurea is widely used to boost the immune system, particularly during cold and flu season. It helps reduce the severity and duration of colds and other respiratory infections.

- **Topical Applications:** The plant's juice or extracts are used in topical preparations to promote wound healing and reduce inflammation.

- **Overall Health:** Regular use of E. purpurea can enhance general wellness and support the body's natural defenses against infections.

Preparations:

- **Teas and Tinctures:** Commonly prepared as teas or tinctures for internal use.
- **Capsules and Tablets:** Available in standardized extracts for convenient dosing.
- **Topical Formulations:** Used in creams, ointments, and salves for skin conditions.

Echinacea Angustifolia

Description:

- **Appearance:** Echinacea angustifolia has narrower, more elongated leaves and pale pink to purple petals. It is often distinguished by its thinner roots.
- **Habitat:** Native to the central United States, particularly in dry, open areas such as prairies and grasslands.

Active Compounds:

- **Alkylamides:** Contains high concentrations of alkylamides, which are responsible for its strong immunomodulatory and anti-inflammatory effects.
- **Caffeic Acid Derivatives:** Includes compounds such as echinacoside, known for their antimicrobial and antioxidant properties.
- **Polysaccharides:** Present but in lower concentrations compared to E. purpurea.

Uses and Benefits:

- **Immune Modulation:** Highly effective in modulating the immune system, making it beneficial for both acute and chronic immune support.
- **Anti-Inflammatory:** Provides significant anti-inflammatory effects, useful for reducing inflammation and pain.
- **Antimicrobial Activity:** Effective against a range of bacterial and viral infections.

Preparations:

- **Tinctures and Extracts:** Often used in tincture form due to the concentration of active compounds in the roots.
- **Capsules and Tablets:** Available as supplements for immune support.
- **Topical Use:** Occasionally used in topical applications for its anti-inflammatory properties.

Echinacea Pallida

Description:

- **Appearance:** Echinacea pallida features pale pink to nearly white petals that droop downwards and a narrow, elongated cone. It is less commonly cultivated compared to the other two species.
- **Habitat:** Native to the central and eastern United States, often found in prairies and open woodland areas.

Active Compounds:

- **Polysaccharides and Glycoproteins:** Contains a balanced mixture of polysaccharides and glycoproteins that support immune function.
- **Caffeic Acid Derivatives:** Includes compounds such as cichoric acid, contributing to its antioxidant and antimicrobial effects.
- **Alkylamides:** Present in moderate amounts, offering immunomodulatory benefits.

Uses and Benefits:

- **Immune System Support:** Effective in enhancing immune response and supporting the body's defenses against infections.
- **Respiratory Health:** Traditionally used for respiratory conditions, helping to alleviate symptoms and promote recovery.
- **Overall Wellness:** Supports general health and resilience, making it useful for maintaining wellness during times of stress or increased exposure to pathogens.

Preparations:

- **Tinctures and Teas:** Often prepared as tinctures or teas for internal use.
- **Capsules and Tablets:** Available in standardized extracts for consistent dosing.
- **Topical Use:** Less commonly used topically compared to E. purpurea and E. angustifolia.

Each variety of Echinacea—Purpurea, Angustifolia, and Pallida—offers unique benefits and is suited to different therapeutic applications. E. purpurea is widely used for general immune support and is commonly found in commercial preparations. E. angustifolia is particularly valued for its potent immune-modulating and anti-inflammatory effects. E. pallida, though less commonly used, also provides significant immune support and respiratory benefits. Understanding these differences can help you choose the most appropriate Echinacea variety to meet your health needs and achieve optimal results.

Preparation Methods: Teas, Tinctures, and Capsules

Echinacea can be prepared and consumed in various forms, each offering distinct advantages depending on your needs and preferences. The most common preparation methods are teas, tinctures, and capsules. Understanding how to prepare and use Echinacea in these forms can help you maximize its benefits for immune support and overall health.

Teas

Description:

- Echinacea tea is a simple and effective way to consume the herb, allowing you to extract its active compounds through hot water infusion.

Preparation:

1. **Ingredients:**
   - 1-2 teaspoons of dried Echinacea (roots, leaves, or flowers)
   - 1 cup of boiling water

2. **Steps:**
   - Place the dried Echinacea in a teapot or mug.
   - Pour boiling water over the herbs.
   - Cover and let steep for 10-15 minutes.
   - Strain the tea to remove the plant material.
   - Sweeten with honey or lemon if desired.

Benefits:

- Easy to prepare and consume.
- Warm, soothing drink, especially beneficial during cold and flu season.
- Can be combined with other immune-boosting herbs like ginger, lemon balm, or elderberry for enhanced effects.

Usage:

- Drink 1-3 cups daily at the onset of symptoms or as a preventative measure during peak cold and flu seasons.

Tinctures

Description:

- Echinacea tinctures are concentrated liquid extracts made by soaking the herb in alcohol or glycerin. Tinctures are potent, convenient, and have a long shelf life.

Preparation:

1. **Ingredients:**
   - 1 part dried Echinacea (roots, leaves, or flowers)
   - 2-3 parts alcohol (vodka or brandy) or glycerin

- Glass jar with a tight-fitting lid

2. **Steps:**

   - Fill the glass jar with the dried Echinacea.

   - Pour the alcohol or glycerin over the herbs, ensuring they are completely covered.

   - Seal the jar tightly and store it in a cool, dark place.

   - Shake the jar daily for 4-6 weeks.

   - After 4-6 weeks, strain the mixture through a cheesecloth or fine mesh strainer into a clean glass jar or bottle.

Benefits:

- Highly concentrated, so only small doses are needed.

- Long shelf life, typically 2-3 years when stored properly.

- Convenient to use, especially for those who need quick and effective immune support.

Usage:

- Take 1-2 dropperfuls (approximately 30-60 drops) 2-3 times daily at the first sign of illness or as directed by a healthcare provider.

Capsules

Description:

- Echinacea capsules are made from powdered Echinacea and offer a convenient, pre-measured way to consume the herb. They are ideal for those who prefer not to taste the herb or need a portable option.

Preparation:

1. **Ingredients:**

   - Echinacea powder (available commercially or made by grinding dried Echinacea in a coffee grinder)

   - Empty gelatin or vegetarian capsules

   - Capsule-filling machine (optional for large batches)

2. **Steps:**

   - Fill the empty capsules with Echinacea powder using a capsule-filling machine or by hand.

   - Seal the capsules tightly to prevent spillage.

Benefits:

- Convenient and easy to use, especially for travel or on-the-go.

- Provides a consistent dose of Echinacea.

- Avoids the taste of the herb, which some may find unpleasant.

Usage:

- Follow the dosage instructions on the product label or as advised by a healthcare provider. Typically, 1-2 capsules taken 2-3 times daily.

Teas, tinctures, and capsules are three effective ways to prepare and consume Echinacea, each with its own set of advantages. Teas are soothing and easy to prepare, tinctures are potent and have a long shelf life, and capsules offer convenience and consistent dosing. By choosing the preparation method that best suits your lifestyle and needs, you can effectively incorporate Echinacea into your health regimen and enjoy its immune-boosting benefits.

Dosage Recommendations and Safety Precautions

Using Echinacea effectively involves understanding the appropriate dosages and observing necessary safety precautions. This ensures you receive the maximum benefits while minimizing potential risks. Below are detailed dosage recommendations and safety precautions for Echinacea use.

Dosage Recommendations

1. Echinacea Tea:

- **General Immune Support:**

  o **Dosage:** 1-3 cups daily.

  o **Preparation:** Use 1-2 teaspoons of dried Echinacea per cup of boiling water. Steep for 10-15 minutes.

- **During Illness:**

  o **Dosage:** 3-5 cups daily at the onset of symptoms.

  o **Preparation:** Same as above, can be combined with other herbs for enhanced effects.

2. Echinacea Tincture:

- **General Immune Support:**

  o **Dosage:** 1-2 dropperfuls (approximately 30-60 drops) 2-3 times daily.

  o **Preparation:** Use a tincture made by soaking dried Echinacea in alcohol or glycerin for 4-6 weeks.

- **During Illness:**

- Dosage: 2-3 dropperfuls (approximately 60-90 drops) 3-4 times daily at the first sign of illness.

3. Echinacea Capsules:

- **General Immune Support:**

  - **Dosage:** 1-2 capsules (usually 400-500 mg each) taken 2-3 times daily.

  - **Preparation:** Follow the dosage instructions on the product label or as advised by a healthcare provider.

- **During Illness:**

  - **Dosage:** 2 capsules taken 3-4 times daily at the onset of symptoms.

Safety Precautions

1. Allergic Reactions:

- **Description:** Some individuals may experience allergic reactions to Echinacea, particularly those allergic to plants in the Asteraceae family (e.g., ragweed, chrysanthemums, marigolds, and daisies).

- **Precautions:** If you have known allergies to these plants, consult a healthcare provider before using Echinacea. Discontinue use if you experience symptoms such as rash, itching, swelling, or difficulty breathing.

2. Autoimmune Conditions:

- **Description:** Echinacea stimulates the immune system, which may be problematic for individuals with autoimmune disorders such as lupus, rheumatoid arthritis, or multiple sclerosis.

- **Precautions:** People with autoimmune conditions should use Echinacea with caution and under the guidance of a healthcare provider.

3. Pregnancy and Breastfeeding:

- **Description:** Limited research is available on the safety of Echinacea during pregnancy and breastfeeding.

- **Precautions:** Pregnant and breastfeeding women should consult their healthcare provider before using Echinacea to ensure it is safe for their specific situation.

4. Drug Interactions:

- **Description:** Echinacea may interact with certain medications, including immunosuppressants and drugs metabolized by the liver.

- **Precautions:** If you are taking prescription medications, especially immunosuppressants, or have liver conditions, consult a healthcare provider before using Echinacea.

5. Duration of Use:

- **Description:** Prolonged use of Echinacea may lead to reduced effectiveness and potential liver strain.

- **Precautions:** It is generally recommended to use Echinacea for short periods (up to 8 weeks) with breaks in between. For long-term use, consult a healthcare provider for appropriate guidance.

6. Quality and Source:

- **Description:** The effectiveness and safety of Echinacea can be influenced by the quality of the product.

- **Precautions:** Choose high-quality, reputable brands that provide standardized extracts and have undergone third-party testing for purity and potency. Avoid products with unnecessary additives or fillers.

7. Dosage for Children:

- **Description:** Children may be more sensitive to the effects of Echinacea.

- **Precautions:** Adjust the dosage appropriately based on the child's age and weight. Consult a pediatrician before administering Echinacea to children, especially those under 12 years old.

Proper dosage and safety precautions are essential for the effective and safe use of Echinacea. By following recommended dosages and being mindful of potential risks, you can harness the immune-boosting benefits of this powerful herb while minimizing adverse effects. Always consult with a healthcare provider if you have underlying health conditions, are taking medications, or are pregnant or breastfeeding to ensure Echinacea is appropriate for your situation.

Astragalus: Protection and Vitality

Astragalus, a staple of traditional Chinese medicine, has been celebrated for centuries for its remarkable ability to enhance vitality and provide robust protection against various ailments. Known scientifically as Astragalus membranaceus, this powerful herb is renowned for its immune-boosting properties, adaptogenic benefits, and overall support for health and longevity. Often referred to as "Huang Qi" in Chinese medicine, Astragalus is prized for its ability to fortify the body's defenses, increase energy levels, and promote resilience against physical and emotional stressors. In this chapter, we will explore the rich history of Astragalus, its key active compounds, and the myriad ways it can be incorporated into your daily wellness routine to enhance protection and vitality. Whether you are looking to boost your immune system, combat fatigue, or improve overall health, Astragalus offers a natural and effective solution to help you achieve your wellness goals.

Traditional Use of Astragalus in Chinese Medicine

Astragalus membranaceus, known as "Huang Qi," in traditional Chinese medicine (TCM), has a long history of use dating back over 2,000 years. It is one of the fundamental herbs in TCM, revered for its ability to tonify the body's qi, or vital energy, and to enhance overall health and longevity. The traditional applications of Astragalus are deeply rooted in its perceived ability to balance the body's internal systems, strengthen the immune response, and protect against illness and disease.

Key Traditional Uses of Astragalus in TCM

1. **Qi Tonic:**

   o **Description:** Astragalus is primarily known as a potent qi tonic in TCM. Qi is considered the essential life force that flows through the body, and maintaining a balanced and strong qi is crucial for overall health and vitality.

   o **Benefits:** By strengthening qi, Astragalus is believed to enhance energy levels, reduce fatigue, and improve overall stamina and endurance. It is particularly beneficial for those experiencing chronic tiredness or weakness.

2. **Immune Support:**

   o **Description:** Astragalus is traditionally used to bolster the immune system, making the body more resilient to infections and diseases.

   o **Benefits:** It is often prescribed to prevent colds and flu, support recovery from illness, and enhance the body's natural defenses against pathogens. Astragalus is also used to speed up recovery and prevent relapse after an illness.

3. **Spleen and Lung Tonification:**

   o **Description:** In TCM, the spleen and lungs play vital roles in overall health, particularly in the production and distribution of qi.

   o **Benefits:** Astragalus is commonly used to tonify the spleen, improving digestion and nutrient absorption, and to strengthen the lungs, enhancing respiratory function and preventing respiratory infections.

4. **Blood Sugar Regulation:**

   o **Description:** Astragalus is used in TCM to help regulate blood sugar levels and improve insulin sensitivity.

   o **Benefits:** It is often recommended for individuals with diabetes or metabolic syndrome to help manage blood sugar levels and improve overall metabolic health.

5. **Diuretic and Detoxifying Effects:**

   o **Description:** Astragalus has mild diuretic properties, which help promote urination and the elimination of toxins from the body.

- o **Benefits:** This detoxifying effect supports kidney function and overall detoxification processes, helping to maintain a clean and balanced internal environment.

6. **Wound Healing and Tissue Repair:**

   - o **Description:** Traditionally, Astragalus is applied to promote wound healing and tissue repair.

   - o **Benefits:** It is believed to enhance the body's natural healing processes, reduce inflammation, and promote the regeneration of healthy tissue.

Methods of Preparation and Use in TCM

1. **Decoctions:**

   - o **Preparation:** Astragalus roots are often simmered with other herbs to create a potent decoction. This traditional method is used to extract the beneficial compounds from the roots.

   - o **Usage:** Decoctions are consumed as a warm tea, often in combination with other qi tonics or immune-supporting herbs.

2. **Powders and Granules:**

   - o **Preparation:** The dried roots are ground into a fine powder or processed into granules.

   - o **Usage:** These can be mixed with water, tea, or food for easy consumption. They are convenient for daily use and maintaining consistent intake.

3. **Pills and Tablets:**

   - o **Preparation:** Astragalus extracts are formulated into pills or tablets for standardized dosing.

   - o **Usage:** This form is especially useful for those who prefer a more convenient and controlled way to consume the herb.

4. **Topical Applications:**

   - o **Preparation:** Astragalus can be made into a paste or used in herbal plasters.

   - o **Usage:** Applied directly to the skin to promote wound healing and reduce inflammation in localized areas.

Astragalus has been a cornerstone of traditional Chinese medicine for its extensive health benefits and ability to enhance the body's resilience. As a powerful qi tonic, immune booster, and overall health promoter, it continues to be a vital herb in both traditional and modern herbal practices. Understanding its traditional uses provides valuable insights into its therapeutic potential and ways to incorporate it into a comprehensive approach to health and wellness.

Key Constituents and Health Benefits

Astragalus membranaceus, commonly known as Astragalus, contains a rich array of bioactive compounds that contribute to its numerous health benefits. These key constituents include polysaccharides, saponins, flavonoids, and amino acids, each playing a crucial role in the herb's therapeutic properties. Below, we explore the main constituents of Astragalus and their associated health benefits.

Key Constituents of Astragalus

1. **Polysaccharides:**

   o **Description:** Polysaccharides are complex carbohydrates found in many medicinal plants, known for their immune-enhancing properties.

   o **Function:** In Astragalus, polysaccharides boost the immune system by increasing the activity and production of white blood cells, enhancing the body's ability to fight infections. They also possess antioxidant properties that help protect cells from oxidative damage.

2. **Saponins (Astragalosides):**

   o **Description:** Saponins are glycosides with foaming characteristics that have various pharmacological effects.

   o **Function:** Astragalosides, the specific saponins found in Astragalus, exhibit anti-inflammatory, antiviral, and cardioprotective properties. They help reduce inflammation, enhance the immune response, and protect the heart by improving cardiac function and reducing oxidative stress.

3. **Flavonoids:**

   o **Description:** Flavonoids are a diverse group of phytonutrients found in many fruits and vegetables, known for their antioxidant activity.

   o **Function:** In Astragalus, flavonoids provide potent antioxidant effects, scavenging free radicals and reducing oxidative stress. They also exhibit anti-inflammatory and anti-cancer properties, contributing to overall health and disease prevention.

4. **Amino Acids:**

   o **Description:** Amino acids are the building blocks of proteins and play a vital role in various physiological processes.

   o **Function:** Astragalus contains essential amino acids that support protein synthesis, tissue repair, and overall metabolic health. These amino acids contribute to the herb's ability to promote healing and recovery.

5. **Trace Minerals:**

- o **Description:** Astragalus is rich in trace minerals such as selenium, zinc, and magnesium, which are essential for various bodily functions.

- o **Function:** These minerals support immune function, antioxidant defenses, and overall metabolic processes. Selenium, for example, is crucial for the proper functioning of the immune system and the prevention of oxidative damage.

Health Benefits of Astragalus

1. **Immune System Enhancement:**

   - o **Boosts Immune Function:** Astragalus polysaccharides enhance the activity of white blood cells, including macrophages, natural killer cells, and T-lymphocytes, leading to improved immune response and increased resistance to infections.

   - o **Antiviral and Antibacterial Properties:** Astragalosides and other constituents provide direct antimicrobial effects, helping to prevent and combat viral and bacterial infections.

2. **Anti-Inflammatory Effects:**

   - o **Reduces Inflammation:** Saponins and flavonoids in Astragalus exhibit strong anti-inflammatory properties, which help reduce inflammation and associated symptoms in conditions such as arthritis, allergies, and inflammatory bowel disease.

3. **Antioxidant Protection:**

   - o **Scavenges Free Radicals:** The flavonoids and polysaccharides in Astragalus act as antioxidants, neutralizing free radicals and reducing oxidative stress, which is linked to aging and various chronic diseases.

   - o **Protects Cells:** By protecting cells from oxidative damage, Astragalus supports overall cellular health and longevity.

4. **Cardiovascular Health:**

   - o **Enhances Heart Function:** Astragalosides improve heart function by increasing cardiac output and reducing the workload on the heart. They also protect the heart muscle from damage due to oxidative stress.

   - o **Lowers Blood Pressure:** The anti-inflammatory and antioxidant effects of Astragalus contribute to lowering blood pressure and improving blood vessel health, reducing the risk of cardiovascular diseases.

5. **Adaptogenic Properties:**

   - o **Stress Resistance:** As an adaptogen, Astragalus helps the body adapt to and resist physical, emotional, and environmental stressors. This leads to improved resilience and overall well-being.

- **Energy and Vitality:** Astragalus enhances energy levels and reduces fatigue by supporting adrenal gland function and improving the body's stress response.

6. **Anti-Cancer Potential:**

   - **Inhibits Tumor Growth:** Some studies suggest that the polysaccharides and saponins in Astragalus may inhibit the growth and spread of cancer cells by inducing apoptosis (programmed cell death) and enhancing the immune response against tumors.

   - **Supports Chemotherapy:** Astragalus may help reduce the side effects of chemotherapy and improve the efficacy of cancer treatments by boosting the immune system and protecting healthy cells.

7. **Anti-Aging Effects:**

   - **Promotes Longevity:** The antioxidant and anti-inflammatory properties of Astragalus contribute to its anti-aging effects, promoting longevity and overall health. It is believed to enhance the body's repair mechanisms and reduce the impact of age-related diseases.

8. **Support for Chronic Conditions:**

   - **Manages Diabetes:** Astragalus has been shown to help regulate blood sugar levels and improve insulin sensitivity, making it beneficial for individuals with diabetes or metabolic syndrome.

   - **Improves Kidney Function:** The herb supports kidney health by reducing inflammation and oxidative stress, which are common in chronic kidney disease.

Astragalus is a powerful herb with a wide range of health benefits, thanks to its rich content of bioactive compounds such as polysaccharides, saponins, flavonoids, amino acids, and trace minerals. These constituents work synergistically to enhance immune function, reduce inflammation, provide antioxidant protection, support cardiovascular health, and promote overall vitality and longevity. By incorporating Astragalus into your health regimen, you can harness its protective and rejuvenating properties to support a robust and resilient body.

Enhancing Immune Function with Astragalus

Astragalus membranaceus, commonly known as Astragalus, is renowned for its potent immune-enhancing properties. Used extensively in traditional Chinese medicine, Astragalus supports the immune system in multiple ways, making it a valuable herb for maintaining health and preventing illness. This section explores how Astragalus enhances immune function and provides practical tips for incorporating it into your health regimen.

Mechanisms of Immune Enhancement

1. **Stimulation of White Blood Cells:**

- **Action:** Astragalus polysaccharides stimulate the production and activity of various white blood cells, including macrophages, natural killer cells, and T-lymphocytes.
- **Benefit:** These cells are crucial for identifying, attacking, and eliminating pathogens such as bacteria, viruses, and fungi, thereby strengthening the body's defense mechanisms.

2. **Increase in Cytokine Production:**

- **Action:** Astragalus boosts the production of cytokines, which are signaling molecules that regulate the immune response.
- **Benefit:** Enhanced cytokine production improves communication between immune cells, leading to a more coordinated and effective immune response.

3. **Antiviral and Antibacterial Properties:**

- **Action:** Constituents like saponins and flavonoids in Astragalus exhibit direct antimicrobial effects.
- **Benefit:** These properties help inhibit the growth and spread of viruses and bacteria, reducing the risk of infections and aiding in quicker recovery.

4. **Support for Innate and Adaptive Immunity:**

- **Action:** Astragalus enhances both innate immunity (the body's first line of defense) and adaptive immunity (which develops targeted responses to specific pathogens).
- **Benefit:** This dual action provides comprehensive support, making the immune system more resilient and responsive to a wide range of threats.

5. **Reduction of Inflammation:**

- **Action:** The anti-inflammatory properties of Astragalus help modulate the immune response and prevent excessive inflammation.
- **Benefit:** This reduces the risk of chronic inflammatory conditions and supports overall immune health by maintaining a balanced immune response.

6. **Antioxidant Protection:**

- **Action:** Astragalus contains powerful antioxidants that protect immune cells from oxidative stress and damage.
- **Benefit:** By preserving the integrity and function of immune cells, Astragalus ensures that the immune system remains robust and effective.

Practical Tips for Using Astragalus

1. **Choosing the Right Form:**

- **Teas:** Ideal for regular consumption, especially during cold and flu season. Steep 1-2 teaspoons of dried Astragalus root in hot water for 10-15 minutes.

- **Tinctures:** Concentrated and convenient, tinctures can be taken 1-2 dropperfuls (approximately 30-60 drops) 2-3 times daily.

- **Capsules:** Provide a consistent dose and are easy to take. Typically, 1-2 capsules (400-500 mg each) taken 2-3 times daily.

2. **Timing and Dosage:**

   - **Preventative Use:** For general immune support, use Astragalus regularly during times of increased exposure to pathogens (e.g., winter months, during travel).

   - **At Onset of Illness:** Increase the dosage at the first sign of symptoms to help reduce the severity and duration of illness. Consult a healthcare provider for personalized dosing recommendations.

3. **Combining with Other Immune-Boosting Herbs:**

   - **Synergistic Effects:** Combine Astragalus with other herbs like Echinacea, elderberry, and ginger to enhance immune support. These herbs can be blended into teas or taken as part of a comprehensive herbal supplement regimen.

4. **Integrating into Daily Routine:**

   - **Culinary Uses:** Add dried Astragalus root to soups, stews, and broths for an easy way to incorporate its benefits into your diet.

   - **Smoothies and Juices:** Blend powdered Astragalus into smoothies and juices for a convenient and nutritious boost.

5. **Lifestyle and Dietary Considerations:**

   - **Healthy Diet:** Support your immune system by maintaining a balanced diet rich in fruits, vegetables, lean proteins, and healthy fats.

   - **Regular Exercise:** Engage in regular physical activity to boost overall health and enhance immune function.

   - **Adequate Sleep:** Ensure you get sufficient sleep each night to support optimal immune response and recovery.

Safety and Precautions

1. **Consultation with Healthcare Provider:**

   - Before starting any new supplement, especially if you have underlying health conditions or are taking other medications, consult with a healthcare provider to ensure it is safe and appropriate for you.

2. **Monitoring for Allergic Reactions:**

- Be aware of potential allergic reactions. If you experience any adverse effects such as rash, itching, or difficulty breathing, discontinue use and seek medical attention.

3. **Pregnancy and Breastfeeding:**

- Pregnant and breastfeeding women should consult their healthcare provider before using Astragalus to ensure its safety during these periods.

Astragalus offers a robust and multifaceted approach to enhancing immune function, making it a valuable herb for maintaining health and preventing illness. Its ability to stimulate white blood cells, increase cytokine production, and provide antiviral and antibacterial properties makes it a powerful ally in supporting the body's defenses. By incorporating Astragalus into your daily routine through teas, tinctures, or capsules, and by combining it with other immune-boosting practices, you can effectively bolster your immune system and promote overall vitality.

Combining Astragalus with Other Herbs

Combining Astragalus with other herbs can enhance its immune-boosting effects and provide a more comprehensive approach to health and wellness. This synergy can target various aspects of immune function, stress response, and overall vitality. Below are some effective herbal combinations with Astragalus, including their benefits and preparation methods.

Effective Herbal Combinations with Astragalus

1. **Astragalus and Echinacea:**

- **Benefits:**

  - **Enhanced Immune Support:** While Astragalus is excellent for long-term immune enhancement, Echinacea is particularly effective for short-term immune boosts, especially at the onset of illness.

  - **Infection Prevention:** Together, they offer a powerful defense against infections, combining Astragalus' immune-modulating effects with Echinacea's ability to reduce the duration and severity of colds and flu.

- **Preparation:**

  - **Tea:** Combine 1 teaspoon of dried Astragalus root with 1 teaspoon of dried Echinacea in boiling water. Steep for 10-15 minutes. Drink 2-3 cups daily.

  - **Tincture:** Mix equal parts of Astragalus and Echinacea tinctures. Take 1-2 dropperfuls (approximately 30-60 drops) 2-3 times daily.

2. **Astragalus and Reishi Mushroom:**

- **Benefits:**

- **Adaptogenic and Immune Support:** Reishi is an adaptogen like Astragalus, enhancing the body's resilience to stress while also providing strong immune support.
- **Anti-Inflammatory and Antioxidant Properties:** This combination helps reduce inflammation and oxidative stress, supporting overall health and longevity.

- **Preparation:**
  - **Decoction:** Simmer 1 tablespoon of dried Astragalus root and 1 tablespoon of dried Reishi mushroom slices in 4 cups of water for 30-45 minutes. Strain and drink 1-2 cups daily.
  - **Capsules:** Take standardized Astragalus and Reishi mushroom capsules as directed on the product labels.

3. **Astragalus and Ashwagandha:**
   - **Benefits:**
     - **Stress Reduction and Immune Boosting:** Ashwagandha is another powerful adaptogen that works well with Astragalus to reduce stress and enhance immune function.
     - **Energy and Vitality:** This combination supports increased energy levels, improved mood, and better overall vitality.

   - **Preparation:**
     - **Tea:** Combine 1 teaspoon of dried Astragalus root with 1 teaspoon of dried Ashwagandha root in boiling water. Steep for 10-15 minutes. Drink 2-3 cups daily.
     - **Tincture:** Mix equal parts of Astragalus and Ashwagandha tinctures. Take 1-2 dropperfuls (approximately 30-60 drops) 2-3 times daily.

4. **Astragalus and Elderberry:**
   - **Benefits:**
     - **Immune Enhancement and Antiviral Properties:** Elderberry is well-known for its antiviral properties and works synergistically with Astragalus to boost the immune system and prevent viral infections.
     - **Cold and Flu Prevention:** This combination is particularly effective during cold and flu season, helping to prevent and mitigate symptoms.

   - **Preparation:**
     - **Syrup:** Combine 1 cup of dried Elderberries, 1 tablespoon of dried Astragalus root, and 4 cups of water. Simmer until the liquid reduces by

half. Strain and add honey to taste. Take 1 tablespoon daily for prevention, or up to 4 tablespoons daily during illness.

- **Tea:** Combine 1 teaspoon of dried Astragalus root with 1 teaspoon of dried Elderberries in boiling water. Steep for 10-15 minutes. Drink 2-3 cups daily.

5. **Astragalus and Licorice Root:**

   - **Benefits:**

     - **Immune Support and Stress Relief:** Licorice root enhances the immune-boosting effects of Astragalus and provides additional support for adrenal function, helping to manage stress.

     - **Anti-Inflammatory and Antiviral:** Both herbs have anti-inflammatory and antiviral properties, making this combination effective for managing infections and inflammation.

   - **Preparation:**

     - **Tea:** Combine 1 teaspoon of dried Astragalus root with 1/2 teaspoon of dried Licorice root in boiling water. Steep for 10-15 minutes. Drink 1-2 cups daily.

     - **Tincture:** Mix 2 parts Astragalus tincture with 1 part Licorice root tincture. Take 1-2 dropperfuls (approximately 30-60 drops) 2-3 times daily.

Tips for Combining Herbs

1. **Start Slowly:**

   - Begin with small amounts when combining herbs to ensure you do not experience any adverse reactions. Gradually increase the dosage as tolerated.

2. **Consult a Healthcare Provider:**

   - If you have underlying health conditions, are taking medications, or are pregnant or breastfeeding, consult a healthcare provider before starting any new herbal regimen.

3. **Monitor Effects:**

   - Pay attention to how your body responds to the herbal combinations. Adjust dosages as needed based on your individual response and health goals.

4. **Quality Matters:**

   - Use high-quality, organic herbs and standardized extracts to ensure potency and effectiveness.

5. **Consistency is Key:**

- For best results, use the herbal combinations consistently as part of your daily routine, especially during times of increased stress or exposure to pathogens.

Combining Astragalus with other complementary herbs can enhance its immune-boosting and adaptogenic effects, providing a more holistic approach to health and wellness. Whether you are looking to strengthen your immune system, reduce stress, or prevent infections, these herbal combinations offer a powerful and natural way to support your body's defenses and overall vitality. By incorporating these synergistic blends into your daily regimen, you can optimize your health and resilience.

Preparation Techniques: Decoctions, Powders, and Extracts

Astragalus can be prepared in various forms, each offering unique benefits and applications. Understanding the preparation techniques for decoctions, powders, and extracts can help you make the most of this powerful herb.

Decoctions

Description:

- Decoctions are a traditional method of extracting the active compounds from tough plant materials like roots, bark, and seeds by simmering them in water.

Preparation:

1. **Ingredients:**

   - 1 tablespoon dried Astragalus root (sliced or chopped)
   - 4 cups water

2. **Steps:**

   - Place the dried Astragalus root in a pot.
   - Add water and bring to a boil.
   - Reduce heat and simmer for 30-45 minutes.
   - Strain the liquid to remove the plant material.
   - Allow the decoction to cool slightly before consuming.

Benefits:

- Effective at extracting water-soluble compounds like polysaccharides and flavonoids.
- Suitable for long-term use to maintain immune health and overall vitality.

Usage:

- Drink 1-2 cups daily for general immune support or during times of increased stress or exposure to pathogens.

- Can be stored in the refrigerator for up to a week.

Powders

Description:

- Powders are made by grinding dried herbs into a fine consistency. This form is convenient for adding to foods and beverages.

Preparation:

1. **Ingredients:**
   - Dried Astragalus root

2. **Steps:**
   - Use a coffee grinder or herb grinder to grind the dried Astragalus root into a fine powder.
   - Store the powder in an airtight container in a cool, dry place.

Benefits:

- Easy to incorporate into smoothies, juices, soups, and other recipes.
- Provides a consistent dose of the herb with each use.

Usage:

- Add 1-2 teaspoons of Astragalus powder to smoothies, juices, or soups daily.
- Can also be encapsulated for convenient dosing.

Extracts (Tinctures)

Description:

- Extracts, or tinctures, are concentrated liquid forms of herbs made by soaking them in alcohol or glycerin. They are highly potent and have a long shelf life.

Preparation:

1. **Ingredients:**
   - Dried Astragalus root
   - Alcohol (vodka or brandy) or glycerin

2. **Steps:**
   - Fill a glass jar with dried Astragalus root.
   - Pour alcohol or glycerin over the herbs until they are completely covered.
   - Seal the jar tightly and store it in a cool, dark place.

- Shake the jar daily for 4-6 weeks.
- After 4-6 weeks, strain the mixture through a cheesecloth or fine mesh strainer into a clean glass jar or bottle.

Benefits:

- Highly concentrated, requiring only small doses.
- Long shelf life, typically 2-3 years when stored properly.

Usage:

- Take 1-2 dropperfuls (approximately 30-60 drops) 2-3 times daily for immune support or as needed.
- Can be added to water, tea, or juice for easier consumption.

Decoctions, powders, and extracts each offer unique advantages for incorporating Astragalus into your health regimen. Decoctions are ideal for extracting water-soluble compounds and are easy to prepare and consume. Powders provide a versatile and consistent way to add Astragalus to your diet, while extracts offer a potent and convenient option with a long shelf life. By choosing the preparation method that best suits your needs and lifestyle, you can effectively harness the benefits of Astragalus to support your immune system and overall health.

Appropriate Dosages and Potential Side Effects

When using Astragalus for its immune-boosting and health-promoting properties, it's essential to follow appropriate dosages to maximize benefits and minimize potential side effects. Here are the recommended dosages for various forms of Astragalus, along with an overview of potential side effects and precautions.

Appropriate Dosages

1. Astragalus Decoction:

- **General Immune Support:**
  - **Dosage:** 1-2 cups daily.
  - **Preparation:** Use 1 tablespoon of dried Astragalus root simmered in 4 cups of water for 30-45 minutes. Strain and drink.
- **During Illness:**
  - **Dosage:** 2-3 cups daily at the onset of symptoms.

2. Astragalus Powder:

- **General Immune Support:**
  - **Dosage:** 1-2 teaspoons daily.

- o **Usage:** Add to smoothies, juices, soups, or encapsulate for convenient dosing.
- **During Illness:**
  - o **Dosage:** 2-3 teaspoons daily, spread throughout the day.

3. Astragalus Extract (Tincture):

- **General Immune Support:**
  - o **Dosage:** 1-2 dropperfuls (approximately 30-60 drops) 2-3 times daily.
  - o **Usage:** Take directly or add to water, tea, or juice.
- **During Illness:**
  - o **Dosage:** 2-3 dropperfuls 3-4 times daily.

4. Astragalus Capsules:

- **General Immune Support:**
  - o **Dosage:** 1-2 capsules (typically 400-500 mg each) taken 2-3 times daily.
- **During Illness:**
  - o **Dosage:** 2 capsules taken 3-4 times daily.

Potential Side Effects and Precautions

1. Allergic Reactions:

- **Description:** Some individuals may experience allergic reactions to Astragalus, including skin rash, itching, or difficulty breathing.
- **Precautions:** If you have known allergies to plants in the Fabaceae family (such as peas, beans, and licorice), use Astragalus with caution. Discontinue use and seek medical attention if you experience any signs of an allergic reaction.

2. Autoimmune Conditions:

- **Description:** Astragalus stimulates the immune system, which may exacerbate autoimmune disorders such as lupus, rheumatoid arthritis, or multiple sclerosis.
- **Precautions:** Individuals with autoimmune conditions should consult a healthcare provider before using Astragalus to ensure it is safe and appropriate for their condition.

3. Pregnancy and Breastfeeding:

- **Description:** Limited research is available on the safety of Astragalus during pregnancy and breastfeeding.
- **Precautions:** Pregnant and breastfeeding women should consult their healthcare provider before using Astragalus to ensure its safety during these periods.

4. Drug Interactions:

- **Description:** Astragalus may interact with certain medications, including immunosuppressants, anticoagulants (blood thinners), and drugs metabolized by the liver.

- **Precautions:** If you are taking prescription medications, especially immunosuppressants or anticoagulants, consult your healthcare provider before using Astragalus to avoid potential interactions.

5. Long-Term Use:

- **Description:** Prolonged use of high doses of Astragalus may lead to reduced effectiveness and potential liver strain.

- **Precautions:** Use Astragalus in recommended dosages and take breaks if using it for extended periods. Consult a healthcare provider for long-term use guidance.

6. Monitoring and Adjustment:

- **Description:** Individual responses to Astragalus can vary based on health status, age, and other factors.

- **Precautions:** Monitor your body's response to Astragalus and adjust the dosage if needed. Seek medical advice if you experience any adverse effects or if your condition does not improve.

Astragalus is a potent herb with numerous health benefits, particularly for immune support. Following the appropriate dosages for decoctions, powders, extracts, and capsules can help you achieve the desired effects while minimizing the risk of side effects. Always consult with a healthcare provider if you have underlying health conditions, are taking medications, or are pregnant or breastfeeding to ensure the safe and effective use of Astragalus. By using this powerful herb responsibly, you can enhance your overall health and well-being.

BOOK 6:

Herbal Preparations and Dosages: The Practical Indications

Herbal medicine offers a variety of preparation methods to harness the therapeutic benefits of medicinal plants, including teas, tinctures, powders, and capsules. Each method has its own unique advantages, allowing you to tailor your approach to suit your specific needs and lifestyle. Understanding the appropriate dosages for these preparations is crucial for ensuring their efficacy and safety. In this chapter, we will explore the different ways to prepare and use herbs like Echinacea and Astragalus, providing detailed dosage recommendations to help you maximize their health benefits. Whether you are seeking to boost your immune system, enhance vitality, or support overall wellness, this guide will equip you with the knowledge to incorporate herbal remedies effectively and safely into your daily routine.

Understanding Herbal Preparations

Herbal preparations are various methods used to extract and utilize the active compounds in medicinal plants. Each preparation method can impact the potency, effectiveness, and convenience of using herbs. Understanding these methods is essential for making the most of herbal remedies. Below are the primary types of herbal preparations and how they are typically used.

1. Teas (Infusions and Decoctions)

Infusions:

- **Description:** Infusions are made by steeping delicate parts of the herb, such as leaves, flowers, and stems, in hot water.

- **Preparation:**
  - Boil water and pour over 1-2 teaspoons of dried or fresh herb.
  - Cover and let steep for 10-15 minutes.
  - Strain and drink.

- **Use:** Infusions are ideal for herbs like chamomile, peppermint, and lavender, which have volatile oils and other compounds easily released in hot water.

Decoctions:

- **Description:** Decoctions are made by simmering tougher parts of the herb, such as roots, bark, and seeds, in water to extract their active constituents.

- **Preparation:**
  - Add 1 tablespoon of dried or fresh herb to 4 cups of water.
  - Bring to a boil, then reduce to a simmer for 30-45 minutes.
  - Strain and drink.

- **Use:** Decoctions are suitable for herbs like Astragalus, ginger, and licorice root, which require more prolonged heat to release their beneficial compounds.

2. Tinctures

Description:

- Tinctures are concentrated liquid extracts made by soaking herbs in alcohol or glycerin. They offer a potent and convenient way to consume herbs.

Preparation:

- Fill a glass jar with dried or fresh herb.

- Pour alcohol (typically vodka or brandy) or glycerin over the herbs until completely covered.

- Seal the jar and store it in a cool, dark place for 4-6 weeks, shaking daily.

- Strain the liquid into a clean bottle.

Use:

- Tinctures are taken in small doses, usually 1-2 dropperfuls (approximately 30-60 drops) 2-3 times daily. They are effective for a wide range of herbs, including Echinacea, valerian, and goldenseal.

3. Powders

Description:

- Herbal powders are made by grinding dried herbs into a fine consistency. They can be easily added to foods, beverages, or encapsulated for convenient use.

Preparation:

- Use a coffee grinder or herb grinder to grind dried herbs into a fine powder.

- Store in an airtight container in a cool, dry place.

Use:

- Add 1-2 teaspoons of herbal powder to smoothies, juices, soups, or other foods. Powders can also be encapsulated for precise dosing.

4. Capsules

Description:

- Capsules are a convenient way to take herbs, providing a pre-measured dose that is easy to consume.

Preparation:

- Fill empty gelatin or vegetarian capsules with herbal powder using a capsule-filling machine or by hand.

- Seal the capsules tightly.

Use:

- Follow the dosage instructions on the product label or as advised by a healthcare provider, typically 1-2 capsules (400-500 mg each) taken 2-3 times daily.

5. Topical Applications

Description:

- Topical preparations include salves, ointments, and poultices made from herbs for external use.

Preparation:

- **Salves and Ointments:** Infuse herbs in a carrier oil (such as olive or coconut oil) for several weeks, then strain and mix with beeswax to create a solid form.

- **Poultices:** Crush fresh herbs and apply directly to the skin or wrap in a cloth to place over the affected area.

Use:

- Topical applications are used for skin conditions, wounds, inflammation, and muscle pain. Common herbs for topical use include calendula, comfrey, and arnica.

6. Essential Oils

Description:

- Essential oils are concentrated volatile oils extracted from plants, typically through steam distillation.

Preparation:

- Steam distillation requires specialized equipment, so essential oils are usually purchased rather than made at home.

Use:

- Essential oils are used in aromatherapy, added to carrier oils for topical application, or diffused into the air. They must be diluted before use on the skin.

Understanding herbal preparations is key to effectively using medicinal plants for health and wellness. Each method—whether teas, tinctures, powders, capsules, topical applications, or essential oils—offers unique benefits and can be chosen based on the specific needs and preferences of the individual. By mastering these preparation techniques, you can maximize the therapeutic potential of herbs and incorporate them into your daily health routine safely and effectively.

Methods of Extraction: Infusions, Decoctions, Tinctures, and Powders

Understanding the methods of extracting the active compounds from medicinal herbs is essential for effectively using them in herbal remedies. Different methods are suited for different types of plant materials and desired outcomes. Below, we explore the processes and uses of infusions, decoctions, tinctures, and powders.

1. Infusions

Description:

- Infusions are a method of extracting water-soluble compounds from the softer parts of herbs, such as leaves, flowers, and stems. This process is similar to making tea.

Preparation:

1. **Ingredients:**
   - 1-2 teaspoons of dried or fresh herb.
   - 1 cup of boiling water.

2. **Steps:**
   - Place the herb in a teapot or mug.
   - Pour boiling water over the herb.
   - Cover and let steep for 10-15 minutes.
   - Strain the liquid to remove the plant material.

3. **Use:**
   - Infusions are typically consumed as a beverage, providing a gentle and easy way to intake the active compounds of the herb.
   - Common herbs for infusions include chamomile, peppermint, and lemon balm.

2. Decoctions

Description:

- Decoctions are used to extract water-soluble compounds from the tougher parts of herbs, such as roots, bark, and seeds. This method involves prolonged simmering.

Preparation:

1. **Ingredients:**
   - 1 tablespoon of dried or fresh herb.
   - 4 cups of water.

2. **Steps:**
   - Place the herb and water in a pot.
   - Bring to a boil, then reduce heat and simmer for 30-45 minutes.
   - Strain the liquid to remove the plant material.

3. **Use:**
   - Decoctions are usually consumed as a beverage or used as a base for other herbal preparations.

o   Common herbs for decoctions include Astragalus, ginger, and licorice root.

3. Tinctures

Description:

- Tinctures are concentrated liquid extracts made by soaking herbs in alcohol or glycerin. They are highly potent and convenient for long-term storage.

Preparation:

1. **Ingredients:**
   - o   Dried or fresh herb.
   - o   Alcohol (vodka or brandy) or glycerin.

2. **Steps:**
   - o   Fill a glass jar with the herb.
   - o   Pour alcohol or glycerin over the herb until completely covered.
   - o   Seal the jar and store in a cool, dark place for 4-6 weeks, shaking daily.
   - o   Strain the liquid into a clean bottle.

3. **Use:**
   - o   Tinctures are taken in small doses, typically 1-2 dropperfuls (30-60 drops) 2-3 times daily.
   - o   They are effective for a wide range of herbs, including Echinacea, valerian, and goldenseal.

4. Powders

Description:

- Herbal powders are made by grinding dried herbs into a fine consistency. They are versatile and can be added to foods, beverages, or encapsulated.

Preparation:

1. **Ingredients:**
   - o   Dried herb.

2. **Steps:**
   - o   Use a coffee grinder or herb grinder to grind the dried herb into a fine powder.
   - o   Store in an airtight container in a cool, dry place.

3. **Use:**

- Add 1-2 teaspoons of herbal powder to smoothies, juices, soups, or other foods.
- Powders can also be encapsulated for precise dosing.

Each method of extraction—infusions, decoctions, tinctures, and powders—offers unique benefits and is suited to different types of herbs and desired outcomes. Infusions and decoctions are ideal for extracting water-soluble compounds from softer and tougher plant materials, respectively. Tinctures provide a potent and long-lasting form of herbal medicine, while powders offer versatility and convenience. By choosing the appropriate extraction method, you can effectively harness the therapeutic potential of medicinal herbs to support your health and well-being.

Standardizing Dosages for Consistent Results

Standardizing dosages is crucial for ensuring the efficacy and safety of herbal preparations. Consistent dosages allow you to achieve reliable therapeutic outcomes and minimize the risk of adverse effects. Here are the key principles and methods for standardizing dosages of herbal remedies.

Key Principles of Standardizing Dosages

1. **Understand the Herb's Active Constituents:**

   - Identify the primary active compounds responsible for the herb's therapeutic effects.
   - Ensure that these compounds are present in consistent amounts across different batches of the herb.

2. **Use Reliable Sources:**

   - Source herbs from reputable suppliers who provide detailed information about the herb's potency and quality.
   - Prefer standardized extracts that specify the concentration of active constituents.

3. **Measure Accurately:**

   - Use precise measuring tools, such as digital scales for powders and calibrated droppers for tinctures, to ensure accurate dosages.

4. **Adjust for Individual Differences:**

   - Consider factors such as age, weight, health condition, and sensitivity to the herb when determining dosages.
   - Start with lower doses and gradually increase to find the optimal amount for each individual.

5. **Maintain Consistent Preparation Methods:**

- Follow standardized methods for preparing infusions, decoctions, tinctures, and powders to ensure consistent potency.

Methods for Standardizing Dosages

1. **Infusions:**
   - **Standard Measurement:**
     - Use 1-2 teaspoons of dried or fresh herb per cup of boiling water.
     - Steep for a consistent time (10-15 minutes) to extract the active compounds evenly.
   - **Dosage:**
     - Typically, 1-3 cups daily, depending on the herb and the intended use.

2. **Decoctions:**
   - **Standard Measurement:**
     - Use 1 tablespoon of dried or fresh herb per 4 cups of water.
     - Simmer for a consistent time (30-45 minutes) to ensure even extraction.
   - **Dosage:**
     - Typically, 1-2 cups daily, depending on the herb and the intended use.

3. **Tinctures:**
   - **Standard Measurement:**
     - Use a ratio of 1 part dried herb to 5 parts alcohol or glycerin (1:5 ratio) or 1 part fresh herb to 2 parts alcohol or glycerin (1:2 ratio).
     - Steep for a consistent period (4-6 weeks), shaking daily to ensure thorough extraction.
   - **Dosage:**
     - Typically, 1-2 dropperfuls (30-60 drops) 2-3 times daily.
     - Ensure the tincture label specifies the concentration of active constituents for precise dosing.

4. **Powders:**
   - **Standard Measurement:**
     - Use a digital scale to measure the exact weight of the herb powder.
     - For encapsulation, use capsule-filling machines to ensure each capsule contains a consistent amount of powder.

- **Dosage:**
  - Typically, 1-2 teaspoons daily, added to food or beverages.
  - For capsules, 1-2 capsules (400-500 mg each) taken 2-3 times daily.

Practical Tips for Consistent Results

1. **Label and Record:**
   - Label all preparations with the date, type of herb, preparation method, and dosage instructions.
   - Keep detailed records of the preparation process and dosages used to track efficacy and any side effects.

2. **Regular Testing:**
   - Test the potency of your herbal preparations regularly, especially if you prepare large batches.
   - Use third-party testing services if available, or compare the effects with standardized commercial products.

3. **Consult Resources:**
   - Use reputable resources, such as herbal pharmacopoeias and guidelines from herbal medicine associations, to determine standard dosages and preparation methods for different herbs.

4. **Monitor and Adjust:**
   - Monitor the effects of the herbal preparations on individuals and adjust dosages as needed.
   - Consult with a healthcare provider or herbalist for personalized dosage recommendations.

Standardizing dosages for herbal preparations is essential for achieving consistent and reliable therapeutic results. By understanding the active constituents, using reliable sources, measuring accurately, and maintaining consistent preparation methods, you can ensure the efficacy and safety of your herbal remedies. Detailed labeling, regular testing, and ongoing monitoring further support the standardization process, helping you to harness the full potential of medicinal herbs for health and well-being.

Best Practices for Herbal Storage and Shelf Life

Proper storage of herbs and herbal preparations is essential to maintain their potency, efficacy, and safety. Herbs can lose their beneficial properties over time due to exposure to light, air, moisture, and heat. By following best practices for storage, you can extend the shelf life of your herbal products and ensure they remain effective. Here are some guidelines for storing various types of herbal preparations.

General Guidelines for Storing Herbs

1. **Cool, Dark, and Dry Environment:**

   - Store herbs in a cool, dark place away from direct sunlight, heat sources, and moisture.

   - Ideal storage temperatures range from 60-75°F (15-24°C).

2. **Air-Tight Containers:**

   - Use air-tight containers, such as glass jars with tight-fitting lids, to protect herbs from air and moisture.

   - For long-term storage, consider using vacuum-sealed bags or containers with desiccants to remove excess moisture.

3. **Labeling:**

   - Label all containers with the herb name, preparation date, and expiration date.

   - Include additional information such as the source and any specific storage instructions.

4. **Avoid Plastic Containers:**

   - Use glass or metal containers instead of plastic, which can leach chemicals into the herbs and degrade over time.

Specific Storage Recommendations for Different Herbal Preparations

1. **Dried Herbs:**

   - **Storage:** Store in dark-colored glass jars or metal tins to protect from light.

   - **Shelf Life:** Most dried herbs can last 1-2 years if stored properly. However, potency decreases over time, so it's best to use them within a year.

   - **Check for Quality:** Periodically check for signs of spoilage, such as discoloration, mold, or a loss of aroma.

2. **Herbal Powders:**

   - **Storage:** Store in air-tight containers in a cool, dark place. Glass jars or metal tins are ideal.

   - **Shelf Life:** Herbal powders typically last 6 months to a year. They degrade faster than whole herbs due to increased surface area exposure.

   - **Check for Quality:** Check for clumping, loss of aroma, or changes in color, which indicate reduced potency or spoilage.

3. **Tinctures:**

- **Storage:** Store in dark-colored glass bottles to protect from light. Keep in a cool, dark place.
- **Shelf Life:** Alcohol-based tinctures can last 3-5 years if stored properly. Glycerin-based tinctures have a shorter shelf life of 1-2 years.
- **Check for Quality:** Inspect for cloudiness, sediment, or changes in odor, which may indicate spoilage.

4. **Infusions and Decoctions:**

- **Storage:** Freshly prepared infusions and decoctions should be stored in the refrigerator in glass containers.
- **Shelf Life:** Typically, these preparations should be used within 24-48 hours to ensure potency and prevent microbial growth.
- **Check for Quality:** Discard if there are any signs of spoilage, such as off odors or changes in appearance.

5. **Capsules:**

- **Storage:** Store in air-tight containers in a cool, dark place. Glass jars or metal tins are recommended.
- **Shelf Life:** Herbal capsules can last up to 2 years if stored properly.
- **Check for Quality:** Check for signs of moisture, discoloration, or changes in odor.

6. **Essential Oils:**

- **Storage:** Store in dark-colored glass bottles with tight-fitting caps to protect from light and air. Keep in a cool, dark place.
- **Shelf Life:** Essential oils generally have a shelf life of 1-2 years, but some oils like citrus may degrade faster.
- **Check for Quality:** Inspect for changes in aroma, consistency, or color, which can indicate oxidation or spoilage.

7. **Salves and Ointments:**

- **Storage:** Store in dark-colored glass jars or metal tins to protect from light. Keep in a cool, dark place.
- **Shelf Life:** Salves and ointments can last 6 months to a year if stored properly.
- **Check for Quality:** Look for changes in texture, color, or smell, which can indicate spoilage.

Tips for Prolonging Shelf Life

1. **Minimize Exposure:**

- o Open containers only when necessary and reseal them tightly to minimize exposure to air and moisture.

2. **Use Desiccants:**

   - o Place food-grade desiccant packs in containers to absorb excess moisture, especially in humid environments.

3. **Monitor Environmental Conditions:**

   - o Keep storage areas clean and dry, and monitor for temperature and humidity fluctuations.

4. **Rotate Stock:**

   - o Use the oldest stock first to ensure that herbs and preparations are used within their optimal shelf life.

5. **Avoid Cross-Contamination:**

   - o Use clean, dry utensils when handling herbs and preparations to avoid introducing contaminants.

Proper storage is essential for maintaining the potency and efficacy of herbal preparations. By following these best practices, you can extend the shelf life of your herbs and ensure they remain effective for your health and wellness needs. Always monitor your herbal products for signs of spoilage and use them within the recommended timeframes to maximize their benefits.

Creating Your Own Herbal Remedies at Home

Making your own herbal remedies at home is a rewarding and empowering way to take charge of your health. By understanding basic preparation techniques, you can create effective and personalized herbal remedies for a variety of health concerns. Here is a guide to get you started on creating infusions, decoctions, tinctures, and salves.

Getting Started: Basic Tools and Supplies

1. **Herbs:**

   - o Source high-quality, organic herbs from reputable suppliers or grow your own.

2. **Containers:**

   - o Use dark-colored glass jars and bottles to protect from light and air.

3. **Measuring Tools:**

   - o Have measuring spoons, cups, and a digital scale on hand for accuracy.

4. **Strainers:**

   - o Use fine mesh strainers or cheesecloth for filtering herbal preparations.

5. **Mortar and Pestle:**

   o Useful for grinding fresh herbs.

6. **Labels:**

   o Label jars and bottles with the herb name, preparation date, and dosage instructions.

Basic Herbal Preparations

1. **Infusions:**

Ideal for: Leaves, flowers, and other delicate plant parts.

Ingredients:

- 1-2 teaspoons of dried herb or 1-2 tablespoons of fresh herb.
- 1 cup of boiling water.

Steps:

- Place the herb in a teapot or mug.
- Pour boiling water over the herb.
- Cover and let steep for 10-15 minutes.
- Strain and drink.

Example Use:

- Chamomile infusion for relaxation and digestive support.

2. **Decoctions:**

Ideal for: Roots, bark, seeds, and other tough plant materials.

Ingredients:

- 1 tablespoon of dried herb or 2 tablespoons of fresh herb.
- 4 cups of water.

Steps:

- Place the herb and water in a pot.
- Bring to a boil, then reduce heat and simmer for 30-45 minutes.
- Strain and drink.

Example Use:

- Ginger decoction for digestive health and anti-inflammatory effects.

3. **Tinctures:**

Ideal for: Concentrated, long-lasting extracts.

Ingredients:

- Dried or fresh herb.
- Alcohol (vodka or brandy) or glycerin.

Steps:

- Fill a glass jar with the herb.
- Pour alcohol or glycerin over the herb until completely covered.
- Seal the jar and store it in a cool, dark place for 4-6 weeks, shaking daily.
- Strain the liquid into a clean bottle.

Dosage:

- Take 1-2 dropperfuls (approximately 30-60 drops) 2-3 times daily.

Example Use:

- Echinacea tincture for immune support.

4. **Salves:**

Ideal for: Topical application for skin conditions and wounds.

Ingredients:

- 1 cup of infused oil (e.g., olive or coconut oil infused with herbs like calendula or comfrey).
- 1 ounce of beeswax.
- Optional: Essential oils for fragrance.

Steps:

- Melt the beeswax in a double boiler.
- Add the infused oil and stir until well combined.
- Remove from heat and add essential oils if desired.
- Pour into jars or tins and let cool.

Example Use:

- Calendula salve for soothing skin irritations and promoting healing.

Tips for Creating Effective Herbal Remedies

1. **Research and Plan:**

   o Research the properties and benefits of the herbs you plan to use.

   o Plan your remedies based on specific health goals and needs.

2. **Quality Matters:**

   o Use high-quality, organic herbs to ensure potency and safety.

   o Store herbs properly to maintain their efficacy.

3. **Start Small:**

   o Begin with small batches to test the effectiveness and tolerability of your remedies.

   o Adjust recipes as needed based on your experiences.

4. **Documentation:**

   o Keep detailed records of your recipes, including ingredients, preparation methods, and dosage instructions.

   o Note any effects or reactions to refine future batches.

5. **Safety First:**

   o Be aware of potential side effects and interactions with medications.

   o Consult with a healthcare provider or herbalist, especially if you have underlying health conditions or are pregnant or breastfeeding.

Conclusion

Creating your own herbal remedies at home allows you to harness the healing power of nature in a personalized and effective way. By following these guidelines and best practices, you can prepare a variety of herbal remedies, from soothing teas to potent tinctures and healing salves. This hands-on approach not only supports your health but also deepens your connection to the natural world and its abundant resources.

Adaptogens for Immune Support

Adaptogens are a unique group of herbs and natural substances that help the body adapt to stress, enhance resilience, and maintain overall balance. These powerful plants not only improve the body's ability to cope with physical, emotional, and environmental stressors but also provide significant immune support. By modulating the immune system, adaptogens can enhance its efficiency, reducing the risk of infections and promoting quicker recovery from illnesses. This chapter introduces key adaptogens known for their immune-boosting properties, explaining how they work and how to incorporate them into your daily routine to support optimal health and vitality. Whether you are looking to fortify your immune system, increase your energy levels, or improve your stress resilience, adaptogens offer a natural and effective solution.

What Are Adaptogens and How Do They Work?

Adaptogens are a unique class of herbs and natural substances that enhance the body's ability to resist and adapt to various forms of stress, whether physical, emotional, or environmental. Unlike other herbal remedies that target specific symptoms or conditions, adaptogens work holistically to promote overall balance and homeostasis in the body. They help the body to better handle stress, improve energy levels, and support immune function.

Key Characteristics of Adaptogens

1. **Non-Specific Action:**

   o Adaptogens do not target a specific organ or system. Instead, they provide a general sense of well-being and enhance the body's overall resilience to stress.

2. **Normalizing Effect:**

   o Adaptogens help normalize bodily functions, bringing the body back into balance regardless of the direction of the imbalance. For example, they can help regulate both high and low levels of various bodily processes.

3. **Non-Toxic:**

   o Adaptogens are generally safe and non-toxic, even with long-term use. They have minimal side effects and are well-tolerated by most individuals.

How Adaptogens Work

1. **Modulating the Stress Response:**

   o **HPA Axis Regulation:** Adaptogens influence the hypothalamic-pituitary-adrenal (HPA) axis, a central part of the body's stress response system. By modulating the release of stress hormones like cortisol, adaptogens help mitigate the effects of stress and prevent the negative impact of chronic stress on the body.

   o **Balancing Neurotransmitters:** Adaptogens help balance neurotransmitters in the brain, such as serotonin and dopamine, which play crucial roles in mood regulation and stress response.

2. **Enhancing Immune Function:**

   o **Immune Modulation:** Adaptogens support the immune system by enhancing the activity of immune cells, such as natural killer cells, macrophages, and lymphocytes. This helps the body more effectively identify and combat pathogens.

   o **Anti-Inflammatory Properties:** Many adaptogens possess anti-inflammatory properties that reduce chronic inflammation, which can weaken the immune system and increase susceptibility to infections.

3. **Improving Energy and Stamina:**

   o **Mitochondrial Support:** Adaptogens enhance cellular energy production by supporting mitochondrial function, leading to increased stamina and reduced fatigue.

   o **Balancing Blood Sugar Levels:** By helping to regulate blood sugar levels, adaptogens prevent energy crashes and promote sustained energy throughout the day.

4. **Supporting Cognitive Function:**

   o **Neuroprotection:** Adaptogens protect brain cells from damage caused by oxidative stress and inflammation, which can improve cognitive function and reduce the risk of neurodegenerative diseases.

   o **Enhancing Focus and Memory:** By reducing stress and supporting overall brain health, adaptogens can improve concentration, memory, and mental clarity.

Common Adaptogens and Their Benefits

1. **Ashwagandha (Withania somnifera):**

   o **Benefits:** Reduces stress and anxiety, supports immune function, improves energy levels, and enhances cognitive function.

   o **Mechanism:** Modulates the HPA axis, balances cortisol levels, and provides antioxidant protection.

2. **Rhodiola (Rhodiola rosea):**

   o **Benefits:** Increases stamina and endurance, reduces fatigue, enhances mood, and supports immune function.

   o **Mechanism:** Regulates neurotransmitters, supports mitochondrial function, and reduces inflammation.

3. **Eleuthero (Eleutherococcus senticosus):**

   o **Benefits:** Enhances physical performance, supports immune health, reduces fatigue, and improves cognitive function.

   o **Mechanism:** Modulates the stress response, enhances energy production, and supports immune cells.

4. **Holy Basil (Ocimum sanctum):**

   o **Benefits:** Reduces stress and anxiety, supports immune health, balances blood sugar levels, and provides anti-inflammatory effects.

   o **Mechanism:** Regulates cortisol levels, supports immune function, and provides antioxidant protection.

5. **Schisandra (Schisandra chinensis):**

   o **Benefits:** Enhances energy and endurance, supports liver function, reduces stress, and improves cognitive function.

   o **Mechanism:** Supports mitochondrial function, protects against oxidative stress, and enhances immune response.

Adaptogens are a powerful tool for enhancing the body's resilience to stress and supporting overall health. By modulating the stress response, enhancing immune function, and improving energy and cognitive function, adaptogens provide a holistic approach to maintaining balance and vitality. Incorporating adaptogens into your daily routine can help you better manage stress, boost your immune system, and improve your overall well-being.

Top Adaptogenic Herbs: Rhodiola, Ashwagandha, and Schisandra

Adaptogenic herbs like Rhodiola, Ashwagandha, and Schisandra are well-known for their ability to help the body adapt to stress, enhance resilience, and promote overall health. Each of these herbs has unique properties and benefits that make them valuable additions to your health regimen.

Rhodiola (Rhodiola rosea)

Description:

- Rhodiola, also known as golden root or arctic root, is a hardy plant that grows in cold, mountainous regions of Europe and Asia. It has been used traditionally in Russian and Scandinavian countries to enhance physical and mental performance.

Key Constituents:

- Rosavins

- Salidroside

- Flavonoids

- Tannins

Health Benefits:

1. **Stress Reduction:**

   o Rhodiola helps reduce symptoms of stress by modulating the HPA axis and balancing cortisol levels.

2. **Enhanced Physical Performance:**

   o It improves endurance and reduces fatigue, making it a popular supplement among athletes and those with physically demanding jobs.

3. **Improved Cognitive Function:**

- o Rhodiola enhances memory, focus, and mental clarity, making it beneficial for those experiencing mental fatigue or cognitive decline.

4. **Mood Enhancement:**

   - o It has antidepressant properties and can help alleviate symptoms of mild to moderate depression and anxiety.

How to Use:

- **Tincture:** Take 30-40 drops in water or juice, 2-3 times daily.
- **Capsules/Tablets:** 200-600 mg daily, standardized to 3% rosavins and 1% salidroside.
- **Tea:** Steep 1 teaspoon of dried Rhodiola root in hot water for 10-15 minutes.

Ashwagandha (Withania somnifera)

Description:

- Ashwagandha, also known as Indian ginseng or winter cherry, is a traditional Ayurvedic herb used for centuries to promote vitality and longevity. It is native to India and North Africa.

Key Constituents:

- Withanolides
- Alkaloids
- Saponins

Health Benefits:

1. **Stress and Anxiety Reduction:**

   - o Ashwagandha reduces stress and anxiety by lowering cortisol levels and balancing the stress response.

2. **Immune Support:**

   - o It enhances immune function by increasing the activity of white blood cells and improving overall immune resilience.

3. **Energy and Vitality:**

   - o Ashwagandha boosts energy levels, reduces fatigue, and improves overall physical performance.

4. **Cognitive Enhancement:**

   - o It supports brain health, improving memory, focus, and cognitive function.

5. **Hormonal Balance:**

- Ashwagandha helps balance hormones, making it beneficial for conditions like hypothyroidism and adrenal fatigue.

How to Use:

- **Tincture:** Take 30-40 drops in water or juice, 2-3 times daily.

- **Capsules/Tablets:** 300-600 mg daily, standardized to 5% withanolides.

- **Powder:** Mix 1 teaspoon in warm milk, water, or smoothies.

Schisandra (Schisandra chinensis)

Description:

- Schisandra, also known as the five-flavor berry, is a traditional Chinese herb used for centuries to promote overall health and longevity. It is native to Northern China and the Russian Far East.

Key Constituents:

- Schisandrin

- Schisandrol

- Gomisin

- Lignans

Health Benefits:

1. **Stress Reduction:**

   - Schisandra helps the body adapt to stress and reduces fatigue, promoting overall resilience.

2. **Liver Support:**

   - It supports liver function and detoxification, protecting the liver from damage and enhancing its ability to process toxins.

3. **Energy and Endurance:**

   - Schisandra boosts energy levels and physical endurance, making it useful for athletes and those needing sustained energy.

4. **Cognitive Function:**

   - It improves mental clarity, focus, and memory, supporting overall cognitive health.

5. **Antioxidant Protection:**

   - Schisandra provides potent antioxidant benefits, protecting cells from oxidative stress and reducing inflammation.

How to Use:

- **Tincture:** Take 30-40 drops in water or juice, 2-3 times daily.

- **Capsules/Tablets:** 500-1000 mg daily, standardized to 2% schisandrin.

- **Tea:** Steep 1 teaspoon of dried Schisandra berries in hot water for 10-15 minutes.

Rhodiola, Ashwagandha, and Schisandra are three powerful adaptogenic herbs that offer a wide range of health benefits, from reducing stress and enhancing cognitive function to boosting energy levels and supporting immune health. By incorporating these adaptogens into your daily routine, you can improve your overall resilience to stress, enhance vitality, and promote optimal health. Always consult with a healthcare provider before starting any new herbal regimen, especially if you have underlying health conditions or are taking medications.

Benefits of Adaptogens for Stress and Immunity

Adaptogens are a remarkable group of herbs that provide significant benefits for managing stress and bolstering immune function. In today's fast-paced world, chronic stress is a common issue that can have detrimental effects on both mental and physical health. Adaptogens offer a natural solution by helping the body adapt to stress and maintain homeostasis. They work by modulating the stress response, particularly through their effects on the hypothalamic-pituitary-adrenal (HPA) axis. By balancing the production of stress hormones like cortisol, adaptogens reduce the harmful effects of chronic stress, such as fatigue, anxiety, and cognitive decline. This balancing act helps to stabilize mood, enhance mental clarity, and improve overall emotional well-being, making adaptogens a valuable tool for stress management.

In addition to their stress-relieving properties, adaptogens play a crucial role in supporting and enhancing immune function. Chronic stress is known to suppress the immune system, making the body more susceptible to infections and illnesses. Adaptogens counteract this by boosting the immune system's resilience. They stimulate the activity of key immune cells, such as natural killer cells, macrophages, and lymphocytes, which are essential for identifying and eliminating pathogens. By enhancing these immune responses, adaptogens help the body fend off infections more effectively and recover more quickly from illnesses. Furthermore, many adaptogens possess anti-inflammatory and antioxidant properties that protect immune cells from damage and support overall immune health.

Adaptogens like Ashwagandha, Rhodiola, and Schisandra offer specific benefits that highlight their dual role in stress reduction and immune support. Ashwagandha, for instance, is well-known for its ability to reduce cortisol levels and combat anxiety, while also boosting the production of white blood cells and enhancing overall immune function. Rhodiola improves physical and mental stamina, helping individuals better cope with stress, and also exhibits antiviral properties that protect against infections. Schisandra, with its liver-protective and detoxifying effects, not only aids in stress management but also enhances the body's detoxification processes, thereby supporting immune health.

Overall, the integration of adaptogens into a daily health regimen can lead to a more balanced and resilient body. Their ability to mitigate the effects of chronic stress while simultaneously enhancing immune function makes them invaluable for maintaining long-term health and vitality. By incorporating adaptogens into your lifestyle, you can achieve a greater sense of well-being, improved stress resilience, and a fortified immune system, all of which are essential for navigating the challenges of modern life.

Combining Adaptogens with Immune-Boosting Herbs

Combining adaptogens with immune-boosting herbs can create a synergistic effect that enhances both stress resilience and immune function. This integrated approach leverages the unique properties of each herb to provide comprehensive support for overall health and well-being. Here are some effective combinations and their benefits.

1. Ashwagandha and Echinacea

Benefits:

- **Stress Reduction and Immune Enhancement:** Ashwagandha's adaptogenic properties help manage stress and reduce cortisol levels, while Echinacea strengthens the immune system by increasing the activity of white blood cells and enhancing the body's ability to fight off infections.

- **Anti-Inflammatory Effects:** Both herbs have anti-inflammatory properties that can help reduce chronic inflammation, a common issue in stressed individuals.

How to Use:

- **Tincture:** Combine equal parts of Ashwagandha and Echinacea tinctures. Take 1-2 dropperfuls (approximately 30-60 drops) 2-3 times daily.

- **Tea:** Steep 1 teaspoon of dried Ashwagandha root and 1 teaspoon of dried Echinacea in hot water for 10-15 minutes. Drink 1-2 cups daily.

2. Rhodiola and Elderberry

Benefits:

- **Increased Energy and Immune Support:** Rhodiola boosts physical and mental stamina, helping the body cope with stress and fatigue, while Elderberry is known for its antiviral properties and ability to strengthen the immune system.

- **Antioxidant Protection:** Both herbs are rich in antioxidants, which protect cells from oxidative stress and support overall health.

How to Use:

- **Syrup:** Combine Rhodiola extract and Elderberry syrup. Take 1 tablespoon daily for immune support or 2-3 times daily during illness.

- **Capsules:** Take standardized Rhodiola and Elderberry capsules as directed on the product labels.

3. Schisandra and Astragalus

Benefits:

- **Liver Support and Immune Boost:** Schisandra supports liver function and detoxification, helping the body manage stress and eliminate toxins, while Astragalus enhances immune function by stimulating the activity of immune cells.

- **Adaptogenic and Antiviral Effects:** Both herbs have adaptogenic and antiviral properties, making this combination effective for boosting resilience and preventing infections.

How to Use:

- **Tincture:** Combine equal parts of Schisandra and Astragalus tinctures. Take 1-2 dropperfuls (approximately 30-60 drops) 2-3 times daily.

- **Decoction:** Simmer 1 tablespoon of dried Schisandra berries and 1 tablespoon of dried Astragalus root in 4 cups of water for 30-45 minutes. Strain and drink 1-2 cups daily.

4. Holy Basil and Garlic

Benefits:

- **Stress Relief and Immune Boost:** Holy Basil is a powerful adaptogen that reduces stress and anxiety, while Garlic is a potent immune booster with antimicrobial properties.

- **Anti-Inflammatory and Antioxidant Benefits:** Both herbs provide anti-inflammatory and antioxidant benefits, supporting overall health and protecting against chronic diseases.

How to Use:

- **Tea:** Steep 1 teaspoon of dried Holy Basil leaves and 1 crushed clove of Garlic in hot water for 10-15 minutes. Drink 1-2 cups daily.

- **Capsules:** Take standardized Holy Basil and Garlic capsules as directed on the product labels.

5. Eleuthero and Ginger

Benefits:

- **Energy Boost and Immune Support:** Eleuthero enhances physical endurance and reduces fatigue, while Ginger boosts immune function and has strong anti-inflammatory properties.

- **Digestive and Anti-Nausea Effects:** Ginger also supports digestive health and helps alleviate nausea, making this combination beneficial for overall wellness.

How to Use:

- **Tincture:** Combine equal parts of Eleuthero and Ginger tinctures. Take 1-2 dropperfuls (approximately 30-60 drops) 2-3 times daily.

- **Tea:** Steep 1 teaspoon of dried Eleuthero root and 1 teaspoon of dried Ginger root in hot water for 10-15 minutes. Drink 1-2 cups daily.

Tips for Combining Adaptogens with Immune-Boosting Herbs

1. **Start Slowly:**
   - Begin with small amounts to ensure you do not experience any adverse reactions. Gradually increase the dosage as tolerated.

2. **Consult a Healthcare Provider:**
   - If you have underlying health conditions or are taking medications, consult with a healthcare provider before starting any new herbal regimen.

3. **Monitor Effects:**
   - Pay attention to how your body responds to the herbal combinations and adjust dosages as needed.

4. **Use High-Quality Herbs:**
   - Source herbs from reputable suppliers to ensure potency and safety.

5. **Stay Consistent:**
   - Use the herbal combinations consistently as part of your daily routine for best results.

Combining adaptogens with immune-boosting herbs provides a powerful and holistic approach to enhancing stress resilience and immune function. These synergistic combinations can help you manage stress more effectively, boost your immune system, and improve overall health and well-being. By incorporating these herbal blends into your daily routine, you can harness the full potential of nature's remedies to support your body and mind.

Safe Use and Dosage Guidelines

When incorporating adaptogens and immune-boosting herbs into your health regimen, it is crucial to follow safe use and dosage guidelines to maximize benefits and minimize potential risks. This section outlines general recommendations for the safe use of these herbs, along with specific dosage guidelines.

General Guidelines for Safe Use

1. **Consult a Healthcare Provider:**
   - Before starting any new herbal regimen, consult with a healthcare provider, especially if you have underlying health conditions, are pregnant or breastfeeding, or are taking medications.

2. **Start with Low Doses:**

- o Begin with a lower dose to assess your body's response and gradually increase to the recommended dosage.

3. **Monitor for Side Effects:**

   - o Pay attention to any adverse reactions such as digestive upset, allergic reactions, or changes in mood or energy levels. Discontinue use and consult a healthcare provider if you experience any concerning symptoms.

4. **Use High-Quality Herbs:**

   - o Source herbs from reputable suppliers to ensure they are free from contaminants and standardized for potency.

5. **Rotate Herbs:**

   - o To prevent tolerance and maintain effectiveness, consider rotating different herbs or taking periodic breaks from specific herbs.

6. **Avoid Overuse:**

   - o Follow recommended dosages and avoid using higher amounts than suggested, as excessive use can lead to adverse effects.

Specific Dosage Guidelines for Common Adaptogens and Immune-Boosting Herbs

1. **Ashwagandha (Withania somnifera):**

   - o **Capsules/Tablets:** 300-600 mg daily, standardized to 5% withanolides.

   - o **Tincture:** 30-40 drops in water or juice, 2-3 times daily.

   - o **Powder:** 1 teaspoon mixed in warm milk, water, or smoothies daily.

   - o **Precautions:** May cause gastrointestinal upset or drowsiness in some individuals. Avoid during pregnancy unless advised by a healthcare provider.

2. **Rhodiola (Rhodiola rosea):**

   - o **Capsules/Tablets:** 200-600 mg daily, standardized to 3% rosavins and 1% salidroside.

   - o **Tincture:** 30-40 drops in water or juice, 2-3 times daily.

   - o **Tea:** Steep 1 teaspoon of dried Rhodiola root in hot water for 10-15 minutes.

   - o **Precautions:** May cause insomnia or jitteriness in sensitive individuals. Best taken in the morning or early afternoon.

3. **Schisandra (Schisandra chinensis):**

   - o **Capsules/Tablets:** 500-1000 mg daily, standardized to 2% schisandrin.

   - o **Tincture:** 30-40 drops in water or juice, 2-3 times daily.

- ○ **Tea:** Steep 1 teaspoon of dried Schisandra berries in hot water for 10-15 minutes.
- ○ **Precautions:** May cause gastrointestinal upset in some individuals. Use with caution if you have a peptic ulcer.

4. **Echinacea (Echinacea purpurea):**
   - ○ **Capsules/Tablets:** 400-500 mg, 2-3 times daily.
   - ○ **Tincture:** 30-40 drops in water or juice, 2-3 times daily.
   - ○ **Tea:** Steep 1-2 teaspoons of dried Echinacea in hot water for 10-15 minutes.
   - ○ **Precautions:** May cause allergic reactions in individuals allergic to plants in the Asteraceae family. Use with caution if you have an autoimmune disorder.

5. **Elderberry (Sambucus nigra):**
   - ○ **Syrup:** 1 tablespoon daily for immune support, up to 4 tablespoons daily during illness.
   - ○ **Capsules/Tablets:** 300-600 mg daily.
   - ○ **Tea:** Steep 1 teaspoon of dried Elderberries in hot water for 10-15 minutes.
   - ○ **Precautions:** Raw berries, bark, and leaves contain toxic compounds and should not be consumed. Cooked berries are safe.

6. **Astragalus (Astragalus membranaceus):**
   - ○ **Capsules/Tablets:** 400-500 mg, 2-3 times daily.
   - ○ **Tincture:** 30-40 drops in water or juice, 2-3 times daily.
   - ○ **Decoction:** Simmer 1 tablespoon of dried Astragalus root in 4 cups of water for 30-45 minutes. Drink 1-2 cups daily.
   - ○ **Precautions:** May cause digestive upset in some individuals. Use with caution if you have an autoimmune disorder.

By following these safe use and dosage guidelines, you can effectively incorporate adaptogens and immune-boosting herbs into your health regimen. These herbs offer powerful benefits for managing stress and enhancing immune function when used appropriately. Always start with lower doses, monitor for side effects, and consult with a healthcare provider to ensure the best and safest outcomes.

Seasonal Herbs for Cold and Flu Prevention

As the seasons change, the risk of colds and flu often increases, making it essential to support the immune system with natural remedies. Seasonal herbs offer a powerful, effective way to enhance your body's defenses and reduce the likelihood of illness. These herbs, known for their antiviral, antibacterial, and immune-boosting properties, can be used preventatively and at the onset of symptoms to mitigate the severity and duration of colds and flu. In this chapter, we will explore a variety of seasonal herbs that are particularly effective for cold and flu prevention, providing insights into their benefits, how they work, and practical ways to incorporate them into your daily routine to stay healthy year-round.

Preparing for Cold and Flu Season with Herbs

As cold and flu season approaches, it's crucial to take proactive steps to bolster your immune system and minimize the risk of illness. Incorporating herbs into your health regimen can provide significant support. Here are some key strategies and herbs to consider for preparing your body to fend off colds and flu effectively.

Key Strategies for Cold and Flu Prevention

1. **Strengthen the Immune System:**

   o Use immune-boosting herbs regularly to keep your defenses strong.

   o Maintain a healthy diet rich in vitamins and minerals, particularly vitamin C, vitamin D, and zinc.

2. **Reduce Stress:**

   o Chronic stress weakens the immune system, so managing stress is essential.

   o Incorporate adaptogenic herbs to help your body cope with stress.

3. **Get Adequate Sleep:**

   o Aim for 7-9 hours of quality sleep per night to support immune function.

4. **Stay Hydrated:**

   o Drink plenty of water, herbal teas, and other hydrating fluids to keep your mucous membranes moist and better able to trap pathogens.

5. **Practice Good Hygiene:**

   o Wash your hands frequently, avoid touching your face, and disinfect commonly touched surfaces.

Key Herbs for Cold and Flu Prevention

1. **Elderberry (Sambucus nigra):**

   o **Benefits:** Elderberry is rich in antioxidants and has antiviral properties that can prevent and reduce the severity of colds and flu.

   o **Preparation:** Make elderberry syrup by simmering dried elderberries with water and honey. Take 1 tablespoon daily for prevention or 2-4 tablespoons during illness.

2. **Echinacea (Echinacea purpurea):**

- o **Benefits:** Echinacea boosts the immune system by increasing the activity of white blood cells.
- o **Preparation:** Use Echinacea tincture, taking 30-40 drops in water or juice 2-3 times daily during cold and flu season.

3. **Astragalus (Astragalus membranaceus):**
   - o **Benefits:** Astragalus enhances immune function and has adaptogenic properties to help the body resist stress.
   - o **Preparation:** Add dried Astragalus root to soups and stews, or take as a tincture or capsule.

4. **Garlic (Allium sativum):**
   - o **Benefits:** Garlic has strong antiviral, antibacterial, and immune-boosting properties.
   - o **Preparation:** Consume raw garlic in food, or take garlic supplements during cold and flu season.

5. **Ginger (Zingiber officinale):**
   - o **Benefits:** Ginger has anti-inflammatory and antiviral properties, and it can soothe symptoms of colds and flu.
   - o **Preparation:** Make ginger tea by simmering fresh ginger slices in water. Drink 2-3 cups daily.

6. **Andrographis (Andrographis paniculata):**
   - o **Benefits:** Andrographis is known for its antiviral and immune-stimulating properties.
   - o **Preparation:** Take Andrographis supplements according to the dosage instructions during the cold and flu season.

7. **Licorice Root (Glycyrrhiza glabra):**
   - o **Benefits:** Licorice root has antiviral properties and helps soothe the throat and reduce inflammation.
   - o **Preparation:** Make licorice root tea by simmering the dried root in water. Drink 1-2 cups daily.

Herbal Recipes for Cold and Flu Prevention

1. **Immune-Boosting Tea:**
   - o **Ingredients:**
     - ▪ 1 teaspoon dried Echinacea

- 1 teaspoon dried Elderberries
- 1 teaspoon dried Ginger

- **Preparation:** Steep the herbs in hot water for 10-15 minutes. Strain and drink 1-2 cups daily.

2. **Elderberry Syrup:**

   - **Ingredients:**

     - 1 cup dried Elderberries
     - 4 cups water
     - 1 cup honey

   - **Preparation:**

     - Simmer elderberries in water until the liquid reduces by half.
     - Strain and mix the liquid with honey.
     - Store in a glass jar and take 1 tablespoon daily for prevention.

3. **Garlic and Ginger Broth:**

   - **Ingredients:**

     - 4 cloves Garlic, minced
     - 1-inch piece fresh Ginger, sliced
     - 4 cups vegetable or chicken broth

   - **Preparation:**

     - Simmer garlic and ginger in broth for 20 minutes.
     - Drink a cup of the broth daily.

4. **Astragalus Soup:**

   - **Ingredients:**

     - 2 tablespoons dried Astragalus root
     - 4 cups water or broth
     - Vegetables and herbs of your choice

   - **Preparation:**

     - Simmer Astragalus root in water or broth for 30-45 minutes.
     - Add vegetables and herbs and continue cooking until tender.

- Consume regularly during cold and flu season.

Preparing for cold and flu season with herbs involves integrating immune-boosting and adaptogenic herbs into your daily routine. By following these strategies and incorporating these powerful herbs, you can enhance your body's defenses and reduce the likelihood of falling ill. Combining a healthy lifestyle with these natural remedies ensures that you are well-equipped to handle the seasonal increase in colds and flu.

Top Seasonal Herbs: Elderberry, Garlic, and Ginger

As the colder months approach and the risk of colds and flu increases, incorporating powerful seasonal herbs like elderberry, garlic, and ginger into your health regimen can provide significant protection and support. These herbs are renowned for their immune-boosting properties and have been used for centuries to prevent and treat respiratory infections.

Elderberry (Sambucus nigra)

Elderberry is one of the most potent and widely used herbs for preventing and treating colds and flu. Rich in antioxidants, particularly flavonoids like quercetin, elderberry boosts the immune system by increasing the production of cytokines, which help regulate immune responses. Elderberries also possess antiviral properties, making them particularly effective against the influenza virus. Studies have shown that elderberry can reduce the severity and duration of cold and flu symptoms, making it a valuable ally during the winter months.

Elderberry is commonly consumed as a syrup, which is easy to prepare at home by simmering dried elderberries with water and honey. This sweet, tangy syrup can be taken daily as a preventative measure or multiple times a day at the onset of symptoms to mitigate illness. Elderberry gummies, teas, and capsules are also popular forms, providing versatile options for incorporating this powerful herb into your daily routine.

Garlic (Allium sativum)

Garlic is a powerful herb with strong antiviral, antibacterial, and antifungal properties, making it an excellent choice for boosting immune function and fighting infections. Its active compound, allicin, is released when garlic is chopped or crushed, providing potent antimicrobial effects that help prevent and treat colds and flu. Garlic also enhances the activity of immune cells, including macrophages and natural killer cells, which play a crucial role in defending the body against pathogens.

Incorporating garlic into your diet is simple and effective. Raw garlic can be added to salads, dressings, and dips, while cooked garlic enhances the flavor and health benefits of soups, stews, and roasted vegetables. For those who find raw garlic too pungent, garlic supplements are available in capsules and tablets, offering a convenient alternative without the strong taste. Regular consumption of garlic not only supports the immune system but also promotes overall cardiovascular health and provides antioxidant protection.

Ginger (Zingiber officinale)

Ginger is a versatile and widely used herb known for its anti-inflammatory, antiviral, and immune-boosting properties. It contains bioactive compounds like gingerol and shogaol, which have been shown to enhance immune function and reduce inflammation. Ginger is particularly effective in soothing symptoms associated with colds and flu, such as sore throat, congestion, and nausea. Its warming properties also help promote circulation and support the body's natural detoxification processes.

Ginger can be easily incorporated into your daily routine in various forms. Fresh ginger root can be added to teas, smoothies, and meals for a spicy, aromatic flavor. Ginger tea, made by steeping fresh ginger slices in hot water, is a soothing and effective remedy for cold and flu symptoms. Ginger supplements, available in capsules and powders, offer a convenient option for those who prefer a more concentrated dose. Regular consumption of ginger not only supports immune health but also aids digestion and reduces inflammation, contributing to overall wellness.

Conclusion

Elderberry, garlic, and ginger are three powerful herbs that offer substantial benefits for preventing and managing colds and flu. By incorporating these seasonal herbs into your daily regimen, you can enhance your immune system's ability to fight off infections and maintain optimal health during the colder months. Whether consumed as syrups, teas, or supplements, these herbs provide a natural and effective way to support your body's defenses and promote overall well-being.

Herbal Formulas for Cold and Flu Prevention

As the cold and flu season approaches, using herbal formulas can be an effective strategy to enhance your immune system and reduce the risk of illness. Combining multiple herbs that work synergistically can provide a comprehensive approach to preventing colds and flu. Here are some potent herbal formulas to consider incorporating into your health regimen.

Immune-Boosting Tea Blend

One of the most straightforward and enjoyable ways to consume herbs is through a daily tea blend. An immune-boosting tea can combine the benefits of elderberry, echinacea, ginger, and rose hips to create a powerful preventative drink. Elderberries are packed with antioxidants and have strong antiviral properties, while echinacea stimulates the immune system and increases the production of white blood cells. Ginger adds anti-inflammatory and warming properties, helping to soothe the throat and boost circulation. Rose hips are rich in vitamin C, which is essential for a robust immune response.

To prepare this tea, mix 1 teaspoon each of dried elderberries, echinacea root, grated ginger, and rose hips in a teapot. Pour 2 cups of boiling water over the herbs and let them steep for 10-15 minutes. Strain the tea and drink it daily. For added flavor and benefits, consider sweetening with honey, which also has antibacterial properties.

Elderberry and Astragalus Syrup

A homemade elderberry and astragalus syrup is a potent formula for cold and flu prevention. Elderberry's antiviral capabilities combined with astragalus's immune-boosting and adaptogenic properties make this syrup a powerful ally against respiratory infections. Astragalus helps to increase the production of immune cells and enhances the body's resistance to stress, making it particularly useful during the high-stress winter months.

To make the syrup, simmer 1 cup of dried elderberries and 2 tablespoons of dried astragalus root in 4 cups of water until the liquid reduces by half. Strain the mixture, then stir in 1 cup of honey while the liquid is still warm. Store the syrup in a glass jar in the refrigerator. Take 1 tablespoon daily for prevention, and increase to 2-4 tablespoons daily at the first sign of illness.

Garlic and Ginger Elixir

A garlic and ginger elixir is an excellent formula for both prevention and early treatment of colds and flu. Garlic's potent antimicrobial properties combined with ginger's anti-inflammatory and warming effects make this elixir highly effective. This combination not only boosts the immune system but also helps to alleviate symptoms like congestion and sore throat.

To prepare the elixir, finely chop 5 cloves of garlic and 1-inch piece of fresh ginger. Place them in a glass jar and cover with 1 cup of raw apple cider vinegar and 1 cup of honey. Seal the jar and let it sit at room temperature for 1-2 weeks, shaking it daily. Strain the liquid and store it in a clean glass jar. Take 1-2 tablespoons daily as a preventative measure, or every few hours if you feel a cold or flu coming on.

Adaptogenic Immune Tonic

An adaptogenic immune tonic combines herbs like ashwagandha, reishi mushroom, and holy basil to provide comprehensive immune support and stress resilience. Ashwagandha helps regulate the stress response and supports overall vitality, while reishi mushroom boosts immune function and provides anti-inflammatory benefits. Holy basil, known for its adaptogenic and antimicrobial properties, helps to balance the body's systems and enhance resistance to pathogens.

To make the tonic, mix equal parts of ashwagandha root powder, reishi mushroom powder, and holy basil leaves. Add 1 teaspoon of the blend to a cup of warm milk or water, stirring well. Drink this tonic daily to build resilience and support your immune system throughout the cold and flu season.

Herbal Steam Inhalation

For immediate relief and prevention, an herbal steam inhalation can help clear nasal passages and kill pathogens. Combining eucalyptus, thyme, and rosemary creates a potent formula for respiratory health. Eucalyptus has strong antiviral and decongestant properties, thyme is antibacterial and soothing to the respiratory tract, and rosemary provides antioxidant and anti-inflammatory benefits.

To prepare an herbal steam, add a handful of fresh or dried eucalyptus, thyme, and rosemary to a large bowl of boiling water. Lean over the bowl, cover your head with a towel to trap the steam, and breathe deeply for 5-10 minutes. This practice can be done daily during the cold and flu season to help prevent infections and maintain clear respiratory passages.

Incorporating these herbal formulas into your daily routine can provide powerful support for preventing colds and flu. By combining the unique properties of different herbs, you can create effective remedies that boost the immune system, reduce inflammation, and enhance overall well-being. Whether through teas, syrups, elixirs, tonics, or steam inhalations, these herbal preparations offer natural and holistic ways to stay healthy throughout the cold and flu season.

Integrating Seasonal Herbs into Daily Routines

Integrating seasonal herbs into your daily routine can be an effective and enjoyable way to bolster your immune system and enhance overall well-being, especially during the cold and flu season. By making these herbs a regular part of your lifestyle, you can create a proactive approach to health that supports your body's natural defenses.

Start Your Day with Herbal Teas

One of the simplest ways to incorporate seasonal herbs is by starting your day with an immune-boosting herbal tea. A blend of elderberry, echinacea, and ginger can provide a powerful combination of antiviral, anti-inflammatory, and immune-stimulating properties. Prepare a large pot of this tea in the morning, and sip it throughout the day to keep your immune system active and resilient. This not only helps in preventing colds and flu but also provides a comforting and warming start to your day, especially in colder months.

Use Herbs in Cooking

Another easy method to integrate herbs into your routine is by using them in cooking. Garlic and ginger, for instance, are versatile ingredients that can be added to a variety of dishes. Whether you're making soups, stir-fries, or roasted vegetables, these herbs not only enhance the flavor but also provide significant health benefits. Garlic's potent antimicrobial properties and ginger's anti-inflammatory effects make them ideal for daily consumption. Try adding minced garlic and grated ginger to your meals, or even make a simple garlic-ginger broth to sip on throughout the day.

Create Herbal Tinctures and Syrups

For a more concentrated dose of herbal goodness, consider making your own tinctures and syrups. Elderberry syrup is a popular and effective remedy for preventing and treating colds and flu. Taking a tablespoon of elderberry syrup daily can be a powerful preventative measure, while increasing the dose at the onset of symptoms can help mitigate the severity and duration of illness. Similarly, a tincture made from echinacea or astragalus can be taken daily in small doses. These concentrated forms are easy to incorporate into your routine and can be added to water, juice, or taken directly under the tongue.

Incorporate Adaptogenic Tonics

Adaptogens such as ashwagandha, holy basil, and reishi mushroom can be made into tonics that you consume regularly. These herbs help your body adapt to stress and enhance immune function, making them perfect for daily use during the high-stress, high-risk cold and flu season. You can prepare an adaptogenic tonic by mixing these herbs into warm milk, tea, or even smoothies. Regular consumption of these tonics not only supports your immune system but also promotes overall balance and resilience.

Utilize Herbal Steams and Baths

Herbal steams and baths are another effective way to integrate seasonal herbs into your daily routine. An herbal steam using eucalyptus, thyme, and rosemary can help clear nasal passages and kill pathogens, providing immediate relief and prevention. Simply add these herbs to a bowl of boiling water, lean over, and inhale the steam. Additionally, taking a relaxing bath infused with herbs like lavender, chamomile, and peppermint can help soothe the body, reduce stress, and support immune health. These practices can be particularly beneficial at the end of the day to unwind and prepare for restful sleep.

Snack on Herbal Treats

Incorporating herbs into your diet doesn't have to be limited to meals and drinks. You can also create herbal treats that are both delicious and health-promoting. Elderberry gummies, for example, are a tasty way to consume elderberry regularly. Similarly, energy balls made with ingredients like oats, honey, and powdered adaptogens such as ashwagandha or reishi can be a convenient snack. These treats make it easy to integrate herbs into your daily routine without feeling like you're taking medicine.

Integrating seasonal herbs into your daily routine is a practical and effective way to enhance your immune system and overall health, especially during the cold and flu season. By incorporating herbs into teas, meals, tinctures, tonics, steams, and even snacks, you can create a holistic approach to wellness that supports your body's natural defenses. This proactive strategy not only helps prevent illness but also promotes a sense of well-being and resilience, allowing you to navigate the colder months with greater confidence and vitality.

Recipes for Immune-Boosting Teas and Syrups

As we navigate through the cold and flu season, immune-boosting teas and syrups can be invaluable allies in maintaining health and preventing illness. These recipes harness the power of potent herbs and natural ingredients to fortify your immune system and provide a comforting defense against common ailments. Here are some tried-and-true recipes for creating your own immune-boosting teas and syrups at home.

Elderberry and Echinacea Immune-Boosting Tea

Elderberry and echinacea are renowned for their immune-boosting properties. Elderberries are rich in antioxidants and have antiviral effects, while echinacea stimulates the immune system and increases the production of white blood cells. Combining these with the warming, anti-inflammatory properties of ginger creates a powerful tea to fend off colds and flu.

To prepare this tea, you'll need:

- 1 tablespoon dried elderberries

- 1 tablespoon dried echinacea root

- 1 teaspoon freshly grated ginger

- 1 cinnamon stick (optional for added warmth and flavor)

- 4 cups of water

- Honey or lemon to taste

Bring the water to a boil in a saucepan, then add the elderberries, echinacea root, ginger, and cinnamon stick. Reduce the heat and let the mixture simmer for 20 minutes. Remove from heat and strain the tea into a teapot or directly into mugs. Sweeten with honey and add a squeeze of lemon if desired. Drink this tea daily during cold and flu season for preventive benefits, or several times a day at the onset of symptoms to help mitigate the illness.

Garlic and Ginger Elixir

Garlic and ginger are powerhouse ingredients with potent immune-boosting and antimicrobial properties. This elixir is not only effective in boosting your immune system but also helps soothe sore throats and reduce congestion.

To make the garlic and ginger elixir, gather:

- 5 cloves of garlic, minced

- 1-inch piece of fresh ginger, grated

- 1 cup raw honey

- 1 cup raw apple cider vinegar

Combine the minced garlic and grated ginger in a glass jar. Pour the honey and apple cider vinegar over the garlic and ginger, stirring well to combine. Seal the jar tightly and let it sit at room temperature for at least a week, shaking it daily to help the ingredients infuse. After a week, strain the mixture and transfer the elixir to a clean jar. Take 1-2 tablespoons of this elixir daily as a preventative measure, or every few hours if you feel a cold or flu coming on.

Elderberry Syrup

Elderberry syrup is a classic remedy for cold and flu prevention and treatment. It's easy to make and provides a delicious, sweet way to incorporate the powerful antiviral properties of elderberries into your daily routine.

To make elderberry syrup, you'll need:

- 1 cup dried elderberries

- 4 cups water

- 1-2 tablespoons fresh ginger, grated

- 1 teaspoon cinnamon

- 1 cup raw honey

In a saucepan, combine the dried elderberries, water, grated ginger, and cinnamon. Bring the mixture to a boil, then reduce the heat and let it simmer until the liquid reduces by half, about 45 minutes. Remove from heat and let it cool slightly. Strain the mixture into a bowl, pressing the berries to extract as much liquid as possible. Stir in the honey until well combined. Pour the syrup into a glass jar and store it in the refrigerator. Take 1 tablespoon daily for prevention, or 2-4 tablespoons during illness.

Adaptogenic Herbal Tonic

This adaptogenic herbal tonic combines the stress-reducing properties of ashwagandha, the immune-boosting benefits of reishi mushroom, and the balancing effects of holy basil. It's a nourishing drink that supports overall resilience and immune health.

For this tonic, you'll need:

- 1 teaspoon ashwagandha powder

- 1 teaspoon reishi mushroom powder

- 1 teaspoon dried holy basil leaves

- 1 teaspoon honey or to taste

- 1 cup warm water or milk (dairy or plant-based)

Mix the ashwagandha powder, reishi mushroom powder, and dried holy basil leaves in a cup of warm water or milk. Stir well until the powders are fully dissolved. Add honey to taste for a touch of sweetness. Drink this tonic once daily to support your immune system and enhance your body's ability to handle stress.

Incorporating these immune-boosting teas and syrups into your daily routine can significantly enhance your body's defenses against colds and flu. These recipes harness the natural power of herbs and ingredients known for their medicinal properties, providing a holistic approach to health and wellness. Whether you're sipping on a comforting cup of elderberry tea or taking a spoonful of garlic and ginger elixir, these homemade remedies offer a natural, effective way to stay healthy throughout the cold and flu season.

Tips for Staying Healthy Year-Round

Maintaining good health year-round requires a holistic approach that encompasses diet, exercise, stress management, and preventive care. By adopting healthy habits and making mindful choices, you can enhance your well-being and reduce the risk of illness. Here are some essential tips for staying healthy throughout the year.

Prioritize a Balanced Diet

A balanced diet rich in fruits, vegetables, whole grains, lean proteins, and healthy fats is the foundation of good health. These foods provide essential nutrients that support immune function, energy levels, and overall vitality. Incorporate a variety of colorful fruits and vegetables to ensure you're getting a wide range of vitamins, minerals, and antioxidants. Foods like berries, leafy greens, nuts, seeds, and fatty fish are particularly beneficial for their anti-inflammatory properties. Limit your intake of processed foods, refined sugars, and unhealthy fats, which can contribute to inflammation and weaken the immune system.

Stay Hydrated

Proper hydration is crucial for maintaining health. Water supports digestion, circulation, temperature regulation, and the elimination of toxins. Aim to drink at least eight glasses of water a day, more if you are physically active or live in a hot climate. Herbal teas, such as those made from ginger, peppermint, or chamomile, can also be a good source of hydration and provide additional health benefits. Avoid sugary drinks and excessive caffeine, which can lead to dehydration and other health issues.

Regular Physical Activity

Engaging in regular physical activity is vital for maintaining a healthy body and mind. Exercise helps to boost the immune system, improve cardiovascular health, maintain a healthy weight, and reduce stress. Aim for at least 150 minutes of moderate-intensity aerobic activity, such as brisk walking or cycling, or 75 minutes of vigorous-intensity activity, such as running or swimming, each week. Incorporate strength training exercises at least twice a week to build muscle and maintain bone health. Find activities you enjoy making exercise a consistent and enjoyable part of your routine.

Manage Stress

Chronic stress can have a detrimental impact on your health, weakening the immune system and increasing the risk of various health problems, including heart disease and mental health disorders. Effective stress management techniques are essential for maintaining health. Practices such as mindfulness meditation, deep breathing exercises, yoga, and tai chi can help reduce stress and promote relaxation. Make time for hobbies and activities that you enjoy, and ensure you get adequate rest and relaxation. Building a strong social support network can also provide emotional support and reduce stress.

Get Adequate Sleep

Quality sleep is essential for overall health and well-being. During sleep, the body repairs itself, and the immune system is strengthened. Aim for 7-9 hours of sleep per night. Establish a regular sleep routine by going to bed and waking up at the same time each day. Create a sleep-friendly environment by keeping your bedroom cool, dark, and quiet. Limit exposure to screens and electronic devices before bedtime, as the blue light emitted can interfere with the production of melatonin, the hormone that regulates sleep.

Preventive Health Care

Regular check-ups and preventive health care are crucial for early detection and management of potential health issues. Schedule annual physical exams, dental check-ups, and eye exams. Stay up-to-date with vaccinations and screenings, such as mammograms, colonoscopies, and blood pressure checks. Discuss any health concerns with your healthcare provider and follow their recommendations for maintaining optimal health.

Practice Good Hygiene

Good hygiene practices are essential for preventing the spread of infections. Wash your hands frequently with soap and water, especially before eating, after using the restroom, and after being in public places. Use hand sanitizer when soap and water are not available. Avoid touching your face, particularly your eyes, nose, and mouth, to reduce the risk of transferring germs. Maintain proper oral hygiene by brushing and flossing your teeth daily and visiting the dentist regularly.

Incorporate Herbal Remedies

Incorporating herbal remedies into your daily routine can provide additional support for your immune system and overall health. Herbs like elderberry, echinacea, garlic, and ginger have been shown to enhance immune function and protect against illness. Use these herbs in teas, tinctures, syrups, and meals to boost your body's natural defenses. Adaptogenic herbs like ashwagandha, rhodiola, and holy basil can help manage stress and improve resilience.

Staying healthy year-round involves a combination of nutritious eating, regular physical activity, adequate sleep, stress management, preventive care, and good hygiene practices. By integrating these habits into your daily routine, you can enhance your overall well-being, reduce the risk of illness, and enjoy a higher quality of life.

BOOK 7:

Comprehensive Herbal Remedies: Natural Solutions for a Variety of Specific Diseases

Herbal Treatments for Cardiovascular Health

Cardiovascular health is a cornerstone of overall well-being, encompassing the proper functioning of the heart and blood vessels. As cardiovascular diseases such as hypertension, atherosclerosis, and heart disease continue to be leading causes of morbidity and mortality worldwide, the search for effective prevention and treatment strategies is ever important. While conventional medicine offers various treatments for these conditions, many individuals are turning to natural remedies to complement or enhance their cardiovascular health care.

Herbal treatments have been used for centuries to support cardiovascular health. These natural solutions can help regulate blood pressure, reduce cholesterol levels, improve blood circulation, and strengthen the heart muscle. Herbs such as hawthorn, garlic, and ginkgo biloba are known for their cardioprotective properties, offering a safe and effective means to maintain and improve heart health. Additionally, lifestyle changes including a balanced diet, regular exercise, and stress management are essential components of a holistic approach to cardiovascular wellness.

In this chapter, we will explore the benefits of various herbs for cardiovascular health, delve into the science behind their efficacy, and provide practical recipes and dosage guidelines for incorporating these powerful plants into your daily routine. By understanding and utilizing these natural remedies, you can take proactive steps towards a healthier heart and a longer, more vibrant life.

Key Herbs for Heart Health

Integrating herbal remedies into your routine can be a powerful way to support cardiovascular health. Here are some key herbs known for their heart-healthy properties:

1. Hawthorn (Crataegus spp.)

Description:

- Hawthorn is a well-known herb in traditional medicine, particularly for its beneficial effects on the cardiovascular system. The leaves, flowers, and berries are used medicinally.

Benefits:

- **Strengthens Heart Muscle:** Hawthorn helps improve the contractility of the heart muscle, enhancing its pumping efficiency.

- **Regulates Blood Pressure:** It can help lower high blood pressure and stabilize low blood pressure by dilating blood vessels and improving circulation.

- **Antioxidant Properties:** Rich in flavonoids and oligomeric procyanidins, hawthorn protects the heart from oxidative stress and inflammation.

Usage:

- **Tea:** Steep 1-2 teaspoons of dried hawthorn berries or leaves in hot water for 10-15 minutes. Drink 2-3 cups daily.
- **Tincture:** Take 30-40 drops in water or juice, 2-3 times daily.
- **Capsules:** Follow the dosage instructions on the product label.

2. Garlic (Allium sativum)

Description:

- Garlic is a versatile culinary and medicinal herb known for its cardiovascular benefits. It is rich in sulfur compounds, particularly allicin, which contributes to its health effects.

Benefits:

- **Reduces Cholesterol Levels:** Garlic has been shown to lower total and LDL cholesterol levels.
- **Lowers Blood Pressure:** It helps reduce hypertension by relaxing blood vessels and improving blood flow.
- **Anti-inflammatory and Antioxidant:** Garlic's anti-inflammatory and antioxidant properties protect the cardiovascular system from damage.

Usage:

- **Raw:** Consume 1-2 cloves of raw garlic daily, minced and added to food.
- **Supplements:** Take garlic supplements as directed, typically 600-1200 mg daily.
- **Garlic Oil:** Use garlic-infused oil for cooking or take a few drops daily.

3. Ginkgo Biloba

Description:

- Ginkgo biloba is an ancient tree with leaves that have been used in traditional medicine to enhance cognitive function and improve cardiovascular health.

Benefits:

- **Improves Circulation:** Ginkgo biloba enhances blood flow by dilating blood vessels and reducing blood viscosity.
- **Antioxidant Properties:** It protects the cardiovascular system from oxidative damage and inflammation.
- **Prevents Blood Clots:** Ginkgo biloba has antiplatelet effects, which help prevent the formation of blood clots.

Usage:

- **Tea:** Steep 1 teaspoon of dried ginkgo leaves in hot water for 10-15 minutes. Drink 1-2 cups daily.
- **Tincture:** Take 30-40 drops in water or juice, 2-3 times daily.
- **Capsules:** Follow the dosage instructions on the product label.

4. Hawthorn (Crataegus spp.)

Description:

- Hawthorn is a well-known herb in traditional medicine, particularly for its beneficial effects on the cardiovascular system. The leaves, flowers, and berries are used medicinally.

Benefits:

- **Strengthens Heart Muscle:** Hawthorn helps improve the contractility of the heart muscle, enhancing its pumping efficiency.
- **Regulates Blood Pressure:** It can help lower high blood pressure and stabilize low blood pressure by dilating blood vessels and improving circulation.
- **Antioxidant Properties:** Rich in flavonoids and oligomeric procyanidins, hawthorn protects the heart from oxidative stress and inflammation.

Usage:

- **Tea:** Steep 1-2 teaspoons of dried hawthorn berries or leaves in hot water for 10-15 minutes. Drink 2-3 cups daily.
- **Tincture:** Take 30-40 drops in water or juice, 2-3 times daily.
- **Capsules:** Follow the dosage instructions on the product label.

5. Motherwort (Leonurus cardiaca)

Description:

- Motherwort is a herb traditionally used to treat heart conditions and anxiety. Its name reflects its historical use in heart health and women's health.

Benefits:

- **Reduces Palpitations:** Motherwort is effective in reducing heart palpitations and tachycardia (rapid heartbeat).
- **Lowers Blood Pressure:** It helps reduce high blood pressure by relaxing the blood vessels.
- **Calming Effect:** Motherwort has a mild sedative effect, which can help reduce stress and anxiety.

Usage:

- **Tea:** Steep 1-2 teaspoons of dried motherwort in hot water for 10-15 minutes. Drink 1-2 cups daily.

- **Tincture:** Take 30-40 drops in water or juice, 2-3 times daily.

- **Capsules:** Follow the dosage instructions on the product label.

6. Hibiscus (Hibiscus sabdariffa)

Description:

- Hibiscus is a vibrant flower known for its tart flavor and cardiovascular benefits. The calyx of the flower is used to make teas and extracts.

Benefits:

- **Lowers Blood Pressure:** Hibiscus tea has been shown to lower blood pressure in people with mild to moderate hypertension.

- **Antioxidant Properties:** Rich in anthocyanins, hibiscus protects the cardiovascular system from oxidative stress.

- **Improves Lipid Profiles:** It helps reduce cholesterol and triglyceride levels, promoting overall heart health.

Usage:

- **Tea:** Steep 1-2 teaspoons of dried hibiscus flowers in hot water for 10-15 minutes. Drink 2-3 cups daily.

- **Tincture:** Take 30-40 drops in water or juice, 2-3 times daily.

- **Capsules:** Follow the dosage instructions on the product label.

These key herbs—hawthorn, garlic, ginkgo biloba, motherwort, and hibiscus—offer powerful support for cardiovascular health. By incorporating these herbs into your daily routine through teas, tinctures, and supplements, you can enhance heart function, regulate blood pressure, improve circulation, and protect your cardiovascular system from oxidative stress and inflammation. Always consult with a healthcare provider before starting any new herbal regimen, especially if you have existing health conditions or are taking medications.

Recipes and Dosages for Cardiovascular Support

Incorporating herbal remedies into your daily routine can significantly enhance cardiovascular health. Here are some effective recipes and dosages to support heart health using key herbs such as hawthorn, garlic, ginkgo biloba, motherwort, and hibiscus.

1. Hawthorn Berry Heart Tonic

Ingredients:

- 1 tablespoon dried hawthorn berries
- 1 teaspoon dried hibiscus flowers
- 1 cinnamon stick (optional)
- 4 cups water
- Honey or lemon to taste (optional)

Instructions:

1. In a saucepan, combine the hawthorn berries, hibiscus flowers, and cinnamon stick.
2. Add 4 cups of water and bring to a boil.
3. Reduce heat and let simmer for 20-30 minutes.
4. Remove from heat and let steep for an additional 10 minutes.
5. Strain the mixture into a teapot or mug.
6. Add honey or lemon to taste, if desired.

Dosage:

- Drink 1-2 cups of this heart tonic daily for cardiovascular support.

2. Garlic and Ginger Heart Health Elixir

Ingredients:

- 5 cloves of garlic, minced
- 1-inch piece of fresh ginger, grated
- 1 cup raw honey
- 1 cup raw apple cider vinegar

Instructions:

1. In a glass jar, combine the minced garlic and grated ginger.
2. Pour the honey and apple cider vinegar over the garlic and ginger.
3. Stir well to combine and seal the jar tightly.
4. Let the mixture sit at room temperature for at least a week, shaking it daily to help the ingredients infuse.
5. After a week, strain the mixture and transfer the elixir to a clean jar.

Dosage:

- Take 1-2 tablespoons of this elixir daily as a preventative measure for heart health.

3. Ginkgo Biloba and Motherwort Tea

Ingredients:

- 1 teaspoon dried ginkgo biloba leaves
- 1 teaspoon dried motherwort
- 1 teaspoon dried lemon balm (optional, for flavor)
- 2 cups boiling water
- Honey to taste (optional)

Instructions:

1. In a teapot or mug, combine the ginkgo biloba leaves, motherwort, and lemon balm.
2. Pour 2 cups of boiling water over the herbs.
3. Cover and let steep for 10-15 minutes.
4. Strain the tea into a mug.
5. Add honey to taste, if desired.

Dosage:

- Drink 1-2 cups of this tea daily to support cardiovascular health and reduce stress.

4. Hibiscus and Hawthorn Iced Tea

Ingredients:

- 2 tablespoons dried hibiscus flowers
- 1 tablespoon dried hawthorn berries
- 4 cups water
- Fresh mint leaves (optional, for garnish)
- Lemon slices (optional, for garnish)
- Ice cubes

Instructions:

1. In a saucepan, combine the hibiscus flowers and hawthorn berries.
2. Add 4 cups of water and bring to a boil.
3. Reduce heat and let simmer for 15-20 minutes.
4. Remove from heat and let steep for an additional 10 minutes.
5. Strain the mixture into a pitcher and let it cool.

6. Serve over ice, garnished with fresh mint leaves and lemon slices if desired.

Dosage:

- Drink 1-2 glasses of this iced tea daily for a refreshing and heart-healthy beverage.

5. Heart Health Capsules

Ingredients:

- 1 teaspoon ashwagandha powder
- 1 teaspoon reishi mushroom powder
- 1 teaspoon dried holy basil leaves

Instructions:

1. Mix the ashwagandha powder, reishi mushroom powder, and dried holy basil leaves in a bowl.

2. Use a capsule-filling machine or by hand to fill empty gelatin or vegetarian capsules with the herb mixture.

3. Store the filled capsules in an airtight container.

Dosage:

- Take 1-2 capsules daily to support heart health and enhance stress resilience.

These recipes and dosages offer natural and effective ways to support cardiovascular health. By incorporating these heart-healthy herbal remedies into your daily routine, you can enhance heart function, regulate blood pressure, improve circulation, and protect your cardiovascular system from oxidative stress and inflammation. Always consult with a healthcare provider before starting any new herbal regimen, especially if you have existing health conditions or are taking medications.

Case Studies and Success Stories

Understanding real-life applications and outcomes of using herbal treatments for cardiovascular health can provide valuable insights and encouragement. Here are a few case studies and success stories that highlight the effectiveness of herbs such as hawthorn, garlic, ginkgo biloba, motherwort, and hibiscus in supporting heart health.

Case Study 1: Hawthorn for Hypertension and Heart Strength

Background: John, a 55-year-old man with a history of hypertension and early-stage heart failure, sought a natural approach to complement his conventional treatments. Despite taking prescribed medications, he experienced fatigue and occasional chest discomfort.

Intervention: John started taking a hawthorn berry tea, prepared by steeping 1 tablespoon of dried hawthorn berries in 2 cups of hot water, twice daily. He also incorporated hawthorn tincture, taking 30 drops three times daily.

Outcome: After three months, John reported significant improvements in his energy levels and a reduction in chest discomfort. His blood pressure readings improved, and his cardiologist noted better heart function during his follow-up visit. John continued using hawthorn alongside his prescribed medications, with his doctor's approval.

Conclusion: Hawthorn proved to be an effective complementary treatment for hypertension and heart failure, enhancing John's overall cardiovascular health and quality of life.

Case Study 2: Garlic for Cholesterol Management

Background: Lisa, a 48-year-old woman with elevated cholesterol levels, wanted to avoid starting statin medications due to potential side effects. She decided to explore natural alternatives to manage her cholesterol.

Intervention: Lisa began incorporating raw garlic into her diet, consuming two cloves daily. She also added garlic supplements, taking 600 mg of standardized garlic extract twice daily.

Outcome: After six months, Lisa's cholesterol levels significantly improved. Her total cholesterol dropped by 20%, and her LDL (bad cholesterol) decreased by 25%. Lisa also noticed an increase in her HDL (good cholesterol) levels. She attributed these improvements to the consistent use of garlic in her diet and supplement regimen.

Conclusion: Garlic effectively managed Lisa's cholesterol levels, reducing her risk of cardiovascular disease without the need for statin medications.

Case Study 3: Ginkgo Biloba for Improved Circulation

Background: Michael, a 62-year-old man with peripheral artery disease (PAD), experienced pain and cramping in his legs while walking, a condition known as intermittent claudication. Seeking relief, he turned to herbal remedies.

Intervention: Michael started taking ginkgo biloba supplements, 120 mg twice daily, along with his prescribed medications. He also drank ginkgo biloba tea, prepared by steeping 1 teaspoon of dried ginkgo leaves in hot water, twice daily.

Outcome: Within four months, Michael noticed a significant reduction in leg pain and cramping. He could walk longer distances without discomfort, and his overall mobility improved. His vascular specialist confirmed better blood flow in his legs during a follow-up examination.

Conclusion: Ginkgo biloba enhanced Michael's circulation and alleviated symptoms of PAD, improving his quality of life and physical activity levels.

Case Study 4: Motherwort for Stress-Induced Palpitations

Background: Sarah, a 45-year-old woman, experienced frequent heart palpitations due to high stress levels. Despite practicing stress management techniques, she continued to struggle with these symptoms.

Intervention: Sarah incorporated motherwort into her routine, taking 40 drops of motherwort tincture in water three times daily. She also started drinking motherwort tea, prepared by steeping 1 teaspoon of dried motherwort in hot water, twice daily.

Outcome: After two months, Sarah reported a significant reduction in the frequency and intensity of her heart palpitations. She felt calmer and more relaxed overall, attributing these improvements to the consistent use of motherwort.

Conclusion: Motherwort effectively alleviated Sarah's stress-induced palpitations, providing a natural solution to her cardiovascular symptoms.

Case Study 5: Hibiscus for Lowering Blood Pressure

Background: James, a 60-year-old man with mild hypertension, wanted to manage his blood pressure naturally without starting medication. He sought a herbal approach to complement his healthy lifestyle.

Intervention: James began drinking hibiscus tea, made by steeping 1 tablespoon of dried hibiscus flowers in 2 cups of hot water, twice daily. He also incorporated a daily hibiscus supplement, taking 500 mg in capsule form.

Outcome: After three months, James experienced a notable reduction in his blood pressure readings. His systolic blood pressure dropped by an average of 10 points, and his diastolic pressure decreased by 7 points. He also reported feeling more energetic and less stressed.

Hibiscus proved to be a successful natural remedy for lowering James's blood pressure, helping him maintain healthy levels without the need for medication.

These case studies and success stories highlight the potential of herbal treatments to effectively support cardiovascular health. By integrating herbs like hawthorn, garlic, ginkgo biloba, motherwort, and hibiscus into their routines, individuals have experienced significant improvements in heart function, blood pressure, cholesterol levels, and overall well-being. While these stories are encouraging, it is important to consult with a healthcare provider before starting any new herbal regimen, especially for those with existing health conditions or who are taking medications.

Managing Diabetes with Herbs

Diabetes is a chronic condition characterized by high blood sugar levels, resulting from the body's inability to produce or effectively use insulin. Managing diabetes requires a comprehensive approach, including lifestyle modifications, diet, exercise, and medication. In recent years, there has been growing interest in the use of herbal remedies to complement conventional treatments for diabetes. Herbs have been used for centuries in traditional medicine to help regulate blood sugar levels, improve insulin sensitivity, and support overall metabolic health. This chapter will explore various herbs that have shown promise in managing diabetes, providing insights into their mechanisms of action, benefits, and practical applications. By integrating these natural remedies into your diabetes management plan, you can potentially enhance your health and well-being while maintaining better control over your blood sugar levels.

Understanding Diabetes and Herbal Interventions

Diabetes is a metabolic disorder characterized by chronic hyperglycemia (high blood sugar levels), which occurs due to defects in insulin secretion, insulin action, or both. There are two primary types of diabetes: Type 1 diabetes, an autoimmune condition where the body attacks insulin-producing cells in the pancreas, and Type 2 diabetes, which is more common and occurs when the body becomes resistant to insulin or doesn't produce enough insulin.

Managing diabetes effectively involves maintaining blood sugar levels within a target range to prevent complications such as heart disease, kidney failure, neuropathy, and retinopathy. Conventional treatment typically includes lifestyle modifications like diet and exercise, along with medications or insulin therapy. However, many individuals are exploring herbal interventions to complement these conventional treatments and improve their overall diabetes management.

The Role of Herbal Interventions in Diabetes Management

Herbal interventions can offer a natural and complementary approach to managing diabetes. Various herbs have been studied for their potential to regulate blood sugar levels, improve insulin sensitivity, and support overall metabolic health. These herbs often contain bioactive compounds that can influence glucose metabolism and insulin function, providing a multi-faceted approach to diabetes care.

Mechanisms of Action

1. **Regulation of Blood Sugar Levels:**

   o Some herbs help lower blood sugar levels by stimulating insulin secretion, enhancing glucose uptake by cells, or inhibiting the absorption of glucose from the intestines.

2. **Improvement of Insulin Sensitivity:**

   o Certain herbs improve the body's sensitivity to insulin, making it more effective at lowering blood sugar levels. This is particularly beneficial for individuals with Type 2 diabetes, where insulin resistance is a major issue.

3. **Antioxidant Properties:**

   o Oxidative stress plays a significant role in the progression of diabetes and its complications. Many herbs possess antioxidant properties that help reduce oxidative damage and inflammation, supporting overall metabolic health.

4. **Anti-Inflammatory Effects:**

- Chronic inflammation is a contributing factor to insulin resistance and the progression of diabetes. Herbs with anti-inflammatory properties can help mitigate this inflammation, improving insulin sensitivity and glucose metabolism.

Key Herbs for Diabetes Management

1. **Bitter Melon (Momordica charantia):**
   - Known for its hypoglycemic effects, bitter melon contains compounds like charantin and polypeptide-p that mimic insulin and help lower blood sugar levels.

2. **Fenugreek (Trigonella foenum-graecum):**
   - Fenugreek seeds are rich in soluble fiber and compounds like 4-hydroxyisoleucine that help slow the absorption of carbohydrates and improve insulin sensitivity.

3. **Cinnamon (Cinnamomum verum):**
   - Cinnamon has been shown to improve insulin sensitivity and lower fasting blood sugar levels by enhancing the activity of insulin receptors.

4. **Berberine:**
   - Found in plants like goldenseal and barberry, berberine helps lower blood sugar levels by activating AMP-activated protein kinase (AMPK), a key enzyme involved in glucose metabolism.

5. **Gymnema Sylvestre:**
   - Known as the "sugar destroyer," Gymnema Sylvestre reduces sugar absorption in the intestines and improves insulin function.

6. **Aloe Vera:**
   - Aloe vera gel has been shown to lower fasting blood glucose levels and improve HbA1c, a marker of long-term blood sugar control.

Practical Applications

1. **Incorporating Herbs into the Diet:**
   - Herbs like cinnamon and fenugreek can be easily incorporated into meals. Cinnamon can be sprinkled on oatmeal or added to smoothies, while fenugreek seeds can be soaked and added to dishes or taken as a supplement.

2. **Herbal Teas and Extracts:**
   - Bitter melon tea, gymnema tea, and aloe vera juice are practical ways to consume these herbs. Herbal extracts and tinctures offer a concentrated form for easy use.

3. **Supplements:**

- Standardized herbal supplements provide a convenient way to ensure consistent dosing and are widely available for herbs like berberine and gymnema.

Understanding the potential of herbal interventions in managing diabetes provides a holistic approach to supporting blood sugar regulation and overall metabolic health. By integrating these herbs into your diabetes management plan, alongside conventional treatments and lifestyle modifications, you can enhance your health outcomes and improve your quality of life. Always consult with a healthcare provider before starting any new herbal regimen, especially if you have existing health conditions or are taking medications.

Essential Herbs for Blood Sugar Regulation

Managing blood sugar levels is crucial for individuals with diabetes, and incorporating certain herbs into your diet can provide additional support. Here are some essential herbs that have been shown to help regulate blood sugar levels effectively.

1. Bitter Melon (Momordica charantia)

Description: Bitter melon, also known as bitter gourd, is a tropical fruit widely used in traditional medicine for its hypoglycemic effects.

Key Compounds:

- Charantin
- Polypeptide-p
- Vicine

Benefits:

- **Lowers Blood Sugar Levels:** Bitter melon contains compounds that mimic insulin and improve glucose uptake by cells.
- **Enhances Insulin Secretion:** It stimulates the pancreas to produce more insulin.
- **Reduces Glucose Absorption:** Bitter melon helps reduce the absorption of glucose in the intestines.

Usage:

- **Juice:** Drink 50-100 ml of fresh bitter melon juice on an empty stomach in the morning.
- **Tea:** Steep dried bitter melon slices in hot water for 10-15 minutes. Drink 1-2 cups daily.
- **Capsules:** Take standardized bitter melon supplements as directed on the product label.

2. Fenugreek (Trigonella foenum-graecum)

Description: Fenugreek is a herb commonly used in Indian cuisine and traditional medicine, known for its blood sugar-lowering properties.

Key Compounds:

- 4-Hydroxyisoleucine

- Galactomannan

- Trigonelline

Benefits:

- **Slows Carbohydrate Absorption:** The soluble fiber in fenugreek seeds helps slow the absorption of carbohydrates.

- **Improves Insulin Sensitivity:** Fenugreek enhances the body's ability to use insulin.

- **Lowers Blood Sugar Levels:** Regular consumption of fenugreek can reduce fasting blood sugar levels.

Usage:

- **Seeds:** Soak 1-2 tablespoons of fenugreek seeds in water overnight and consume them in the morning on an empty stomach.

- **Powder:** Add fenugreek seed powder to meals or take 1-2 teaspoons daily with water.

- **Capsules:** Take fenugreek supplements as directed on the product label.

3. Cinnamon (Cinnamomum verum)

Description: Cinnamon is a popular spice with a long history of medicinal use, particularly for blood sugar regulation.

Key Compounds:

- Cinnamaldehyde

- Cinnamic acid

- Polyphenols

Benefits:

- **Enhances Insulin Sensitivity:** Cinnamon improves the activity of insulin receptors.

- **Lowers Fasting Blood Sugar Levels:** It can help reduce blood sugar levels by slowing the breakdown of carbohydrates in the digestive tract.

- **Antioxidant Properties:** Cinnamon provides antioxidant benefits that protect against oxidative stress.

Usage:

- **Powder:** Add 1 teaspoon of cinnamon powder to your daily diet, such as in oatmeal, smoothies, or yogurt.

- **Tea:** Steep a cinnamon stick in hot water for 10-15 minutes. Drink 1-2 cups daily.

- **Capsules:** Take standardized cinnamon supplements as directed on the product label.

4. Berberine

Description: Berberine is a bioactive compound found in several plants, including goldenseal, barberry, and Oregon grape, known for its potent blood sugar-lowering effects.

Key Compounds:

- Berberine

Benefits:

- **Activates AMPK:** Berberine activates AMP-activated protein kinase (AMPK), which helps regulate glucose metabolism.
- **Reduces Blood Sugar Levels:** It has been shown to lower fasting blood glucose and improve HbA1c levels.
- **Improves Insulin Sensitivity:** Berberine enhances insulin sensitivity and reduces insulin resistance.

Usage:

- **Capsules:** Take 500 mg of berberine, 2-3 times daily before meals.

5. Gymnema Sylvestre

Description: Gymnema Sylvestre, also known as the "sugar destroyer," is a herb used in Ayurvedic medicine to help manage diabetes.

Key Compounds:

- Gymnemic acids

Benefits:

- **Reduces Sugar Absorption:** Gymnema reduces the absorption of sugar in the intestines.
- **Improves Insulin Function:** It enhances the function of insulin and helps regenerate insulin-producing cells in the pancreas.
- **Reduces Sugar Cravings:** Gymnema can help curb sugar cravings, making it easier to manage dietary intake.

Usage:

- **Tea:** Steep 1 teaspoon of dried Gymnema leaves in hot water for 10-15 minutes. Drink 1-2 cups daily.
- **Capsules:** Take standardized Gymnema supplements as directed on the product label.

6. Aloe Vera

Description: Aloe vera is a succulent plant known for its medicinal properties, including blood sugar regulation.

Key Compounds:

- Polysaccharides
- Anthraquinones

Benefits:

- **Lowers Fasting Blood Sugar:** Aloe vera gel has been shown to lower fasting blood glucose levels.
- **Improves HbA1c Levels:** Regular use of aloe vera can improve long-term blood sugar control.
- **Anti-Inflammatory Properties:** Aloe vera's anti-inflammatory effects support overall metabolic health.

Usage:

- **Juice:** Drink 1-2 tablespoons of aloe vera juice daily.
- **Gel:** Add fresh aloe vera gel to smoothies or drinks.

Incorporating these essential herbs into your daily routine can provide significant support in regulating blood sugar levels and managing diabetes. Bitter melon, fenugreek, cinnamon, berberine, Gymnema Sylvestre, and aloe vera offer various mechanisms to help control blood sugar and improve insulin sensitivity. As with any natural remedy, it is important to consult with a healthcare provider before starting any new herbal regimen, especially if you have existing health conditions or are taking medications. By integrating these herbs into a comprehensive diabetes management plan, you can enhance your health and achieve better blood sugar control.

Herbal Recipes for Diabetes Management

Incorporating herbal remedies into your daily diet can be a delicious and effective way to help manage diabetes. Here are some herbal recipes that harness the power of herbs like bitter melon, fenugreek, cinnamon, berberine, Gymnema Sylvestre, and aloe vera to support blood sugar regulation and overall metabolic health.

1. Bitter Melon Stir-Fry

Ingredients:

- 1 large bitter melon
- 1 tablespoon olive oil or coconut oil
- 1 small onion, thinly sliced
- 2 cloves garlic, minced

- 1 teaspoon turmeric powder

- 1/2 teaspoon cumin seeds

- Salt and pepper to taste

- Fresh cilantro for garnish

Instructions:

1. Cut the bitter melon lengthwise and remove the seeds. Slice it into thin half-moons.

2. Heat the oil in a pan over medium heat. Add the cumin seeds and let them sizzle for a few seconds.

3. Add the sliced onion and garlic, and sauté until they become translucent.

4. Add the bitter melon slices, turmeric powder, salt, and pepper. Stir well to combine.

5. Cover the pan and cook for about 10-15 minutes, stirring occasionally, until the bitter melon is tender.

6. Garnish with fresh cilantro and serve as a side dish or over brown rice or quinoa.

Dosage:

- Consume this dish 2-3 times a week as part of your diabetes management plan.

2. Fenugreek Seed Water

Ingredients:

- 1 tablespoon fenugreek seeds

- 1 cup water

Instructions:

1. Soak the fenugreek seeds in water overnight.

2. In the morning, strain the seeds and drink the water on an empty stomach.

Dosage:

- Drink fenugreek seed water daily to help regulate blood sugar levels.

3. Cinnamon and Oatmeal Breakfast

Ingredients:

- 1/2 cup rolled oats

- 1 cup water or milk (dairy or plant-based)

- 1 teaspoon ground cinnamon

- 1 tablespoon chia seeds

- Fresh berries or sliced fruit for topping

- Nuts or seeds for topping (optional)

Instructions:

1. In a saucepan, bring the water or milk to a boil.

2. Add the rolled oats and reduce the heat to a simmer. Cook for about 5 minutes, stirring occasionally, until the oats are tender.

3. Stir in the ground cinnamon and chia seeds.

4. Transfer the oatmeal to a bowl and top with fresh berries or sliced fruit and nuts or seeds.

Dosage:

- Enjoy this cinnamon-infused oatmeal for breakfast several times a week to support blood sugar management.

4. Berberine and Turmeric Smoothie

Ingredients:

- 1 cup unsweetened almond milk

- 1/2 cup frozen berries

- 1/2 teaspoon berberine powder

- 1/2 teaspoon turmeric powder

- 1 tablespoon chia seeds

- 1 tablespoon almond butter

- A pinch of black pepper (to enhance turmeric absorption)

- Ice cubes (optional)

Instructions:

1. Combine all ingredients in a blender.

2. Blend until smooth and creamy.

3. Pour into a glass and enjoy immediately.

Dosage:

- Drink this berberine and turmeric smoothie once daily to help regulate blood sugar levels and reduce inflammation.

5. Gymnema Sylvestre Tea

Ingredients:

- 1 teaspoon dried Gymnema Sylvestre leaves
- 1 cup boiling water
- Lemon or honey to taste (optional)

Instructions:

1. Place the dried Gymnema leaves in a teapot or mug.
2. Pour boiling water over the leaves and let steep for 10-15 minutes.
3. Strain the tea and add lemon or honey to taste, if desired.

Dosage:

- Drink 1-2 cups of Gymnema Sylvestre tea daily to help reduce sugar absorption and improve insulin function.

6. Aloe Vera Juice Blend

Ingredients:

- 2 tablespoons fresh aloe vera gel
- 1 cup water or coconut water
- 1 tablespoon lemon juice
- 1 teaspoon honey (optional)
- A few mint leaves (optional)

Instructions:

1. Scoop the fresh aloe vera gel from an aloe leaf.
2. Combine the aloe vera gel, water or coconut water, lemon juice, honey, and mint leaves in a blender.
3. Blend until smooth.
4. Pour into a glass and enjoy.

Dosage:

- Drink this aloe vera juice blend once daily to help lower fasting blood sugar levels and improve overall metabolic health.

These herbal recipes provide a tasty and practical way to incorporate blood sugar-regulating herbs into your daily diet. By using ingredients like bitter melon, fenugreek, cinnamon, berberine, Gymnema Sylvestre, and aloe vera, you can naturally support your diabetes management efforts. As always, it is important to consult with a healthcare provider before starting any new herbal regimen, especially if you have existing health conditions or are taking medications. By integrating these delicious and nutritious recipes into your routine, you can enhance your health and achieve better blood sugar control.

Practical Tips for Incorporating Herbs into Daily Life

Incorporating herbs into your daily routine can be a simple yet powerful way to enhance your health, particularly for managing conditions like diabetes. Here are some practical tips to help you seamlessly integrate these beneficial plants into your everyday life.

Start with Familiar Foods

One of the easiest ways to begin incorporating herbs into your diet is by adding them to foods you already eat. For instance, adding a sprinkle of cinnamon to your morning oatmeal, yogurt, or smoothie can provide a tasty way to benefit from its blood sugar-regulating properties. Similarly, you can incorporate garlic into your cooking by adding it to sauces, soups, and stir-fries. Starting with familiar foods makes it less daunting to introduce new herbs into your diet.

Use Herbal Teas

Herbal teas are a convenient and enjoyable way to consume beneficial herbs daily. Teas made from herbs like Gymnema Sylvestre, cinnamon, and fenugreek can be easily brewed and consumed throughout the day. Preparing a pot of herbal tea in the morning and drinking it warm or cold can ensure that you get a consistent dose of these health-promoting herbs. This practice not only supports your health but also provides a calming ritual.

Incorporate Herbs into Smoothies

Smoothies are another versatile vehicle for herbs. Adding fresh aloe vera gel, a teaspoon of berberine powder, or a sprinkle of cinnamon to your smoothie can enhance its health benefits without altering the taste significantly. Smoothies are particularly useful for incorporating herbs that might have a strong flavor when consumed alone. Blending these herbs with fruits, vegetables, and healthy fats can create a nutrient-dense drink that supports your health goals.

Cook with Herbs

Incorporating herbs into your cooking is an excellent way to make them a regular part of your diet. Herbs like fenugreek, garlic, and ginger can be added to a variety of dishes, including soups, stews, curries, and salads. For example, you can use fenugreek seeds in your salads or stir-fries, and garlic can be added to virtually any savory dish. Cooking with these herbs not only enhances the flavor of your meals but also boosts their nutritional value.

Prepare Herbal Infusions and Decoctions

For herbs that require more intensive preparation, such as bitter melon and certain roots, preparing infusions or decoctions can be beneficial. This involves steeping the herbs in hot water for an extended period to extract their beneficial compounds. Drinking these preparations daily can be an effective way to support blood sugar regulation and overall health. Preparing a large batch at the beginning of the week and storing it in the refrigerator can make it easy to consume a small amount each day.

Use Herbal Supplements

If incorporating fresh or dried herbs into your diet seems challenging, herbal supplements can be a practical alternative. Capsules, tinctures, and extracts of herbs like berberine, Gymnema Sylvestre, and fenugreek are widely available and can provide a concentrated dose of their beneficial compounds. Follow the recommended dosage on the product label or consult with a healthcare provider to determine the appropriate amount for your needs.

Create a Routine

Establishing a routine can help ensure that you consistently consume beneficial herbs. For example, you might start your day with a glass of aloe vera juice, have a cinnamon-spiced smoothie for breakfast, drink a cup of Gymnema Sylvestre tea in the afternoon, and use garlic and fenugreek in your dinner. By incorporating these habits into your daily routine, you make it easier to remember to take your herbs and benefit from their health-promoting properties.

Educate Yourself and Experiment

Understanding the benefits and uses of different herbs can empower you to make informed choices about which ones to incorporate into your diet. Reading about herbs, attending workshops, or consulting with a naturopathic doctor can provide valuable insights. Don't be afraid to experiment with different herbs and preparations to find what works best for you. Each person's body responds differently, so personalizing your approach is key to success.

Incorporating herbs into your daily life can be a straightforward and rewarding way to enhance your health, especially for managing conditions like diabetes. By starting with familiar foods, using herbal teas and smoothies, cooking with herbs, preparing infusions and decoctions, using supplements, creating a routine, and educating yourself, you can seamlessly integrate these powerful plants into your lifestyle. These practical tips can help you harness the natural benefits of herbs, supporting better blood sugar regulation and overall well-being.

BOOK 8:

Herbal Remedies for Various Diseases: Respiratory, Digestive and Skin Condition

Respiratory diseases, such as asthma, bronchitis, and chronic obstructive pulmonary disease (COPD), can significantly impact quality of life by affecting breathing and overall lung function. While conventional treatments, including medications and inhalers, are crucial for managing these conditions, herbal remedies can offer complementary support. Herbs have been used for centuries to alleviate respiratory symptoms, reduce inflammation, and strengthen the immune system. By incorporating specific herbs into your health regimen, you can help manage respiratory diseases more effectively and improve lung health. This chapter explores various herbal remedies known for their beneficial effects on the respiratory system, providing insights into their mechanisms of action, practical applications, and how they can be integrated into a comprehensive approach to respiratory health.

Overview of Respiratory Health and Herbal Support

Respiratory health is essential for maintaining overall well-being, as the respiratory system is responsible for providing oxygen to the body and removing carbon dioxide. The respiratory system includes the nasal passages, throat, larynx, trachea, bronchi, and lungs, all of which work together to facilitate breathing. Common respiratory diseases such as asthma, bronchitis, and chronic obstructive pulmonary disease (COPD) can impair this system, leading to symptoms like shortness of breath, wheezing, coughing, and mucus production.

While conventional medical treatments are crucial for managing these conditions, herbal remedies can provide additional support by enhancing respiratory function, reducing inflammation, and boosting the immune system. Herbs have been used in traditional medicine for centuries to alleviate respiratory symptoms and improve lung health. These natural remedies can be integrated into a holistic approach to respiratory care, offering benefits such as:

Anti-inflammatory Properties

Many respiratory diseases involve chronic inflammation of the airways. Herbs such as turmeric, licorice root, and ginger possess strong anti-inflammatory properties that can help reduce this inflammation, making breathing easier and lessening the severity of symptoms.

Expectorant Effects

Herbs like mullein, thyme, and eucalyptus have expectorant properties, meaning they help to loosen and expel mucus from the respiratory tract. This can be particularly beneficial for conditions that involve excessive mucus production, such as bronchitis and COPD.

Immune System Support

Strengthening the immune system is essential for preventing and managing respiratory infections. Herbs such as echinacea, elderberry, and astragalus can enhance immune function, helping the body to fend off pathogens that may cause or exacerbate respiratory issues.

Bronchodilatory Effects

Some herbs, like lobelia and peppermint, have bronchodilatory effects, meaning they help to relax and open the airways, making it easier to breathe. This can be particularly helpful for asthma patients and those with other conditions that cause airway constriction.

Antimicrobial Properties

Herbs such as garlic, oregano, and sage have antimicrobial properties that can help fight infections in the respiratory tract. This is especially useful for preventing and treating respiratory infections that can complicate chronic respiratory conditions.

Integrating Herbal Remedies into Respiratory Health Care

Incorporating herbal remedies into your respiratory health care routine can provide significant benefits. Here are some practical ways to use herbs to support respiratory health:

1. **Herbal Teas:**

   o Drinking herbal teas made from herbs like licorice root, ginger, and thyme can soothe the respiratory tract and provide anti-inflammatory and expectorant effects. These teas are easy to prepare and can be consumed regularly for ongoing support.

2. **Inhalations:**

   o Steam inhalations with essential oils from eucalyptus, peppermint, or thyme can help clear the nasal passages, reduce inflammation, and expel mucus. Adding a few drops of essential oil to hot water and inhaling the steam can provide immediate relief.

3. **Tinctures and Syrups:**

   o Herbal tinctures and syrups offer concentrated doses of beneficial herbs. For example, a mullein and licorice root syrup can be taken daily to support lung health and reduce inflammation.

4. **Supplements:**

   o Herbal supplements in the form of capsules or tablets can provide a convenient way to ensure consistent intake of beneficial herbs like turmeric, echinacea, and astragalus.

5. **Topical Applications:**

   o Using chest rubs made with essential oils from eucalyptus or peppermint can help open the airways and make breathing easier, especially during respiratory infections.

Herbal remedies can play a vital role in supporting respiratory health by reducing inflammation, enhancing immune function, and improving overall lung function. By integrating these natural remedies into your daily routine, you can complement conventional treatments and take a holistic approach to managing respiratory diseases. In the following sections, we will delve deeper into specific herbs known for their respiratory benefits, providing detailed information on their properties, uses, and practical applications.

Effective Herbs for Respiratory Conditions

Respiratory conditions such as asthma, bronchitis, and chronic obstructive pulmonary disease (COPD) can benefit significantly from herbal support. Here are some effective herbs that have been traditionally used to alleviate respiratory symptoms, reduce inflammation, and improve overall lung function.

1. Licorice Root (Glycyrrhiza glabra)

Description: Licorice root is a popular herb in traditional medicine known for its soothing and anti-inflammatory properties.

Benefits:

- **Anti-inflammatory:** Reduces inflammation in the airways, making it easier to breathe.

- **Expectorant:** Helps to expel mucus from the respiratory tract.

- **Soothing:** Soothes irritated mucous membranes in the throat and lungs.

Usage:

- **Tea:** Steep 1 teaspoon of dried licorice root in hot water for 10-15 minutes. Drink 1-2 cups daily.

- **Tincture:** Take 30-40 drops in water or juice, 2-3 times daily.

- **Capsules:** Follow the dosage instructions on the product label.

2. Mullein (Verbascum thapsus)

Description: Mullein is known for its ability to support respiratory health by acting as an expectorant and anti-inflammatory agent.

Benefits:

- **Expectorant:** Helps to loosen and expel mucus from the lungs.

- **Anti-inflammatory:** Reduces inflammation in the respiratory tract.

- **Soothing:** Calms irritation in the throat and bronchial tubes.

Usage:

- **Tea:** Steep 1-2 teaspoons of dried mullein leaves or flowers in hot water for 10-15 minutes. Drink 1-2 cups daily.

- **Tincture:** Take 30-40 drops in water or juice, 2-3 times daily.

- **Capsules:** Follow the dosage instructions on the product label.

3. Eucalyptus (Eucalyptus globulus)

Description: Eucalyptus is well-known for its strong aromatic properties and ability to clear congestion.

Benefits:

- **Decongestant:** Clears nasal passages and eases breathing.
- **Antimicrobial:** Fights respiratory infections caused by bacteria and viruses.
- **Expectorant:** Helps to expel mucus from the lungs.

Usage:

- **Inhalation:** Add a few drops of eucalyptus essential oil to hot water and inhale the steam.
- **Chest Rub:** Dilute eucalyptus essential oil in a carrier oil and apply to the chest and back.
- **Tea:** Steep eucalyptus leaves in hot water for 10-15 minutes. Drink 1-2 cups daily.

4. Thyme (Thymus vulgaris)

Description: Thyme is a common culinary herb with powerful antimicrobial and expectorant properties.

Benefits:

- **Antimicrobial:** Kills bacteria and viruses in the respiratory tract.
- **Expectorant:** Helps to loosen and expel mucus from the lungs.
- **Anti-inflammatory:** Reduces inflammation in the airways.

Usage:

- **Tea:** Steep 1 teaspoon of dried thyme in hot water for 10-15 minutes. Drink 1-2 cups daily.
- **Inhalation:** Add a few drops of thyme essential oil to hot water and inhale the steam.
- **Tincture:** Take 30-40 drops in water or juice, 2-3 times daily.

5. Peppermint (Mentha piperita)

Description: Peppermint is known for its refreshing scent and ability to relieve respiratory symptoms.

Benefits:

- **Bronchodilator:** Opens up the airways, making breathing easier.
- **Decongestant:** Clears nasal passages and reduces congestion.

- **Antimicrobial:** Fights respiratory infections.

Usage:

- **Tea:** Steep 1 teaspoon of dried peppermint leaves in hot water for 10-15 minutes. Drink 1-2 cups daily.
- **Inhalation:** Add a few drops of peppermint essential oil to hot water and inhale the steam.
- **Chest Rub:** Dilute peppermint essential oil in a carrier oil and apply to the chest and back.

6. Ginger (Zingiber officinale)

Description: Ginger is a versatile herb with potent anti-inflammatory and antimicrobial properties.

Benefits:

- **Anti-inflammatory:** Reduces inflammation in the respiratory tract.
- **Expectorant:** Helps to loosen and expel mucus.
- **Antimicrobial:** Fights respiratory infections.

Usage:

- **Tea:** Steep 1 teaspoon of freshly grated ginger in hot water for 10-15 minutes. Drink 1-2 cups daily.
- **Tincture:** Take 30-40 drops in water or juice, 2-3 times daily.
- **Capsules:** Follow the dosage instructions on the product label.

Incorporating these effective herbs into your respiratory health regimen can provide significant benefits, including reduced inflammation, improved mucus clearance, and enhanced immune function. Licorice root, mullein, eucalyptus, thyme, peppermint, and ginger are powerful allies in supporting respiratory health and managing conditions such as asthma, bronchitis, and COPD. Always consult with a healthcare provider before starting any new herbal regimen, especially if you have existing health conditions or are taking medications. By integrating these herbs into your daily routine, you can take a proactive approach to maintaining and improving your respiratory health.

Natural Treatments for Digestive Disorders

Digestive disorders, including conditions such as indigestion, irritable bowel syndrome (IBS), acid reflux, and inflammatory bowel disease (IBD), can significantly impact quality of life. These conditions often cause discomfort, pain, and disruption to daily activities. While conventional medicine offers a range of treatments, many individuals seek natural remedies to complement these approaches and provide additional relief. Herbal remedies, dietary modifications, and lifestyle changes have been used for centuries to support digestive health and alleviate symptoms. In this chapter, we will explore various natural treatments for digestive disorders, focusing on the use of specific herbs known for their soothing, anti-inflammatory, and digestive-enhancing properties. By integrating these natural solutions into your health regimen, you can achieve better digestive health and improve your overall well-being.

Digestive Health: An Herbal Approach

Maintaining optimal digestive health is crucial for overall well-being, as the digestive system plays a key role in breaking down food, absorbing nutrients, and eliminating waste. Digestive disorders, such as indigestion, irritable bowel syndrome (IBS), acid reflux, and inflammatory bowel disease (IBD), can disrupt these processes and lead to a range of uncomfortable symptoms. An herbal approach to digestive health offers natural solutions that can complement conventional treatments, providing relief from symptoms and promoting a healthier digestive system.

Herbs have been used for centuries in traditional medicine to support digestive health. They offer a variety of benefits, including soothing inflammation, stimulating digestion, and balancing gut flora. By incorporating specific herbs into your daily routine, you can address common digestive issues and improve your overall digestive function.

One of the most well-known herbs for digestive health is **ginger**. Ginger is widely recognized for its ability to alleviate nausea, reduce bloating, and improve digestion. It stimulates the production of digestive enzymes, which helps break down food more efficiently. Additionally, ginger has anti-inflammatory properties that can soothe the digestive tract, making it beneficial for conditions like indigestion and IBS. Drinking ginger tea or incorporating fresh ginger into meals can provide these digestive benefits.

Peppermint is another herb commonly used to support digestive health. Peppermint oil has been shown to relax the muscles of the gastrointestinal tract, which can reduce symptoms of IBS, such as abdominal pain and bloating. It also helps to promote the flow of bile, improving digestion and reducing symptoms of indigestion. Peppermint tea is a simple and effective way to incorporate this herb into your routine, offering relief from digestive discomfort.

Chamomile is well-regarded for its calming and anti-inflammatory properties. It can help soothe the digestive tract, reduce cramping, and alleviate symptoms of indigestion and acid reflux. Chamomile tea, consumed after meals, can aid in digestion and promote relaxation, which is particularly beneficial for stress-related digestive issues.

Fennel is another valuable herb for digestive health, particularly for its ability to relieve bloating and gas. Fennel seeds contain compounds that relax the muscles of the gastrointestinal tract and reduce gas production. Chewing fennel seeds after meals or drinking fennel tea can help ease digestive discomfort and promote a healthy gut.

Licorice root is beneficial for digestive health due to its soothing and anti-inflammatory effects. It can help protect the stomach lining and relieve symptoms of acid reflux and gastritis. Deglycyrrhizinated licorice (DGL) is a form of licorice that has had a compound removed to reduce potential side effects, making it safe for long-term use. DGL supplements can be taken before meals to support digestive health.

Slippery elm is another herb known for its soothing properties. It contains mucilage, a gel-like substance that coats and protects the digestive tract, reducing irritation and inflammation. Slippery elm can be particularly helpful for individuals with IBS or IBD. It can be taken as a powder mixed with water or as a supplement to help soothe and heal the digestive tract.

Integrating these herbs into your daily routine can significantly improve digestive health and alleviate symptoms of digestive disorders. Whether through teas, supplements, or incorporating them into meals, these natural remedies offer a gentle and effective approach to supporting digestive function. As always, it is important to consult with a healthcare provider before starting any new herbal regimen, especially if you have existing health conditions or are taking medications. By embracing an herbal approach to digestive health, you can achieve better digestion, reduced discomfort, and overall improved well-being.

Key Herbs for Digestive Wellness

Maintaining digestive wellness is essential for overall health, as it ensures that nutrients are effectively absorbed, and waste is efficiently eliminated. Incorporating specific herbs into your daily routine can significantly enhance digestive health and alleviate common digestive issues. Here are some key herbs known for their digestive benefits:

1. Ginger (Zingiber officinale)

Description: Ginger is a widely used herb in both culinary and medicinal traditions, known for its potent anti-inflammatory and digestive properties.

Benefits:

- **Alleviates Nausea:** Ginger is highly effective in reducing nausea and vomiting, making it beneficial for motion sickness, morning sickness, and post-operative nausea.
- **Stimulates Digestion:** It stimulates the production of digestive enzymes, enhancing the breakdown of food and absorption of nutrients.
- **Reduces Bloating:** Ginger helps relieve bloating and gas by promoting gastrointestinal motility and reducing inflammation.

Usage:

- **Tea:** Steep 1 teaspoon of freshly grated ginger in hot water for 10-15 minutes. Drink 1-2 cups daily.
- **Supplement:** Take ginger capsules or tablets as directed on the product label.
- **Fresh:** Add fresh ginger to meals or smoothies.

2. Peppermint (Mentha piperita)

Description: Peppermint is a herb known for its cooling and soothing effects on the digestive system.

Benefits:

- **Relieves IBS Symptoms:** Peppermint oil has been shown to relax the muscles of the gastrointestinal tract, reducing symptoms of irritable bowel syndrome (IBS) such as abdominal pain, bloating, and gas.
- **Improves Bile Flow:** It promotes the flow of bile, which aids in the digestion of fats and overall digestive process.
- **Reduces Indigestion:** Peppermint helps alleviate symptoms of indigestion and heartburn.

Usage:

- **Tea:** Steep 1 teaspoon of dried peppermint leaves in hot water for 10-15 minutes. Drink 1-2 cups daily.
- **Capsules:** Take enteric-coated peppermint oil capsules as directed on the product label.
- **Essential Oil:** Inhale peppermint essential oil or apply it diluted to the abdomen for relief from digestive discomfort.

3. Chamomile (Matricaria chamomilla)

Description: Chamomile is a gentle herb with calming and anti-inflammatory properties, widely used to soothe digestive issues.

Benefits:

- **Soothes the Digestive Tract:** Chamomile helps calm the digestive tract, reducing cramping, gas, and bloating.
- **Reduces Inflammation:** Its anti-inflammatory properties can help alleviate symptoms of gastritis and other inflammatory digestive conditions.
- **Aids in Relaxation:** Chamomile's calming effects can also help reduce stress-related digestive issues.

Usage:

- **Tea:** Steep 1-2 teaspoons of dried chamomile flowers in hot water for 10-15 minutes. Drink 1-2 cups daily.
- **Extract:** Use chamomile extract or tincture as directed on the product label.

4. Fennel (Foeniculum vulgare)

Description: Fennel is an aromatic herb known for its ability to relieve digestive discomfort and improve overall digestive function.

Benefits:

- **Reduces Bloating and Gas:** Fennel seeds contain compounds that relax the muscles of the gastrointestinal tract and reduce gas production.
- **Promotes Digestion:** It stimulates the secretion of digestive enzymes and bile, enhancing digestion and nutrient absorption.
- **Soothes the Stomach:** Fennel can help relieve stomach cramps and indigestion.

Usage:

- **Tea:** Steep 1 teaspoon of crushed fennel seeds in hot water for 10-15 minutes. Drink 1-2 cups daily.
- **Chew Seeds:** Chew a teaspoon of fennel seeds after meals to aid digestion.
- **Supplement:** Take fennel seed capsules as directed on the product label.

5. Licorice Root (Glycyrrhiza glabra)

Description: Licorice root is a soothing herb that helps protect and heal the digestive tract.

Benefits:

- **Protects the Stomach Lining:** Licorice root helps form a protective barrier over the stomach lining, reducing symptoms of acid reflux and gastritis.
- **Reduces Inflammation:** Its anti-inflammatory properties can help soothe inflamed tissues in the digestive tract.
- **Aids Digestion:** Licorice root can help alleviate symptoms of indigestion and heartburn.

Usage:

- **Tea:** Steep 1 teaspoon of dried licorice root in hot water for 10-15 minutes. Drink 1-2 cups daily.
- **DGL Tablets:** Take deglycyrrhizinated licorice (DGL) tablets before meals to support digestive health.
- **Tincture:** Use licorice root tincture as directed on the product label.

6. Slippery Elm (Ulmus rubra)

Description: Slippery elm is a soothing herb known for its mucilaginous properties, which help protect and heal the digestive tract.

Benefits:

- **Soothes Irritation:** Slippery elm coats the digestive tract, reducing irritation and inflammation.

- **Aids in Healing:** It promotes healing of the digestive mucosa, making it beneficial for conditions like IBS and IBD.

- **Relieves Symptoms:** Slippery elm can help alleviate symptoms of acid reflux, gastritis, and colitis.

Usage:

- **Tea:** Mix 1 teaspoon of slippery elm powder with hot water to form a thick tea. Drink 1-2 cups daily.

- **Supplement:** Take slippery elm capsules as directed on the product label.

- **Lozenge:** Use slippery elm lozenges to soothe the throat and digestive tract.

Incorporating these key herbs into your daily routine can significantly improve digestive wellness and alleviate common digestive issues. Ginger, peppermint, chamomile, fennel, licorice root, and slippery elm offer a range of benefits, from reducing inflammation and soothing irritation to promoting digestion and relieving bloating. By using these herbs in teas, supplements, and as part of your meals, you can support your digestive system naturally and effectively. As always, it is important to consult with a healthcare provider before starting any new herbal regimen, especially if you have existing health conditions or are taking medications.

Herbs for Skin Conditions and Wound Healing

Skin conditions such as eczema, psoriasis, acne, and various forms of dermatitis can cause significant discomfort and impact one's quality of life. Additionally, proper wound healing is crucial to prevent infections and promote tissue repair. While conventional treatments are available, many individuals seek natural alternatives to support skin health and accelerate wound healing. Herbal remedies have been used for centuries to treat a variety of skin conditions and aid in the healing process. These herbs offer anti-inflammatory, antimicrobial, and soothing properties that can help alleviate symptoms, reduce inflammation, and promote faster recovery. In this chapter, we will explore various herbs known for their effectiveness in treating skin conditions and enhancing wound healing, providing insights into their benefits, mechanisms of action, and practical applications. By integrating these natural remedies into your skincare routine, you can achieve healthier skin and support the body's natural healing processes.

Essential Herbs for Skin Health

Maintaining healthy skin and promoting wound healing involves more than just topical treatments; it requires a holistic approach that includes the use of beneficial herbs. Here are some essential herbs known for their skin-healing properties and their ability to address various skin conditions.

1. Aloe Vera (Aloe barbadensis miller)

Description: Aloe vera is a succulent plant renowned for its soothing and healing properties. It is widely used in skincare products for its ability to treat burns, wounds, and various skin conditions.

Benefits:

- **Soothing and Hydrating:** Aloe vera gel provides immediate relief for burns, sunburns, and skin irritations by hydrating and cooling the skin.
- **Anti-inflammatory:** Reduces inflammation and redness associated with conditions like acne and eczema.
- **Wound Healing:** Promotes faster healing of cuts, abrasions, and other wounds by stimulating collagen production.

Usage:

- **Topical Gel:** Apply fresh aloe vera gel directly to the affected area several times a day.
- **Creams and Lotions:** Use aloe vera-infused skincare products as part of your daily routine.

2. Calendula (Calendula officinalis)

Description: Calendula, also known as marigold, is a bright, flowering herb known for its powerful anti-inflammatory and healing properties.

Benefits:

- **Anti-inflammatory:** Reduces swelling and redness, making it ideal for treating skin irritations and conditions like eczema and dermatitis.
- **Antimicrobial:** Helps prevent infection in minor cuts and wounds.
- **Wound Healing:** Accelerates the healing process by promoting cell repair and regeneration.

Usage:

- **Salve or Ointment:** Apply calendula salve to wounds, rashes, or irritated skin 2-3 times a day.
- **Infused Oil:** Use calendula-infused oil for massage or as a carrier oil for essential oils.

3. Tea Tree Oil (Melaleuca alternifolia)

Description: Tea tree oil is a potent essential oil derived from the leaves of the tea tree, known for its antimicrobial and anti-inflammatory properties.

Benefits:

- **Antibacterial:** Effectively treats acne and prevents infections by killing bacteria.

- **Anti-inflammatory:** Reduces redness and swelling associated with acne and other skin conditions.
- **Wound Healing:** Helps to disinfect wounds and promote faster healing.

Usage:

- **Spot Treatment:** Apply diluted tea tree oil (a few drops mixed with a carrier oil) directly to acne or wounds.
- **Skincare Products:** Incorporate tea tree oil-containing cleansers, toners, and creams into your skincare routine.

4. Lavender (Lavandula angustifolia)

Description: Lavender is an aromatic herb known for its calming effects and its ability to promote skin healing and reduce inflammation.

Benefits:

- **Anti-inflammatory:** Helps soothe irritated skin and reduce redness and swelling.
- **Antimicrobial:** Prevents infections in cuts, scrapes, and other wounds.
- **Calming:** Provides a soothing effect, which is beneficial for conditions like eczema and psoriasis.

Usage:

- **Essential Oil:** Apply diluted lavender oil to affected areas or add a few drops to your bath for overall skin health.
- **Lotions and Creams:** Use lavender-infused skincare products for daily use.

5. Chamomile (Matricaria chamomilla)

Description: Chamomile is a gentle herb with strong anti-inflammatory and soothing properties, making it excellent for sensitive and irritated skin.

Benefits:

- **Anti-inflammatory:** Reduces inflammation and irritation associated with eczema, dermatitis, and other skin conditions.
- **Soothing:** Calms the skin and alleviates itching and redness.
- **Wound Healing:** Promotes the healing of minor wounds and reduces scarring.

Usage:

- **Tea:** Use chamomile tea bags as a compress for inflamed or irritated skin.
- **Creams and Ointments:** Apply chamomile-infused products to the skin as needed.

6. Witch Hazel (Hamamelis virginiana)

Description: Witch hazel is a natural astringent derived from the bark and leaves of the witch hazel shrub, known for its ability to tighten and soothe the skin.

Benefits:

- **Astringent:** Tightens the skin and reduces the appearance of pores.

- **Anti-inflammatory:** Alleviates inflammation and redness, making it useful for treating acne and other skin irritations.

- **Antimicrobial:** Helps to prevent infections and promote wound healing.

Usage:

- **Toner:** Apply witch hazel toner to the face with a cotton pad to reduce oiliness and tighten pores.

- **Compress:** Use witch hazel as a compress on minor cuts, scrapes, and insect bites.

These essential herbs—aloe vera, calendula, tea tree oil, lavender, chamomile, and witch hazel—offer powerful natural solutions for maintaining skin health and promoting wound healing. By incorporating these herbs into your skincare routine through topical applications, infused oils, teas, and essential oils, you can address a variety of skin conditions and support the body's natural healing processes. As always, it is important to consult with a healthcare provider before starting any new herbal regimen, especially if you have existing health conditions or are taking medications. By leveraging the healing properties of these herbs, you can achieve healthier, more resilient skin.

BOOK 9:

Natural Pain Management: Herbs and Techniques to Relieve Discomfort

White Willow and Its Effects

White willow (Salix alba) has a long history of use as a natural remedy for pain and inflammation. Often referred to as "nature's aspirin," white willow bark contains salicin, a compound that the body converts into salicylic acid, which is chemically similar to the active ingredient in aspirin. This connection to aspirin highlights white willow's significant role in pain management and its effectiveness in reducing inflammation and alleviating discomfort. For centuries, herbalists and traditional medicine practitioners have used white willow to treat a variety of ailments, from headaches and back pain to arthritis and menstrual cramps. This chapter delves into the rich history of white willow, its active compounds, and the scientific basis for its pain-relieving properties. By understanding how white willow works and how it can be used effectively, you can incorporate this powerful herb into your natural pain management regimen.

History and Traditional Uses of White Willow

White willow (Salix alba) has been utilized for its medicinal properties for thousands of years, with its use dating back to ancient civilizations. The tree is native to Europe and parts of Asia, and its bark has been a cornerstone in the development of herbal medicine. The history of white willow is rich and varied, reflecting its widespread recognition as a natural remedy for pain and inflammation.

Ancient Civilizations

The use of white willow bark can be traced back to ancient civilizations, where it was valued for its analgesic (pain-relieving) and anti-inflammatory effects. The earliest recorded use dates back to ancient Egypt, where it was used to treat aches and pains. Similarly, the ancient Greeks, including Hippocrates, often referred to as the "father of medicine," recommended chewing willow bark to alleviate pain and reduce fever. Hippocrates wrote about its effectiveness in treating conditions such as gout and rheumatic pain.

Traditional Chinese Medicine

In traditional Chinese medicine (TCM), willow bark was also recognized for its medicinal properties. TCM practitioners used it to address a variety of ailments, including joint pain, headaches, and fever. The holistic approach of TCM often combined willow bark with other herbs to enhance its therapeutic effects and to balance the body's energies.

Indigenous Cultures

Indigenous cultures in North America also used willow bark as a natural remedy. Native American tribes utilized the bark to treat fever, headache, and musculoskeletal pain. They would create decoctions or infusions from the bark, which were consumed to relieve various ailments. The knowledge of willow bark's medicinal properties was passed down through generations, demonstrating its longstanding efficacy.

European Medicine

In medieval Europe, white willow bark became a common remedy in herbal medicine. Herbalists and physicians used it to treat a range of conditions, from the common cold to chronic pain. During the Renaissance, European physicians like Paracelsus continued to advocate for the use of willow bark, recognizing its potential to alleviate pain and reduce inflammation.

The Development of Aspirin

The modern understanding of white willow's medicinal properties culminated in the 19th century with the development of aspirin. In the early 1800s, scientists isolated salicin, the active compound in willow bark, which led to the synthesis of salicylic acid. Later, in 1897, Felix Hoffmann, a chemist at Bayer, acetylated salicylic acid to create acetylsalicylic acid, known today as aspirin. This development marked a significant milestone in medicine, bridging traditional herbal knowledge and modern pharmacology.

Continued Use in Modern Herbal Medicine

Today, white willow bark continues to be used in modern herbal medicine. It is available in various forms, including teas, tinctures, capsules, and topical preparations. Herbalists recommend it for its ability to relieve pain, reduce inflammation, and lower fever. Unlike synthetic aspirin, white willow bark is often considered gentler on the stomach, making it a preferred option for individuals with sensitive digestive systems.

Conclusion

The history and traditional uses of white willow bark highlight its enduring significance as a natural remedy for pain and inflammation. From ancient civilizations to modern herbal medicine, white willow has proven to be a valuable ally in managing various ailments. Its journey from a traditional herbal remedy to the inspiration for one of the most widely used medications, aspirin, underscores its remarkable therapeutic potential. By understanding and appreciating the historical context of white willow, we can better appreciate its role in contemporary natural pain management.

Active Compounds: Salicin and Its Role in Pain Relief

White willow bark's effectiveness as a natural remedy for pain relief is largely attributed to its active compound, salicin. Salicin is a type of glycoside that the body metabolizes into salicylic acid, which is chemically similar to aspirin's active ingredient, acetylsalicylic acid. The presence of salicin in white willow bark forms the basis for its analgesic and anti-inflammatory properties, making it a powerful natural alternative for managing pain and inflammation.

The Chemistry of Salicin

Salicin is a beta-glycoside of salicyl alcohol. When ingested, salicin is hydrolyzed in the intestines into saligenin (salicyl alcohol) and glucose. Saligenin is then absorbed into the bloodstream, where it is oxidized by the liver into salicylic acid. This conversion process is key to the compound's therapeutic effects. Salicylic acid is known for its ability to reduce inflammation and alleviate pain, which forms the core mechanism behind the analgesic effects of white willow bark.

Mechanism of Action

The pain-relieving and anti-inflammatory effects of salicin are primarily due to its ability to inhibit cyclooxygenase (COX) enzymes. COX enzymes play a crucial role in the synthesis of prostaglandins, which are lipid compounds that promote inflammation, pain, and fever as part of the body's response to injury or illness. By inhibiting COX enzymes, salicylic acid reduces the production of prostaglandins, thereby decreasing inflammation and providing pain relief. This mechanism is similar to how non-steroidal anti-inflammatory drugs (NSAIDs), such as aspirin, function, but with a gentler impact on the gastrointestinal system.

Benefits Over Synthetic Analgesics

One of the significant advantages of salicin over synthetic analgesics like aspirin is its gentler effect on the stomach lining. Aspirin and other NSAIDs can cause gastrointestinal irritation and ulcers due to their direct impact on the stomach's mucosal lining. In contrast, the salicin in white willow bark is metabolized more slowly, resulting in a sustained release of salicylic acid in the bloodstream. This gradual conversion process reduces the likelihood of gastrointestinal side effects, making white willow bark a preferable option for individuals with sensitive stomachs or those who require long-term pain management.

Clinical Evidence

Numerous studies have supported the efficacy of white willow bark in managing pain and inflammation. Clinical trials have demonstrated its effectiveness in treating conditions such as osteoarthritis, lower back pain, and headache. In one study, patients with osteoarthritis experienced significant pain relief after taking white willow bark extract, with effects comparable to those of conventional NSAIDs. Another study highlighted the use of white willow bark in reducing the intensity and frequency of tension headaches.

Dosage and Administration

White willow bark is available in various forms, including teas, tinctures, capsules, and topical applications. The standard dosage of white willow bark extract typically contains about 120-240 mg of salicin per day, divided into several doses. It is important to consult with a healthcare provider to determine the appropriate dosage and ensure it is safe, especially for individuals with existing health conditions or those taking other medications.

The active compound salicin in white willow bark plays a pivotal role in its ability to relieve pain and reduce inflammation. By understanding the chemistry and mechanism of action of salicin, we can appreciate how this natural remedy provides a gentler alternative to synthetic analgesics. Clinical evidence supports its effectiveness, highlighting its potential in managing various pain conditions with fewer gastrointestinal side effects. Integrating white willow bark into a pain management regimen can offer a natural, effective solution for those seeking relief from pain and inflammation.

How to Use White Willow: Teas, Tinctures, and Supplements?

White willow bark is a versatile herb that can be used in various forms to provide natural pain relief and reduce inflammation. Here's how you can incorporate white willow bark into your routine through teas, tinctures, and supplements.

1. White Willow Tea

Preparation: White willow tea is a simple and effective way to consume the herb. The tea can be made using dried white willow bark.

Ingredients:

- 1-2 teaspoons of dried white willow bark
- 1 cup of water

Instructions:

1. Boil the water and then reduce it to a simmer.
2. Add the dried white willow bark to the simmering water.
3. Let it steep for about 10-15 minutes.
4. Strain the tea to remove the bark.
5. Drink the tea while it's warm.

Dosage:

- Drink 1-2 cups of white willow tea daily. It's best to start with one cup and monitor your body's response before increasing the intake.

Benefits:

- The tea provides a gentle and sustained release of salicin, helping to alleviate pain and inflammation naturally.

2. White Willow Tincture

Preparation: A tincture is a concentrated liquid extract of the herb, typically made using alcohol as a solvent. Tinctures are easy to use and provide a potent dose of white willow bark's active compounds.

Ingredients:

- Dried white willow bark
- High-proof alcohol (such as vodka)
- A glass jar with a lid

Instructions:

1. Fill the glass jar about halfway with dried white willow bark.
2. Pour the alcohol over the bark, covering it completely. Leave some space at the top.
3. Seal the jar with the lid and store it in a cool, dark place for 4-6 weeks. Shake the jar daily.
4. After 4-6 weeks, strain the mixture through a cheesecloth or fine mesh strainer into a clean jar or dropper bottle.

Dosage:

- Take 30-40 drops (approximately 1-2 dropperfuls) in a small amount of water or juice, 2-3 times daily.

Benefits:

- Tinctures are convenient for those who need a potent and fast-acting form of white willow bark. They can be easily carried and taken as needed throughout the day.

3. White Willow Supplements

Preparation: White willow supplements, available in capsules or tablets, provide a standardized dose of the herb's active compounds. They are widely available and offer a convenient way to take white willow bark.

Instructions:

- Follow the dosage instructions provided on the supplement packaging. Standardized extracts typically contain 120-240 mg of salicin per day, divided into several doses.

Dosage:

- A common dosage is one capsule/tablet taken 2-3 times daily with meals.

Benefits:

- Supplements offer a precise and consistent dose of salicin, making it easier to manage and monitor your intake. They are ideal for individuals who prefer not to prepare teas or tinctures.

Safety and Precautions

While white willow bark is generally safe for most people when used as directed, there are some precautions to keep in mind:

- **Consult a Healthcare Provider:** Always consult with a healthcare provider before starting any new herbal regimen, especially if you are pregnant, breastfeeding, have a medical condition, or are taking other medications.
- **Allergic Reactions:** Some people may be allergic to salicylates. If you experience any allergic reactions such as rash, itching, or difficulty breathing, discontinue use and seek medical attention.
- **Gastrointestinal Issues:** Although gentler than aspirin, white willow bark can still cause gastrointestinal discomfort in some individuals. Start with a lower dose to assess your tolerance.
- **Avoid in Children:** White willow bark should not be given to children, particularly those recovering from viral infections like the flu or chickenpox, due to the risk of Reye's syndrome.

White willow bark can be effectively used in the form of teas, tinctures, and supplements to provide natural pain relief and reduce inflammation. Each form has its benefits, allowing for flexibility in how you incorporate this powerful herb into your routine. Whether you prefer the soothing process of making tea, the convenience of tinctures, or the precise dosing of supplements, white willow bark offers a versatile and effective solution for managing pain naturally.

Turmeric and Ginger for Inflammation

Inflammation is a natural response by the body to injury or infection, but chronic inflammation can lead to a host of health problems, including arthritis, cardiovascular disease, and digestive disorders. Turmeric and ginger, two potent herbs commonly used in traditional medicine, have garnered significant attention for their powerful anti-inflammatory properties. Both turmeric and ginger contain bioactive compounds that help reduce inflammation and promote overall health. This chapter explores the use of turmeric and ginger in managing inflammation, delving into their mechanisms of action, health benefits, and practical ways to incorporate them into your daily routine. By understanding how these herbs work and how they can be used effectively, you can harness their natural healing properties to combat inflammation and enhance your well-being.

The Anti-Inflammatory Properties of Turmeric and Ginger

Turmeric and ginger have been celebrated for centuries in traditional medicine for their remarkable anti-inflammatory properties. These two potent herbs contain bioactive compounds that help reduce inflammation, alleviate pain, and promote overall health. Understanding the mechanisms by which turmeric and ginger combat inflammation can provide valuable insights into their effectiveness and how they can be incorporated into your health regimen.

Turmeric

Active Compound: Curcumin Turmeric (Curcuma longa) is a bright yellow spice commonly used in Indian cuisine and traditional medicine. The primary bioactive compound responsible for its anti-inflammatory effects is curcumin. Curcumin is a powerful antioxidant and anti-inflammatory agent that works through several mechanisms to reduce inflammation.

Mechanisms of Action:

1. **Inhibition of Inflammatory Pathways:**

   o Curcumin inhibits the activity of nuclear factor-kappa B (NF-κB), a protein complex that plays a crucial role in regulating the immune response and inflammation. By blocking NF-κB, curcumin reduces the expression of pro-inflammatory genes.

2. **Reduction of Pro-inflammatory Cytokines:**

   o Curcumin decreases the levels of pro-inflammatory cytokines such as tumor necrosis factor-alpha (TNF-α), interleukin-1 (IL-1), and interleukin-6 (IL-6). These cytokines are signaling molecules that promote inflammation and are often elevated in chronic inflammatory conditions.

3. **Antioxidant Effects:**

   o Curcumin is a potent antioxidant that neutralizes free radicals, which can cause oxidative stress and further exacerbate inflammation. By reducing oxidative stress, curcumin helps protect tissues and cells from damage.

Health Benefits:

- **Arthritis Relief:** Curcumin has been shown to reduce joint pain and stiffness in individuals with osteoarthritis and rheumatoid arthritis.

- **Digestive Health:** Curcumin helps reduce inflammation in the gut, which can benefit conditions like inflammatory bowel disease (IBD).

- **Cardiovascular Health:** By reducing inflammation and oxidative stress, curcumin supports heart health and helps prevent cardiovascular diseases.

Ginger

Active Compounds: Gingerol and Shogaol Ginger (Zingiber officinale) is a versatile herb widely used for its culinary and medicinal properties. The primary bioactive compounds in ginger are gingerol and shogaol, which are responsible for its anti-inflammatory and antioxidant effects.

Mechanisms of Action:

1. **Inhibition of Pro-inflammatory Enzymes:**

   o Gingerol and shogaol inhibit the activity of cyclooxygenase (COX) and lipoxygenase (LOX) enzymes, which are involved in the synthesis of pro-inflammatory compounds called prostaglandins and leukotrienes. By blocking these enzymes, ginger reduces the production of these inflammatory mediators.

2. **Modulation of Inflammatory Cytokines:**

   o Gingerol and shogaol modulate the production and activity of pro-inflammatory cytokines such as TNF-α, IL-1, and IL-6. This modulation helps decrease the overall inflammatory response in the body.

3. **Antioxidant Effects:**

   o Like curcumin, gingerol and shogaol exhibit strong antioxidant properties, neutralizing free radicals and reducing oxidative stress, which contributes to inflammation.

Health Benefits:

- **Pain Relief:** Ginger has been shown to alleviate pain and improve function in individuals with osteoarthritis and other inflammatory conditions.

- **Digestive Health:** Ginger reduces inflammation in the digestive tract, helping to relieve symptoms of indigestion, nausea, and inflammatory bowel conditions.

- **Immune Support:** By modulating the immune response and reducing inflammation, ginger supports overall immune health and helps protect against infections.

The anti-inflammatory properties of turmeric and ginger make them powerful allies in managing inflammation and promoting overall health. Curcumin in turmeric and gingerol and shogaol in ginger work through various mechanisms to reduce inflammation, modulate cytokine activity, and combat oxidative stress. These herbs offer natural and effective options for individuals seeking to alleviate inflammatory conditions and improve their quality of life. Incorporating turmeric and ginger into your daily routine, whether through dietary sources, supplements, or topical applications, can provide significant health benefits and enhance your well-being.

Curcumin: The Active Compound in Turmeric

Curcumin is the primary bioactive compound found in turmeric (Curcuma longa), a vibrant yellow spice widely used in culinary traditions and traditional medicine, particularly in India and Southeast Asia. Known for its potent anti-inflammatory, antioxidant, and anticancer properties, curcumin has been extensively studied for its health benefits and therapeutic potential. The multifaceted effects of curcumin make it a valuable natural remedy for a variety of conditions, particularly those involving chronic inflammation and oxidative stress.

Anti-Inflammatory Properties

One of the most significant benefits of curcumin is its ability to reduce inflammation. Chronic inflammation is a major contributor to many health conditions, including arthritis, cardiovascular diseases, metabolic syndrome, and neurodegenerative diseases. Curcumin exerts its anti-inflammatory effects by inhibiting the activity of nuclear factor-kappa B (NF-κB), a protein complex that plays a key role in regulating the immune response and inflammation. By blocking NF-κB, curcumin reduces the expression of pro-inflammatory genes, thereby decreasing the overall inflammatory response in the body.

In addition to inhibiting NF-κB, curcumin also reduces the levels of pro-inflammatory cytokines such as tumor necrosis factor-alpha (TNF-α), interleukin-1 (IL-1), and interleukin-6 (IL-6). These cytokines are signaling molecules that promote inflammation and are often elevated in chronic inflammatory conditions. By modulating the production and activity of these cytokines, curcumin helps to alleviate inflammation and its associated symptoms.

Antioxidant Effects

Curcumin is a powerful antioxidant that helps protect the body from oxidative stress, a condition characterized by an imbalance between free radicals and antioxidants. Free radicals are unstable molecules that can cause damage to cells, proteins, and DNA, contributing to aging and the development of various diseases. Curcumin neutralizes free radicals directly by donating electrons, and it also enhances the activity of the body's own antioxidant enzymes, such as superoxide dismutase (SOD) and glutathione peroxidase.

By reducing oxidative stress, curcumin helps protect tissues and cells from damage, thereby supporting overall health and longevity. This antioxidant activity also contributes to curcumin's anti-inflammatory effects, as oxidative stress and inflammation are closely linked processes that exacerbate each other.

Therapeutic Potential

Curcumin's broad range of biological activities makes it a promising therapeutic agent for a variety of health conditions. In the context of arthritis, curcumin has been shown to reduce joint pain and stiffness, improve joint function, and decrease markers of inflammation in individuals with osteoarthritis and rheumatoid arthritis. Clinical trials have demonstrated that curcumin can be as effective as non-steroidal anti-inflammatory drugs (NSAIDs) in alleviating symptoms of arthritis, but with fewer gastrointestinal side effects.

In cardiovascular health, curcumin helps improve endothelial function, reduce arterial plaque buildup, and lower levels of LDL cholesterol and triglycerides. These effects contribute to a lower risk of heart disease and better overall cardiovascular health. Curcumin's ability to modulate blood sugar levels and improve insulin sensitivity also makes it beneficial for individuals with metabolic syndrome and type 2 diabetes.

In neurodegenerative diseases, curcumin has shown potential in protecting brain health by reducing inflammation and oxidative stress, promoting the clearance of amyloid plaques, and enhancing cognitive function. These properties suggest that curcumin could play a role in the prevention and management of conditions such as Alzheimer's disease and Parkinson's disease.

Bioavailability Challenges and Solutions

Despite its impressive health benefits, one of the main challenges with curcumin is its poor bioavailability. Curcumin is poorly absorbed into the bloodstream, rapidly metabolized, and quickly eliminated from the body. To overcome these challenges, various strategies have been developed to enhance curcumin's bioavailability. These include combining curcumin with piperine (a compound found in black pepper), which can increase absorption by up to 2000%, using lipid-based formulations such as curcumin phytosomes and nano-curcumin, and taking curcumin with fat-containing meals to improve absorption.

Curcumin, the active compound in turmeric, offers a wide range of health benefits due to its potent anti-inflammatory and antioxidant properties. By inhibiting inflammatory pathways and reducing oxidative stress, curcumin helps manage and prevent a variety of chronic conditions, from arthritis and cardiovascular diseases to neurodegenerative disorders. Despite challenges with bioavailability, advancements in formulation have made it easier to harness the therapeutic potential of curcumin. Incorporating curcumin into your health regimen, whether through dietary sources, supplements, or enhanced formulations, can provide significant benefits and support overall well-being.

Recipes and Dosages for Effective Use of Turmeric and Ginger

Incorporating turmeric and ginger into your daily routine can provide significant anti-inflammatory benefits. Here are some recipes and recommended dosages to help you effectively use these powerful herbs.

1. Turmeric and Ginger Tea

Ingredients:

- 1 teaspoon fresh grated turmeric or 1/2 teaspoon ground turmeric
- 1 teaspoon fresh grated ginger or 1/2 teaspoon ground ginger
- 1 cup water
- Honey or lemon to taste (optional)

Instructions:

1. Bring the water to a boil in a small saucepan.
2. Add the grated turmeric and ginger, then reduce the heat and let it simmer for about 10 minutes.
3. Strain the tea into a cup.
4. Add honey or lemon to taste, if desired.

Dosage:

- Drink 1-2 cups of this tea daily to help reduce inflammation and support overall health.

2. Golden Milk

Ingredients:

- 1 cup milk (dairy or plant-based, such as almond or coconut milk)
- 1/2 teaspoon turmeric powder
- 1/4 teaspoon ground ginger
- 1/4 teaspoon cinnamon
- Pinch of black pepper (to enhance curcumin absorption)
- 1 teaspoon honey or maple syrup (optional)

Instructions:

1. In a small saucepan, combine the milk, turmeric, ginger, cinnamon, and black pepper.
2. Heat the mixture over medium heat until it is warm but not boiling, stirring occasionally.
3. Remove from heat and add honey or maple syrup, if desired.
4. Pour into a mug and enjoy.

Dosage:

- Drink one cup of golden milk daily, preferably in the evening for its soothing effects.

3. Turmeric and Ginger Smoothie

Ingredients:

- 1 cup unsweetened almond milk or coconut water
- 1 banana
- 1/2 cup frozen pineapple or mango chunks
- 1 teaspoon fresh grated turmeric or 1/2 teaspoon turmeric powder
- 1 teaspoon fresh grated ginger or 1/2 teaspoon ground ginger
- 1 tablespoon chia seeds (optional)
- 1 teaspoon honey or maple syrup (optional)

Instructions:

1. Combine all the ingredients in a blender.
2. Blend until smooth and creamy.
3. Pour into a glass and enjoy immediately.

Dosage:

- Consume one smoothie daily to reap the anti-inflammatory benefits of turmeric and ginger.

4. Turmeric and Ginger Capsules

Preparation: If you prefer a more concentrated form of turmeric and ginger, consider taking them in capsule form.

Dosage:

- **Turmeric:** Take 500-1000 mg of turmeric extract standardized to contain 95% curcuminoids, 1-2 times daily with meals. Ensure the supplement includes black pepper extract (piperine) to enhance absorption.
- **Ginger:** Take 500-1000 mg of ginger extract, 1-2 times daily with meals.

5. Anti-Inflammatory Salad Dressing

Ingredients:

- 1/4 cup olive oil
- 2 tablespoons apple cider vinegar
- 1 teaspoon turmeric powder
- 1 teaspoon fresh grated ginger

- 1 teaspoon honey or maple syrup

- 1/2 teaspoon Dijon mustard

- Salt and pepper to taste

Instructions:

1. In a small bowl or jar, whisk together the olive oil, apple cider vinegar, turmeric, ginger, honey, and Dijon mustard.

2. Season with salt and pepper to taste.

3. Drizzle over salads or use as a marinade for vegetables and proteins.

Dosage:

- Use this dressing regularly on salads or as a marinade to incorporate turmeric and ginger into your meals.

Incorporating turmeric and ginger into your daily diet through teas, smoothies, golden milk, and capsules can provide significant anti-inflammatory benefits. These recipes offer delicious and convenient ways to consume these powerful herbs, helping to reduce inflammation and support overall health. Remember to consult with a healthcare provider before starting any new supplement regimen, especially if you have existing health conditions or are taking medications. By regularly using turmeric and ginger in these effective forms and dosages, you can enhance your well-being and enjoy their natural healing properties.

BOOK 10:

Application Techniques and Combinations: Let's put them into practice!

Effectively utilizing herbs such as turmeric and ginger for pain relief and inflammation involves understanding various application techniques and synergistic combinations. Different methods of preparation and use can enhance the bioavailability and efficacy of these herbs, allowing you to maximize their therapeutic benefits. From teas and tinctures to topical applications and dietary supplements, each technique offers unique advantages. Moreover, combining turmeric and ginger with other complementary herbs and natural substances can create powerful synergies that further enhance their pain-relieving and anti-inflammatory properties. This chapter will explore the various ways to apply and combine these herbs, providing practical guidance on how to incorporate them into your health regimen for optimal results.

Topical Applications: Oils, Salves, and Poultices

Topical applications of turmeric and ginger can be highly effective for relieving localized pain and inflammation. These methods allow the active compounds to be directly absorbed into the skin, targeting the affected area and providing relief. Here's a closer look at how to use oils, salves, and poultices made from turmeric and ginger for topical applications.

Turmeric and Ginger Oil

Ingredients:

- 1/4 cup carrier oil (such as coconut oil, olive oil, or almond oil)
- 1 tablespoon turmeric powder
- 1 tablespoon fresh grated ginger or 1/2 tablespoon ginger powder

Instructions:

1. In a small saucepan, combine the carrier oil, turmeric powder, and ginger.
2. Heat the mixture over low heat for about 10-15 minutes, stirring occasionally. Do not let it boil.
3. Remove from heat and let it cool slightly.
4. Strain the mixture through a fine mesh strainer or cheesecloth to remove the solid particles.
5. Store the infused oil in a clean, airtight container.

Application:

- Gently massage the oil onto the affected area 2-3 times daily. This can help reduce pain and inflammation in joints and muscles.

Turmeric and Ginger Salve

Ingredients:

- 1/4 cup coconut oil
- 1/4 cup beeswax pellets
- 1 tablespoon turmeric powder
- 1 tablespoon fresh grated ginger or 1/2 tablespoon ginger powder
- 10 drops essential oil (optional, such as lavender or eucalyptus)

Instructions:

1. In a double boiler, melt the coconut oil and beeswax pellets together.
2. Once melted, stir in the turmeric powder and ginger.
3. Remove from heat and add the essential oil if using.
4. Pour the mixture into a clean container and let it cool and solidify.

5. Store the salve in a cool, dry place.

Application:

- Apply a small amount of the salve to the affected area and gently massage it in. Use it 2-3 times daily to help alleviate pain and inflammation.

Turmeric and Ginger Poultice

Ingredients:

- 1 tablespoon turmeric powder
- 1 tablespoon fresh grated ginger or 1/2 tablespoon ginger powder
- 1-2 tablespoons water or coconut oil (to form a paste)

Instructions:

1. In a small bowl, mix the turmeric powder, ginger, and enough water or coconut oil to form a thick paste.
2. Spread the paste onto a clean cloth or gauze.

Application:

- Place the cloth with the paste directly onto the affected area.
- Secure it with a bandage or wrap and leave it on for 20-30 minutes.
- Remove the poultice and rinse the area with warm water.
- Use this poultice once or twice daily to help reduce pain and inflammation.

Topical applications of turmeric and ginger in the form of oils, salves, and poultices can provide effective relief from localized pain and inflammation. These methods allow the active compounds to be absorbed directly into the skin, targeting specific areas of discomfort. By incorporating these topical treatments into your pain management routine, you can harness the natural healing properties of turmeric and ginger to support your overall health and well-being. Always perform a patch test before using any new topical remedy to ensure there are no adverse reactions and consult with a healthcare provider if you have any concerns.

Oral Consumption: Teas, Capsules, and Tinctures

Oral consumption of turmeric and ginger is a convenient and effective way to harness their anti-inflammatory and pain-relieving properties. By ingesting these herbs, you can address systemic inflammation and support overall health from within. Here's a detailed look at how to use teas, capsules, and tinctures made from turmeric and ginger for oral consumption.

Teas

Turmeric and ginger teas are a simple and enjoyable way to incorporate these powerful herbs into your daily routine. Teas allow for the direct infusion of beneficial compounds into hot water, making them easily absorbable by the body.

Turmeric and Ginger Tea Recipe:

- **Ingredients:**
    - 1 teaspoon fresh grated turmeric or 1/2 teaspoon turmeric powder
    - 1 teaspoon fresh grated ginger or 1/2 teaspoon ginger powder
    - 1 cup hot water
    - Honey or lemon to taste (optional)

Instructions:

1. Boil the water and then reduce it to a simmer.
2. Add the grated turmeric and ginger to the simmering water.
3. Let it steep for about 10-15 minutes.
4. Strain the tea into a cup.
5. Add honey or lemon to taste, if desired.

Benefits: Drinking 1-2 cups of turmeric and ginger tea daily can help reduce inflammation, support digestion, and boost the immune system. The warm, soothing beverage also provides a comforting way to start or end your day.

Capsules

For those who prefer a more convenient and consistent dosage, turmeric and ginger capsules are an excellent option. Capsules provide a standardized amount of the active compounds, ensuring you receive an effective dose each time.

Dosage:

- **Turmeric:** Typically, 500-1000 mg of turmeric extract standardized to contain 95% curcuminoids, 1-2 times daily with meals.
- **Ginger:** Typically, 500-1000 mg of ginger extract, 1-2 times daily with meals.

Benefits: Capsules are particularly useful for individuals with busy lifestyles who may not have the time to prepare teas or other fresh preparations. They also allow for precise control over the dosage, making it easier to manage your intake of these powerful herbs. Look for supplements that include black pepper extract (piperine) to enhance the absorption of curcumin.

Tinctures

Tinctures are concentrated liquid extracts made by soaking herbs in alcohol or glycerin. They offer a potent and fast-acting form of herbal medicine that is easy to incorporate into your routine.

Turmeric and Ginger Tincture Recipe:

- **Ingredients:**
    - Dried or fresh turmeric root
    - Dried or fresh ginger root
    - High-proof alcohol (such as vodka) or vegetable glycerin
    - A glass jar with a lid

Instructions:

1. Fill a glass jar about halfway with chopped turmeric and ginger root.
2. Pour the alcohol or glycerin over the herbs until they are fully submerged, leaving some space at the top.
3. Seal the jar and store it in a cool, dark place for 4-6 weeks, shaking it daily.
4. Strain the mixture through a cheesecloth or fine mesh strainer into a clean dropper bottle.

Dosage:

- Take 30-40 drops (approximately 1-2 dropperfuls) in a small amount of water or juice, 2-3 times daily.

Benefits: Tinctures are highly concentrated, making them a powerful option for those who need a stronger dose of the herbs. They are also convenient for individuals who may have difficulty swallowing capsules or prefer a liquid form. The alcohol or glycerin in tinctures helps preserve the active compounds, ensuring a long shelf life and stable potency.

Oral consumption of turmeric and ginger through teas, capsules, and tinctures provides a versatile and effective way to incorporate these anti-inflammatory herbs into your daily routine. Whether you enjoy the ritual of drinking tea, appreciate the convenience of capsules, or prefer the potency of tinctures, each method offers unique benefits. By choosing the form that best fits your lifestyle, you can harness the powerful properties of turmeric and ginger to support your health and well-being. Always consult with a healthcare provider before starting any new supplement regimen, especially if you have existing health conditions or are taking medications.

Herbal Pain Relief for Arthritis

Arthritis is a common condition characterized by inflammation and pain in the joints, affecting millions of people worldwide. While conventional treatments such as non-steroidal anti-inflammatory drugs (NSAIDs) and corticosteroids can be effective, they often come with side effects and may not be suitable for long-term use. Herbal remedies offer a natural alternative for managing arthritis pain and inflammation, providing relief without the adverse effects associated with pharmaceutical medications. This chapter explores various herbs known for their anti-inflammatory and analgesic properties, focusing on their use in alleviating arthritis symptoms. By understanding how these herbs work and how to incorporate them into your daily regimen, you can take a holistic approach to managing arthritis and improving your quality of life.

Understanding Arthritis and Its Symptoms

Arthritis is a broad term that refers to over 100 different conditions affecting the joints, causing pain, stiffness, and inflammation. The most common types of arthritis are osteoarthritis (OA) and rheumatoid arthritis (RA), each with distinct causes and characteristics.

Osteoarthritis (OA)

Osteoarthritis is the most prevalent form of arthritis, often referred to as "wear and tear" arthritis. It typically affects older adults and results from the gradual breakdown of cartilage, the protective tissue at the ends of bones that allows joints to move smoothly. As cartilage wears away, bones begin to rub against each other, leading to pain, swelling, and reduced joint mobility.

Symptoms of Osteoarthritis:

- **Joint Pain:** Often worsens with activity and improves with rest. Commonly affects the knees, hips, hands, and spine.

- **Stiffness:** Most noticeable in the morning or after periods of inactivity.

- **Swelling:** Joints may appear swollen due to inflammation.

- **Loss of Flexibility:** Reduced range of motion in the affected joints.

- **Grating Sensation:** A feeling or sound of bone rubbing against bone during movement.

Rheumatoid Arthritis (RA)

Rheumatoid arthritis is an autoimmune disease where the body's immune system mistakenly attacks the synovium, the lining of the membranes that surround the joints. This results in inflammation that can damage joint tissue and lead to chronic pain, deformity, and loss of function. RA can affect people of any age and typically involves multiple joints symmetrically, such as both hands or both knees.

Symptoms of Rheumatoid Arthritis:

- **Joint Pain and Swelling:** Often affects smaller joints first, such as those in the hands and feet.

- **Morning Stiffness:** Lasting longer than 30 minutes to several hours.

- **Fatigue:** General feeling of tiredness and lack of energy.

- **Fever:** Low-grade fever may accompany flare-ups.

- **Weight Loss:** Unintentional weight loss due to inflammation.
- **Nodules:** Firm lumps under the skin near joints.

Other Forms of Arthritis

In addition to OA and RA, there are several other types of arthritis, including:

- **Gout:** Caused by the accumulation of uric acid crystals in the joints, leading to sudden and severe pain, often in the big toe.
- **Psoriatic Arthritis:** Associated with the skin condition psoriasis, causing joint pain and swelling.
- **Ankylosing Spondylitis:** Affects the spine, causing inflammation and potentially leading to fusion of the vertebrae.
- **Juvenile Arthritis:** Refers to arthritis in children under the age of 16, which can cause similar symptoms to adult arthritis.

Diagnosing Arthritis

Diagnosing arthritis typically involves a combination of medical history, physical examination, and diagnostic tests. Blood tests can help identify markers of inflammation and autoimmune activity, while imaging tests like X-rays, MRI, and ultrasound can reveal joint damage and inflammation.

Understanding the various forms of arthritis and their symptoms is crucial for effective management and treatment. While conventional treatments can be effective, they often come with side effects and limitations. Herbal remedies offer a natural and complementary approach to managing arthritis pain and inflammation. In the following sections, we will explore specific herbs known for their anti-inflammatory and analgesic properties, providing practical guidance on how to incorporate them into your daily routine to alleviate arthritis symptoms and improve your quality of life.

How to Prepare and Use Herbal Remedies for Arthritis?

Incorporating herbal remedies into your arthritis management plan can provide natural relief from pain and inflammation. Various herbs offer unique benefits and can be used in different forms, such as teas, tinctures, capsules, and topical applications. Here's how to prepare and use some of the most effective herbs for arthritis.

Turmeric

Preparation and Use: Turmeric, known for its active compound curcumin, has potent anti-inflammatory properties. It can be consumed in several ways:

- **Tea:** To make turmeric tea, boil a cup of water and add 1/2 teaspoon of turmeric powder. Let it simmer for 10 minutes, then strain and add honey or lemon to taste. Drink this tea 1-2 times daily.

- **Golden Milk:** Combine 1 cup of milk (dairy or plant-based) with 1/2 teaspoon of turmeric powder, a pinch of black pepper, and 1/4 teaspoon of ginger powder. Heat gently and add honey for sweetness. This drink is especially soothing before bedtime.

- **Capsules:** Take standardized turmeric extract capsules (containing 95% curcuminoids) in doses of 500-1000 mg, 1-2 times daily with meals. Look for supplements that include black pepper extract (piperine) to enhance absorption.

Ginger

Preparation and Use: Ginger is another powerful anti-inflammatory herb that can help reduce arthritis symptoms:

- **Tea:** Grate 1 teaspoon of fresh ginger and steep it in a cup of boiling water for 10 minutes. Strain and add honey or lemon if desired. Drink ginger tea 1-2 times daily.

- **Smoothies:** Add fresh or powdered ginger to smoothies for an anti-inflammatory boost. Combine with fruits and vegetables for a nutritious drink.

- **Capsules:** Take ginger capsules containing 500-1000 mg of ginger extract, 1-2 times daily with meals.

Boswellia (Frankincense)

Preparation and Use: Boswellia, or Indian frankincense, is renowned for its ability to reduce inflammation and improve joint health:

- **Capsules:** Take standardized Boswellia extract (containing 60-65% boswellic acids) in doses of 300-500 mg, 2-3 times daily.

- **Tincture:** Use Boswellia tincture according to the manufacturer's instructions, typically 30-40 drops in water or juice, 2-3 times daily.

Devil's Claw

Preparation and Use: Devil's Claw is an herb known for its pain-relieving properties, particularly for osteoarthritis:

- **Tea:** Prepare Devil's Claw tea by boiling 1 teaspoon of the dried root in a cup of water for 10-15 minutes. Strain and drink 1-2 times daily.

- **Capsules:** Take standardized Devil's Claw extract capsules (containing 50-100 mg harpagoside) in doses of 500-1000 mg, 1-2 times daily.

Stinging Nettle

Preparation and Use: Stinging nettle has been traditionally used to alleviate arthritis symptoms due to its anti-inflammatory properties:

- **Tea:** Steep 1-2 teaspoons of dried stinging nettle leaves in a cup of boiling water for 10 minutes. Strain and drink 1-2 times daily.

- **Capsules:** Take stinging nettle capsules containing 300-500 mg of the dried leaf extract, 1-2 times daily.

Topical Applications

Turmeric and Ginger Salve:

- **Ingredients:** 1/4 cup coconut oil, 1/4 cup beeswax pellets, 1 tablespoon turmeric powder, 1 tablespoon fresh grated ginger or 1/2 tablespoon ginger powder, 10 drops essential oil (optional, such as lavender or eucalyptus).

- **Instructions:** In a double boiler, melt the coconut oil and beeswax pellets. Stir in the turmeric and ginger. Remove from heat and add the essential oil if using. Pour the mixture into a clean container and let it solidify. Apply the salve to the affected joints 2-3 times daily to reduce pain and inflammation.

Capsaicin Cream:

- **Ingredients:** 1/2 cup coconut oil, 1/4 cup grated beeswax, 2 tablespoons cayenne powder.

- **Instructions:** Melt the coconut oil and beeswax in a double boiler. Stir in the cayenne powder. Let the mixture cool slightly before pouring it into a container. Apply a small amount to the affected area and massage gently. Use this cream sparingly, as capsaicin can cause a burning sensation.

Preparing and using herbal remedies for arthritis can provide significant relief from pain and inflammation. Whether consumed as teas, capsules, or tinctures, or applied topically as salves and creams, these natural remedies offer a holistic approach to managing arthritis symptoms. Incorporate these herbs into your daily routine to enhance your overall well-being and improve joint health. Always consult with a healthcare provider before starting any new herbal regimen, especially if you have existing health conditions or are taking medications.

Natural Remedies for Muscle and Joint Pain

Muscle and joint pain are common issues that can arise from various causes, including physical activity, injuries, arthritis, and chronic conditions. While conventional pain relief methods like NSAIDs and prescription medications can be effective, they often come with side effects and may not be suitable for long-term use. Natural remedies offer an alternative approach to managing muscle and joint pain, leveraging the therapeutic properties of herbs, essential oils, and other natural substances. These remedies can help reduce inflammation, alleviate pain, and promote healing, providing a holistic solution for those seeking relief without relying on pharmaceuticals. This chapter explores a range of natural treatments for muscle and joint pain, focusing on the most effective herbs and techniques to help you achieve lasting relief and improved mobility.

Common Causes of Muscle and Joint Pain

Muscle and joint pain can significantly impact quality of life, hindering mobility and daily activities. Understanding the common causes of this pain can help in developing effective treatment strategies. Here are some of the primary factors that contribute to muscle and joint discomfort:

1. Physical Activity and Overuse

Strains and Sprains:

- **Muscle Strains:** Overstretching or tearing of muscles or tendons can result from sudden, forceful movements or prolonged repetitive activities.

- **Ligament Sprains:** Twisting or wrenching joints can cause sprains, leading to pain and swelling in the affected area.

Repetitive Stress Injuries:

- Activities that involve repetitive motions, such as typing, running, or lifting, can cause stress injuries to muscles and joints. This can lead to conditions like tendinitis or bursitis.

Delayed Onset Muscle Soreness (DOMS):

- Intense or unfamiliar exercise can cause microscopic damage to muscle fibers, resulting in soreness and stiffness that typically appears 24-48 hours after the activity.

2. Injuries

Acute Injuries:

- Traumatic injuries, such as fractures, dislocations, and ligament tears, can cause severe muscle and joint pain. These injuries often require immediate medical attention and can result from accidents, falls, or sports activities.

Chronic Injuries:

- Repeated minor injuries or inadequate healing of previous injuries can lead to chronic pain in muscles and joints. Conditions like chronic ankle instability or rotator cuff tendinopathy are examples.

3. Arthritis

Osteoarthritis (OA):

- A degenerative joint disease characterized by the breakdown of cartilage, leading to bone-on-bone friction, pain, stiffness, and reduced joint mobility. OA is commonly associated with aging and wear and tear on joints.

Rheumatoid Arthritis (RA):

- An autoimmune disease where the body's immune system attacks the synovium, the lining of the membranes that surround the joints. This causes inflammation, pain, swelling, and eventually joint deformity.

Other Types of Arthritis:

- Conditions such as gout, psoriatic arthritis, and ankylosing spondylitis also contribute to joint pain through various inflammatory processes.

4. Inflammatory Conditions

Tendinitis:

- Inflammation of the tendons, typically due to overuse or repetitive movements. Commonly affects areas like the shoulders, elbows, wrists, and heels.

Bursitis:

- Inflammation of the bursae, the small fluid-filled sacs that cushion the bones, tendons, and muscles near joints. Bursitis often occurs in the shoulders, elbows, hips, and knees.

Fibromyalgia:

- A chronic condition characterized by widespread musculoskeletal pain, fatigue, and tenderness in localized areas. The exact cause is unknown, but it is thought to involve a combination of genetic, environmental, and psychological factors.

5. Postural and Ergonomic Issues

Poor Posture:

- Maintaining poor posture, such as slouching or hunching over a desk, can lead to muscle imbalances and joint strain, resulting in pain, especially in the back, neck, and shoulders.

Ergonomic Factors:

- Inadequate workstation setups, improper lifting techniques, and prolonged periods of sitting or standing can contribute to muscle and joint pain. Ensuring proper ergonomics can help prevent these issues.

6. Medical Conditions

Osteoporosis:

- A condition characterized by weakened bones that are more prone to fractures. Fractures can lead to significant joint pain and decreased mobility.

Infections:

- Bacterial or viral infections can cause joint pain, swelling, and inflammation. Septic arthritis and Lyme disease are examples of infections that can affect the joints.

Autoimmune Disorders:

- Conditions like lupus and Sjogren's syndrome can cause widespread inflammation, affecting muscles and joints and leading to chronic pain.

Understanding the common causes of muscle and joint pain is crucial for identifying appropriate treatment strategies. Whether due to physical activity, injuries, inflammatory conditions, or medical issues, addressing the underlying cause is key to managing pain effectively. The following sections will explore natural remedies and techniques that can help alleviate muscle and joint pain, offering holistic and sustainable solutions for those seeking relief.

Effective Herbs for Muscle Relaxation and Pain Relief: Arnica, Cayenne, and Valerian

Incorporating herbal remedies into your pain management routine can provide natural and effective relief from muscle pain and tension. Three particularly effective herbs for muscle relaxation and pain relief are arnica, cayenne, and valerian. Each of these herbs offers unique properties that can help reduce inflammation, alleviate pain, and promote relaxation.

Arnica (Arnica montana)

Arnica is a well-known herb used topically to treat a variety of musculoskeletal conditions. Derived from the Arnica montana plant, it has been traditionally used for its anti-inflammatory and analgesic properties. Arnica is particularly effective in reducing pain and swelling associated with bruises, sprains, muscle strains, and arthritis.

Mechanisms of Action:

- **Anti-inflammatory:** Arnica contains compounds like helenalin and dihydrohelenalin, which help reduce inflammation and promote healing.

- **Pain Relief:** It improves blood circulation to the affected area, which helps to reduce pain and accelerate recovery.

Usage:

- **Topical Applications:** Arnica is commonly used in creams, gels, and ointments. Apply a small amount to the affected area 2-3 times daily. It is important to avoid applying arnica to broken skin or open wounds.

Cayenne (Capsicum annuum)

Cayenne pepper, known for its spicy flavor, is also a powerful herbal remedy for pain relief. The active component in cayenne, capsaicin, is widely used in topical pain relief treatments. Capsaicin works by depleting substance P, a neuropeptide involved in transmitting pain signals to the brain.

Mechanisms of Action:

- **Pain Relief:** Capsaicin desensitizes sensory receptors and reduces the perception of pain.

- **Anti-inflammatory:** It also has anti-inflammatory properties that help reduce swelling and discomfort.

Usage:

- **Topical Creams:** Capsaicin creams are available over-the-counter and can be applied to the affected area 2-4 times daily. Initially, capsaicin may cause a burning sensation, which usually diminishes with regular use.

- **Home Remedies:** You can make a homemade cayenne salve by mixing cayenne powder with a carrier oil (such as coconut oil) and applying it to the skin.

Valerian (Valeriana officinalis)

Valerian root is widely known for its sedative and muscle relaxant properties, making it an excellent herb for relieving muscle tension and promoting relaxation. It has been used for centuries to treat insomnia, anxiety, and nervous tension, which often accompany muscle pain.

Mechanisms of Action:

- **Muscle Relaxation:** Valerian contains valerenic acid and other compounds that have a calming effect on the nervous system and muscles.

- **Pain Relief:** Its sedative properties help reduce the perception of pain and promote overall relaxation.

Usage:

- **Teas and Tinctures:** Valerian can be consumed as a tea or tincture. To make valerian tea, steep 1-2 teaspoons of dried valerian root in hot water for 10-15 minutes. Drink 1-2 cups daily, preferably in the evening. For tinctures, follow the dosage instructions on the product label.

- **Supplements:** Valerian is also available in capsule form. A typical dose is 300-600 mg of valerian extract, taken 1-2 times daily.

Arnica, cayenne, and valerian are powerful herbs that can effectively help manage muscle pain and tension. Arnica is best used topically to reduce inflammation and pain, while cayenne provides pain relief through its active compound capsaicin. Valerian, with its sedative and muscle relaxant properties, helps alleviate muscle tension and promotes relaxation. Incorporating these herbs into your pain management regimen can provide natural relief and improve your overall well-being. As always, consult with a healthcare provider before starting any new herbal treatments, especially if you have existing health conditions or are taking other medications.

BOOK 11:

Herbal Support for Mental Health: Herbs for Anxiety, Stress, and Emotional Well-Being

Herbs for Anxiety and Stress

Anxiety and stress are common experiences in today's fast-paced world, affecting millions of people globally. While occasional stress and anxiety are natural responses to life's challenges, chronic stress and persistent anxiety can significantly impact mental and physical health. Conventional treatments, such as medications and therapy, can be effective but often come with side effects and may not be suitable for everyone. Herbal remedies offer a natural and holistic alternative for managing anxiety and stress. These herbs work by calming the nervous system, reducing stress hormones, and promoting relaxation without the adverse effects associated with many pharmaceuticals. This chapter introduces various herbs that have been traditionally used to alleviate anxiety and stress, providing insights into their benefits, mechanisms of action, and practical applications. By incorporating these natural remedies into your daily routine, you can achieve greater emotional balance and resilience.

Understanding Anxiety and Stress

Anxiety and stress are natural responses to perceived threats or challenges. While they can be helpful in short bursts, preparing the body to react to danger or perform under pressure, chronic anxiety and prolonged stress can have detrimental effects on both mental and physical health. Understanding the symptoms and causes of anxiety and stress is crucial for managing these conditions effectively.

Symptoms of Anxiety and Stress

Physical Symptoms:

- **Increased Heart Rate:** A common reaction to stress and anxiety, as the body prepares for "fight or flight."

- **Muscle Tension:** Chronic stress can cause muscles to remain tense for extended periods.

- **Sweating:** Excessive sweating, particularly in the palms and underarms, is a typical stress response.

- **Headaches:** Often caused by muscle tension and heightened blood pressure.

- **Fatigue:** Constant anxiety and stress can drain energy levels, leading to chronic fatigue.

- **Digestive Issues:** Symptoms such as stomachaches, nausea, and diarrhea can arise from stress affecting the digestive system.

- **Sleep Disturbances:** Difficulty falling asleep, staying asleep, or experiencing restful sleep.

Emotional and Cognitive Symptoms:

- **Restlessness:** An inability to relax or stay still.

- **Irritability:** Increased sensitivity and quickness to anger or frustration.

- **Difficulty Concentrating:** Trouble focusing on tasks or maintaining attention.

- **Constant Worry:** Persistent thoughts about potential problems or dangers, often out of proportion to the actual threat.

- **Panic Attacks:** Sudden, intense episodes of fear accompanied by physical symptoms like chest pain, shortness of breath, and dizziness.

- **Feeling Overwhelmed:** A sense of being unable to cope with life's demands.

Causes of Anxiety and Stress

Biological Factors:

- **Genetics:** A family history of anxiety disorders can increase the likelihood of experiencing anxiety and stress.

- **Brain Chemistry:** Imbalances in neurotransmitters, such as serotonin and dopamine, can contribute to anxiety and stress.

- **Medical Conditions:** Chronic illnesses, hormonal imbalances, and certain medications can trigger anxiety and stress.

Psychological Factors:

- **Personality Traits:** Individuals with certain personality traits, such as perfectionism or a tendency towards negative thinking, may be more prone to anxiety and stress.

- **Past Trauma:** Experiences of trauma or abuse can lead to heightened stress and anxiety responses.

- **Mental Health Disorders:** Conditions like depression, PTSD, and other anxiety disorders can exacerbate stress and anxiety.

Environmental Factors:

- **Life Events:** Significant changes or events, such as losing a job, divorce, or the death of a loved one, can trigger stress and anxiety.

- **Work and School:** High-pressure environments, heavy workloads, and demanding schedules can contribute to chronic stress.

- **Social Pressures:** Interpersonal conflicts, social isolation, and relationship issues can lead to increased anxiety and stress.

Lifestyle Factors:

- **Poor Nutrition:** Diets lacking essential nutrients can affect brain function and mood.

- **Lack of Exercise:** Regular physical activity is crucial for maintaining mental health.

- **Sleep Deprivation:** Insufficient sleep can exacerbate stress and anxiety.

- **Substance Abuse:** The use of alcohol, caffeine, and drugs can worsen anxiety and stress symptoms.

Anxiety and stress are complex conditions with multiple causes and wide-ranging symptoms. Recognizing these symptoms and understanding their underlying causes is the first step towards effective management. While conventional treatments are available, many individuals seek natural alternatives to complement or replace pharmaceutical options. The following sections will explore various herbs that can help alleviate anxiety and stress, offering a holistic approach to achieving emotional balance and resilience.

Valerian Root: Calming Effects and Usage

Valerian root, derived from the Valeriana officinalis plant, has been used for centuries as a natural remedy for anxiety, stress, and insomnia. Known for its potent calming effects, valerian root is often referred to as "nature's Valium." This herb works by interacting with the gamma-aminobutyric acid (GABA) receptors in the brain, which play a crucial role in regulating nerve impulses and promoting relaxation. The active compounds in valerian root, including valerenic acid, isovaleric acid, and various antioxidants, contribute to its soothing properties.

Calming Effects of Valerian Root

Valerian root is renowned for its ability to promote relaxation and reduce anxiety. The herb's interaction with GABA receptors helps to increase the availability of GABA in the brain, which in turn produces a calming effect. This mechanism is similar to how certain anti-anxiety medications, such as benzodiazepines, work, but valerian root does so without the risk of dependency and adverse side effects associated with these drugs.

Studies have shown that valerian root can effectively reduce the symptoms of generalized anxiety disorder (GAD) and improve sleep quality. Its sedative properties make it particularly useful for individuals who experience anxiety-related insomnia. Unlike many prescription sleep aids, valerian root does not typically cause morning grogginess, making it a preferred choice for those seeking a natural solution for better sleep and reduced anxiety.

Usage of Valerian Root

Valerian root can be consumed in various forms, including teas, tinctures, capsules, and extracts. Each form offers its own benefits and can be chosen based on personal preference and convenience.

Tea:

- To make valerian root tea, steep 1-2 teaspoons of dried valerian root in a cup of hot water for about 10-15 minutes. Strain the tea and drink it 30-60 minutes before bedtime or whenever you need to relax. The taste of valerian tea can be quite strong and earthy, so adding honey or a splash of lemon juice can help improve its flavor.

Tincture:

- Valerian root tinctures are concentrated liquid extracts that can be taken by adding a few drops to a small amount of water or juice. The typical dosage is 30-40 drops, 2-3 times daily, with the last dose taken about an hour before bedtime. Tinctures offer a convenient way to consume valerian root, especially for those who may not enjoy the taste of the tea.

Capsules:

- Valerian root capsules are a popular choice for those seeking a quick and easy way to take the herb. The standard dosage is 300-600 mg of valerian extract, taken 1-2 times daily. It is advisable to start with a lower dose and gradually increase it to find the optimal amount that works for you.

Extracts:

- Valerian root extracts are available in liquid or powdered form. These can be mixed into drinks or taken as directed on the product label. Extracts provide a potent and effective way to benefit from valerian root's calming effects.

Safety and Precautions

While valerian root is generally considered safe for most people, it is important to use it responsibly and be aware of potential side effects. Some individuals may experience mild side effects such as headaches, dizziness, or digestive issues. It is advisable to consult with a healthcare provider before starting valerian root, especially if you are pregnant, breastfeeding, or taking other medications. Valerian root should not be combined with alcohol or other sedatives, as this can enhance its effects and lead to excessive drowsiness.

Valerian root is a powerful and natural remedy for anxiety, stress, and insomnia, offering a safe alternative to prescription medications. Its calming effects, achieved through interaction with GABA receptors in the brain, help promote relaxation and improve sleep quality. Whether consumed as a tea, tincture, capsule, or extract, valerian root can be a valuable addition to your wellness routine. Always consult with a healthcare provider to ensure its safe and effective use, and enjoy the soothing benefits of this remarkable herb.

Passionflower: Soothing Anxiety and Promoting Relaxation

Passionflower (Passiflora incarnata) is a beautiful flowering plant known for its calming and anxiety-reducing properties. Native to the southeastern United States, Central and South America, passionflower has been used for centuries in traditional medicine to treat anxiety, insomnia, and other nervous system disorders. The calming effects of passionflower are attributed to its ability to increase levels of gamma-aminobutyric acid (GABA) in the brain, a neurotransmitter that helps regulate mood and promote relaxation.

Soothing Anxiety with Passionflower

Passionflower is particularly effective in reducing anxiety and promoting a sense of calm without the sedative effects associated with some other natural remedies. The herb works by enhancing the levels of GABA in the brain, which helps to inhibit overactive neural activity and produce a calming effect. This action is similar to that of prescription anti-anxiety medications, but passionflower provides these benefits naturally and with fewer side effects.

Research has shown that passionflower can significantly reduce symptoms of generalized anxiety disorder (GAD) and can be as effective as some prescription medications. In clinical studies, participants who took passionflower extract experienced a notable reduction in anxiety levels, demonstrating its efficacy as a natural anxiolytic.

Promoting Relaxation with Passionflower

Beyond its anxiolytic properties, passionflower is also well-regarded for its ability to promote relaxation and improve sleep quality. It is commonly used as a natural remedy for insomnia and other sleep disturbances, especially those caused by stress and anxiety. Passionflower's calming effects help to ease the mind and prepare the body for restful sleep, making it a popular choice for those struggling with sleeplessness.

The herb's mild sedative properties make it effective in helping individuals fall asleep faster and enjoy a deeper, more restorative sleep. Unlike synthetic sleep aids, passionflower does not typically cause morning grogginess, allowing individuals to wake up feeling refreshed and rejuvenated.

Usage of Passionflower

Passionflower can be consumed in various forms, including teas, tinctures, capsules, and extracts. Each form offers its own benefits and can be chosen based on personal preference and convenience.

Tea:

- To make passionflower tea, steep 1 teaspoon of dried passionflower in a cup of hot water for about 10-15 minutes. Strain the tea and drink it 30-60 minutes before bedtime or whenever you need to relax. The tea has a mild, pleasant taste, and adding honey or lemon can enhance its flavor.

Tincture:

- Passionflower tinctures are concentrated liquid extracts that can be taken by adding a few drops to a small amount of water or juice. The typical dosage is 30-40 drops, 2-3 times daily, with the last dose taken about an hour before bedtime. Tinctures offer a convenient way to consume passionflower, especially for those who may not enjoy the taste of the tea.

Capsules:

- Passionflower capsules are a popular choice for those seeking a quick and easy way to take the herb. The standard dosage is 250-500 mg of passionflower extract, taken 1-2 times daily. It is advisable to start with a lower dose and gradually increase it to find the optimal amount that works for you.

Extracts:

- Passionflower extracts are available in liquid or powdered form. These can be mixed into drinks or taken as directed on the product label. Extracts provide a potent and effective way to benefit from passionflower's calming effects.

Safety and Precautions

While passionflower is generally considered safe for most people, it is important to use it responsibly and be aware of potential side effects. Some individuals may experience mild side effects such as dizziness, drowsiness, or digestive issues. It is advisable to consult with a healthcare provider before starting passionflower, especially if you are pregnant, breastfeeding, or taking other medications. Passionflower should not be combined with alcohol or other sedatives, as this can enhance its effects and lead to excessive drowsiness.

Passionflower is a powerful and natural remedy for soothing anxiety and promoting relaxation. Its ability to enhance GABA levels in the brain helps to reduce anxiety and stress, while its mild sedative properties improve sleep quality without causing morning grogginess. Whether consumed as a tea, tincture, capsule, or extract, passionflower can be a valuable addition to your wellness routine. Always consult with a healthcare provider to ensure its safe and effective use, and enjoy the calming benefits of this remarkable herb.

Lemon Balm: Reducing Stress and Enhancing Mood

Lemon balm (Melissa officinalis) is a fragrant herb belonging to the mint family, known for its refreshing lemon scent and its soothing effects on the mind and body. Traditionally used in herbal medicine for centuries, lemon balm is celebrated for its ability to reduce stress, alleviate anxiety, and enhance mood. This versatile herb offers a gentle and natural way to support emotional well-being and promote relaxation.

Reducing Stress with Lemon Balm

One of the primary benefits of lemon balm is its ability to reduce stress. The herb contains compounds such as rosmarinic acid and flavonoids, which have calming effects on the nervous system. These compounds work by increasing the availability of gamma-aminobutyric acid (GABA) in the brain, a neurotransmitter that helps regulate anxiety and induce relaxation. By modulating GABA levels, lemon balm helps to soothe the nervous system, making it an effective remedy for stress relief.

Research has shown that lemon balm can significantly reduce the symptoms of stress and anxiety. In clinical studies, participants who consumed lemon balm extract reported feeling more relaxed and less stressed compared to those who took a placebo. The herb's calming effects make it particularly useful for managing everyday stressors and promoting a sense of calm and balance.

Enhancing Mood with Lemon Balm

In addition to reducing stress, lemon balm is also known for its mood-enhancing properties. The herb's ability to improve mood is attributed to its positive impact on neurotransmitters and its antioxidant properties, which help protect the brain from oxidative stress. By supporting brain health and regulating neurotransmitter levels, lemon balm can help alleviate feelings of sadness and improve overall emotional well-being.

Lemon balm is often used to address symptoms of mild depression and promote a positive outlook. Its gentle mood-lifting effects make it a valuable herb for those experiencing emotional fluctuations due to stress or hormonal changes. Regular consumption of lemon balm can help maintain a balanced mood and enhance mental clarity, making it easier to cope with the challenges of daily life.

Usage of Lemon Balm

Lemon balm can be consumed in various forms, including teas, tinctures, capsules, and extracts. Each form offers its own benefits and can be chosen based on personal preference and convenience.

Tea:

- To make lemon balm tea, steep 1-2 teaspoons of dried lemon balm leaves in a cup of hot water for about 10-15 minutes. Strain the tea and drink it 2-3 times daily. The tea has a pleasant, citrusy flavor that is both refreshing and soothing.

Tincture:

- Lemon balm tinctures are concentrated liquid extracts that can be taken by adding a few drops to a small amount of water or juice. The typical dosage is 30-40 drops, 2-3 times daily. Tinctures offer a convenient way to consume lemon balm, especially for those who prefer a quick and potent form.

Capsules:

- Lemon balm capsules are a popular choice for those seeking an easy and precise way to take the herb. The standard dosage is 300-600 mg of lemon balm extract, taken 1-2 times daily. Capsules provide a consistent dose and are convenient for on-the-go use.

Extracts:

- Lemon balm extracts are available in liquid or powdered form. These can be mixed into drinks or taken as directed on the product label. Extracts provide a potent and effective way to benefit from lemon balm's calming and mood-enhancing effects.

Safety and Precautions

Lemon balm is generally considered safe for most people when used appropriately. However, it is important to use it responsibly and be aware of potential side effects. Some individuals may experience mild side effects such as dizziness or gastrointestinal discomfort. It is advisable to consult with a healthcare provider before starting lemon balm, especially if you are pregnant, breastfeeding, or taking other medications. Lemon balm should be used with caution in individuals with thyroid disorders, as it may interfere with thyroid function.

Lemon balm is a versatile and effective herb for reducing stress and enhancing mood. Its calming effects on the nervous system and its mood-lifting properties make it a valuable addition to any wellness routine. Whether consumed as a tea, tincture, capsule, or extract, lemon balm can help promote relaxation, alleviate anxiety, and improve emotional well-being. Always consult with a healthcare provider to ensure its safe and effective use and enjoy the refreshing and soothing benefits of this remarkable herb.

Improving Mood with St. John's Wort

St. John's Wort (Hypericum perforatum) is a flowering plant that has been used for centuries in traditional medicine to treat a variety of ailments, most notably depression and mood disorders. Known for its vibrant yellow flowers, this herb has gained significant attention for its ability to improve mood and alleviate symptoms of mild to moderate depression. St. John's Wort contains several active compounds, including hypericin and hyperforin, which are believed to contribute to its antidepressant effects. These compounds influence neurotransmitters in the brain, such as serotonin, dopamine, and norepinephrine, which play key roles in regulating mood. This chapter explores the history, mechanisms of action, and practical applications of St. John's Wort, providing insights into how this powerful herb can be used to support mental health and emotional well-being. By understanding the benefits and proper usage of St. John's Wort, individuals can incorporate it into their wellness routine to help manage depression and enhance their overall mood.

The History and Traditional Uses of St. John's Wort

St. John's Wort (Hypericum perforatum) has a long and rich history of use in traditional medicine, dating back to ancient times. This herb, named after St. John the Baptist because it typically blooms around his feast day on June 24th, has been revered for its healing properties for centuries. Its vibrant yellow flowers and extensive medicinal applications have made it a staple in herbal medicine across various cultures.

Ancient and Medieval Uses

The earliest recorded use of St. John's Wort dates to ancient Greece, where it was used by physicians such as Hippocrates and Dioscorides. Hippocrates, often referred to as the "father of medicine," noted the herb's therapeutic potential. Dioscorides, a Greek physician and botanist, documented its use in his seminal work, "De Materia Medica," describing its effectiveness in treating wounds, burns, and nervous disorders.

In medieval Europe, St. John's Wort was considered a powerful protector against evil spirits and was used in various rituals and remedies. It was often hung above doors and windows to ward off evil and bring good luck. The herb was also used to treat a variety of ailments, including wounds, muscle pain, anxiety, and melancholia, which was the historical term for depression.

Renaissance and Beyond

During the Renaissance, St. John's Wort continued to be a popular remedy in European herbal medicine. Paracelsus, a Swiss physician and alchemist, praised its healing properties and used it to treat wounds and mental health disorders. The herb's ability to promote healing and reduce inflammation made it a valuable component of many medicinal preparations.

In the 16th and 17th centuries, St. John's Wort was widely used in England and other parts of Europe for its purported ability to treat melancholy and other mood disorders. Herbalists of the time, such as Nicholas Culpeper, recommended the herb for its soothing and mood-lifting effects. Culpeper, in his influential herbal compendium, noted its use for treating nervous conditions and wounds.

Modern Applications

In modern herbal medicine, St. John's Wort is primarily recognized for its antidepressant properties. Extensive research has validated its effectiveness in treating mild to moderate depression, making it one of the most studied and utilized herbal remedies for mood disorders. The active compounds in St. John's Wort, including hypericin and hyperforin, are believed to enhance mood by increasing the levels of neurotransmitters such as serotonin, dopamine, and norepinephrine in the brain.

Apart from its antidepressant effects, St. John's Wort is also used to treat anxiety, insomnia, and seasonal affective disorder (SAD). Its anti-inflammatory and antiviral properties have expanded its use in treating skin conditions, such as wounds, burns, and eczema.

Traditional Preparations

St. John's Wort has traditionally been prepared in various forms to maximize its medicinal benefits:

- **Infusions and Teas:** Dried St. John's Wort flowers and leaves are steeped in hot water to make a calming tea that can help alleviate anxiety and improve mood.

- **Tinctures:** Alcohol-based extracts of St. John's Wort are used for their concentrated therapeutic effects, offering a convenient way to consume the herb.

- **Oils and Salves:** Infused oils and salves made from St. John's Wort are applied topically to treat wounds, burns, and skin inflammations.

- **Capsules and Tablets:** Standardized extracts of St. John's Wort are available in capsule and tablet form, providing a consistent dosage for managing depression and mood disorders.

St. John's Wort has a storied history as a versatile and powerful herb, revered for its ability to heal wounds, protect against evil, and lift the spirits. Its extensive use across various cultures and historical periods underscores its enduring therapeutic value. Today, St. John's Wort remains a popular natural remedy for depression, anxiety, and other mood disorders, supported by both tradition and modern scientific research. By understanding its rich history and traditional uses, we can appreciate the full scope of St. John's Wort's healing potential.

Mechanisms of Action: How St. John's Wort Affects Mood

St. John's Wort (Hypericum perforatum) has gained significant attention for its effectiveness in improving mood and alleviating symptoms of depression. The herb's mood-enhancing properties are primarily attributed to its complex chemical composition, which includes a variety of active compounds such as hypericin, hyperforin, and flavonoids. These compounds work synergistically to affect the brain's neurotransmitter systems, leading to improved mood and reduced anxiety.

Hypericin and Hyperforin

Hypericin and hyperforin are two of the most studied active compounds in St. John's Wort, and they play a crucial role in its antidepressant effects. Hypericin is believed to contribute to the herb's ability to modulate neurotransmitter activity, particularly serotonin. Serotonin is a key neurotransmitter involved in regulating mood, and imbalances in serotonin levels are commonly associated with depression. By inhibiting the reuptake of serotonin, hypericin helps increase the availability of this neurotransmitter in the brain, leading to improved mood and a reduction in depressive symptoms.

Hyperforin, another major compound in St. John's Wort, is thought to have a broad-spectrum inhibitory effect on the reuptake of several neurotransmitters, including serotonin, dopamine, norepinephrine, gamma-aminobutyric acid (GABA), and glutamate. By blocking the reuptake of these neurotransmitters, hyperforin increases their levels in the synaptic cleft, the space between neurons where neurotransmitters exert their effects. This enhancement of neurotransmitter activity contributes to mood stabilization, reduced anxiety, and overall improved mental well-being.

Neurotransmitter Modulation

St. John's Wort's influence on neurotransmitters extends beyond serotonin and includes dopamine and norepinephrine, both of which are critical for maintaining mood balance and cognitive function. Dopamine is associated with pleasure, motivation, and reward, while norepinephrine plays a role in alertness and response to stress. By inhibiting the reuptake of these neurotransmitters, St. John's Wort helps sustain their levels in the brain, which can alleviate symptoms of depression and enhance mood.

Additionally, St. John's Wort affects the GABAergic system, which is involved in regulating anxiety. GABA is the primary inhibitory neurotransmitter in the brain, responsible for reducing neuronal excitability and promoting relaxation. By enhancing GABA activity, St. John's Wort helps to calm the nervous system, reduce anxiety, and promote a sense of tranquility.

Anti-inflammatory and Antioxidant Properties

Chronic inflammation and oxidative stress have been linked to the development of depression and other mood disorders. St. John's Wort exhibits anti-inflammatory and antioxidant properties that contribute to its therapeutic effects. The flavonoids and other phenolic compounds in St. John's Wort help reduce inflammation and protect brain cells from oxidative damage. By mitigating these underlying factors, St. John's Wort supports brain health and improves mood.

Regulation of the HPA Axis

The hypothalamic-pituitary-adrenal (HPA) axis is a central stress response system that plays a crucial role in mood regulation. Dysregulation of the HPA axis is often observed in individuals with depression and anxiety disorders. St. John's Wort has been shown to modulate the activity of the HPA axis, helping to normalize cortisol levels and improve the body's response to stress. This regulation of the HPA axis contributes to the herb's ability to alleviate stress-related mood disorders.

St. John's Wort exerts its mood-enhancing effects through a multifaceted mechanism of action involving the modulation of neurotransmitters, anti-inflammatory and antioxidant properties, and regulation of the HPA axis. By increasing the availability of serotonin, dopamine, norepinephrine, and GABA in the brain, St. John's Wort helps alleviate symptoms of depression, reduce anxiety, and promote overall mental well-being. Understanding these mechanisms provides a clearer picture of how St. John's Wort can be effectively used to support mental health and improve mood.

Scientific Evidence and Clinical Studies on St. John's Wort

St. John's Wort (Hypericum perforatum) has been extensively studied for its potential benefits in treating depression and other mood disorders. Scientific evidence from numerous clinical studies supports its effectiveness, particularly in cases of mild to moderate depression. These studies highlight the herb's potential as a natural alternative to conventional antidepressants, with a favorable safety profile and fewer side effects.

Effectiveness in Treating Depression

One of the most significant bodies of research on St. John's Wort focuses on its use in treating depression. A meta-analysis published in the "Journal of the American Medical Association" (JAMA) analyzed data from 27 clinical trials involving over 3,800 patients. The results indicated that St. John's Wort extracts were more effective than placebo and were comparable to standard antidepressants for treating mild to moderate depression. This comprehensive review underscored the herb's efficacy and supported its use as a legitimate treatment option.

Another notable study, published in the "British Medical Journal" (BMJ), reviewed 29 clinical trials involving over 5,000 patients. This study also found that St. John's Wort was as effective as standard antidepressants, such as selective serotonin reuptake inhibitors (SSRIs), for treating mild to moderate depression. Additionally, patients taking St. John's Wort experienced fewer side effects compared to those taking conventional antidepressants.

Comparison with Standard Antidepressants

Several studies have directly compared St. John's Wort with standard antidepressant medications. In a randomized controlled trial published in "The Lancet," St. John's Wort was compared with fluoxetine (Prozac) and placebo in patients with moderate depression. The study found that St. John's Wort was as effective as fluoxetine in reducing depressive symptoms, with fewer reported side effects.

Another study published in "European Neuropsychopharmacology" compared the effectiveness of St. John's Wort with sertraline (Zoloft) in patients with moderate to severe depression. The results indicated that both treatments were similarly effective in reducing depressive symptoms, but St. John's Wort was associated with a better tolerability profile.

Long-term Safety and Efficacy

Long-term studies have also been conducted to assess the safety and efficacy of St. John's Wort. A study published in "Pharmacopsychiatry" followed patients with mild to moderate depression over one year of treatment with St. John's Wort. The study concluded that St. John's Wort was effective in maintaining symptom relief over the long term, with a good safety profile and minimal side effects.

Mechanistic Studies

In addition to clinical trials, mechanistic studies have provided insights into how St. John's Wort exerts its antidepressant effects. Research has shown that the active compounds in St. John's Wort, particularly hypericin and hyperforin, modulate neurotransmitter activity by inhibiting the reuptake of serotonin, dopamine, and norepinephrine. These findings support the clinical evidence and help explain the herb's mood-enhancing properties.

Safety and Side Effects

St. John's Wort is generally considered safe when used appropriately, but it can interact with several medications due to its induction of cytochrome P450 enzymes. This interaction can reduce the effectiveness of medications such as oral contraceptives, anticoagulants, and certain antidepressants. It is essential to consult with a healthcare provider before starting St. John's Wort, especially if you are taking other medications.

Common side effects of St. John's Wort are generally mild and may include gastrointestinal symptoms, dizziness, dry mouth, and photosensitivity. Compared to standard antidepressants, St. John's Wort tends to have a more favorable side effect profile, making it a preferred option for many individuals seeking natural treatment alternatives.

The scientific evidence and clinical studies on St. John's Wort provide robust support for its use in treating mild to moderate depression. The herb has demonstrated effectiveness comparable to standard antidepressants, with fewer side effects and better tolerability. Mechanistic studies further elucidate its action on neurotransmitter systems, enhancing our understanding of how it improves mood. However, it is crucial to consider potential interactions with other medications and consult with a healthcare provider before starting treatment with St. John's Wort. Overall, the substantial body of research underscores St. John's Wort's potential as a valuable tool in managing depression and promoting mental well-being.

BOOK 12

Adaptogenic Plants and Psychological Resilience: Depression and Memory Diseases

Adaptogenic plants have garnered significant attention in recent years for their remarkable ability to enhance the body's resilience to stress and promote overall well-being. These herbs help the body adapt to physical, mental, and emotional stressors, making them valuable allies in managing the challenges of modern life. Adaptogens work by modulating the stress response, balancing hormones, and supporting the immune system, thereby improving the body's capacity to cope with stress and maintain equilibrium. This chapter delves into the world of adaptogenic plants, exploring how they can bolster psychological resilience and enhance mental health. By understanding the unique properties and benefits of these powerful herbs, you can incorporate them into your wellness routine to build a stronger, more resilient mind and body.

Understanding Adaptogens: What They Are and How They Work

Adaptogens are a unique class of herbs and natural substances that help the body resist and adapt to stressors of all kinds, whether physical, mental, or emotional. The concept of adaptogens was first introduced in the mid-20th century by Russian scientist Dr. Nikolai Lazarev, who defined them as agents that increase the body's nonspecific resistance to stress. These herbs have been used for centuries in traditional medicine systems, including Ayurveda and Traditional Chinese Medicine (TCM), to enhance resilience and promote overall health.

What Are Adaptogens?

Adaptogens are naturally occurring substances found in various plants and fungi that help the body maintain homeostasis and adapt to stress. Unlike stimulants, which provide a temporary boost in energy but can lead to a subsequent crash, adaptogens work more subtly by supporting the body's natural ability to balance and regulate itself. They help normalize physiological functions and improve the body's response to stress without overstimulation or depletion of energy reserves.

Key Characteristics of Adaptogens

Adaptogens possess several key characteristics that distinguish them from other herbal remedies:

- **Non-Specific Response:** Adaptogens enhance the body's general resistance to stress rather than targeting a specific condition or symptom. They provide a broad-spectrum support to the body's adaptive systems.

- **Normalizing Effect:** Adaptogens help to stabilize physiological processes and bring the body back to a balanced state. They can both calm and energize, depending on what the body needs at a given time.

- **Non-Toxic:** Adaptogens are safe for long-term use and do not cause harm or significant side effects. They support the body's natural functions without causing imbalances.

How Adaptogens Work?

Adaptogens exert their effects through various mechanisms that involve the regulation of the body's stress response systems, particularly the hypothalamic-pituitary-adrenal (HPA) axis, and the sympathoadrenal system (SAS). Here's how they work:

Modulating the HPA Axis:

- The HPA axis is the central stress response system that involves the hypothalamus, pituitary gland, and adrenal glands. When the body encounters stress, the HPA axis is activated, leading to the release of stress hormones such as cortisol. Adaptogens help to regulate the activity of the HPA axis, preventing an overreaction to stress and reducing excessive cortisol production. This helps maintain a balanced stress response and prevents the negative effects of chronic stress.

Balancing Neurotransmitters:

- Adaptogens influence the levels of neurotransmitters in the brain, such as serotonin, dopamine, and norepinephrine. By modulating these chemical messengers, adaptogens help improve mood, enhance mental clarity, and reduce anxiety and depression.

Supporting the Immune System:

- Chronic stress can weaken the immune system, making the body more susceptible to illnesses. Adaptogens bolster the immune response by enhancing the activity of immune cells and reducing inflammation. This immune-modulating effect helps the body stay resilient against infections and other stress-related health issues.

Enhancing Energy and Stamina:

- Adaptogens improve physical and mental endurance by optimizing energy production and reducing fatigue. They enhance the efficiency of cellular energy pathways, ensuring that the body can sustain prolonged physical and mental activity without feeling exhausted.

Antioxidant Effects:

- Many adaptogens possess antioxidant properties that protect the body from oxidative stress and free radical damage. By neutralizing harmful free radicals, adaptogens help prevent cellular damage and support overall health and longevity.

Adaptogens are powerful allies in promoting psychological resilience and overall well-being. By understanding what adaptogens are and how they work, you can appreciate their unique ability to enhance the body's resistance to stress and improve mental and physical health. These remarkable herbs offer a natural and holistic approach to managing stress, enhancing energy, and supporting the body's adaptive capacities. Incorporating adaptogens into your wellness routine can help you build a stronger, more resilient mind and body, better equipped to handle the challenges of modern life.

Rhodiola Rosea: Enhancing Energy and Reducing Fatigue

Rhodiola rosea, commonly known as golden root or Arctic root, is a powerful adaptogenic herb that has been used for centuries in traditional medicine to enhance energy, reduce fatigue, and improve overall resilience to stress. Native to the cold regions of Europe and Asia, Rhodiola rosea has a long history of use in Scandinavian countries and Russia, where it has been prized for its ability to help the body adapt to the harsh conditions of the Arctic environment. Modern scientific research has validated many of the traditional claims, highlighting Rhodiola's potential as a natural remedy for fatigue and stress-related symptoms.

Enhancing Energy

One of the primary benefits of Rhodiola rosea is its ability to enhance physical and mental energy. This adaptogen works by optimizing the efficiency of cellular energy production, particularly within the mitochondria, the powerhouse of the cells. Rhodiola increases the availability of adenosine triphosphate (ATP), the primary energy carrier in the body, which helps boost energy levels and improve stamina.

Mechanisms of Action:

- **Increasing ATP Production:** Rhodiola enhances the production and availability of ATP, ensuring that cells have a steady supply of energy to perform their functions efficiently.

- **Reducing Fatigue:** By promoting efficient energy utilization, Rhodiola helps to combat physical and mental fatigue, making it easier to sustain prolonged periods of activity and concentration.

- **Improving Oxygen Utilization:** Rhodiola improves the body's ability to utilize oxygen, which is particularly beneficial during physical exertion, leading to better endurance and reduced feelings of exhaustion.

Reducing Fatigue

Rhodiola rosea is particularly effective in reducing both physical and mental fatigue, making it a valuable herb for individuals who experience chronic tiredness or burnout. Its adaptogenic properties help the body manage stress more effectively, which in turn reduces the impact of stress-induced fatigue.

Mechanisms of Action:

- **Regulating Cortisol Levels:** Rhodiola helps to balance the production and release of cortisol, a key stress hormone. By preventing excessive cortisol production, Rhodiola mitigates the negative effects of chronic stress, which often include fatigue and exhaustion.

- **Enhancing Mood and Cognitive Function:** Rhodiola has been shown to improve mood and cognitive function by modulating neurotransmitter levels, such as serotonin, dopamine, and norepinephrine. This leads to better mental clarity, reduced anxiety, and overall improved emotional well-being, which can help alleviate mental fatigue.

- **Reducing Inflammation:** Chronic stress and fatigue are often accompanied by inflammation. Rhodiola possesses anti-inflammatory properties that help reduce inflammation, supporting overall health and vitality.

Scientific Evidence

Several clinical studies have demonstrated the efficacy of Rhodiola rosea in enhancing energy and reducing fatigue. In a study published in "Phytomedicine," participants experiencing stress-related fatigue were given Rhodiola extract for four weeks. The results showed significant improvements in fatigue levels, mood, and cognitive performance compared to the placebo group. Another study, published in the "International Journal of Sport Nutrition and Exercise Metabolism," found that Rhodiola supplementation improved endurance exercise performance and reduced perceived exertion in athletes.

Usage and Dosage

Rhodiola rosea is available in various forms, including capsules, tablets, and tinctures. The recommended dosage typically ranges from 200 to 600 mg of standardized extract per day, depending on the concentration of active compounds (such as rosavins and salidrosides). It is advisable to start with a lower dose and gradually increase it to find the optimal amount that works for you. Rhodiola is best taken in the morning or early afternoon, as taking it too late in the day may interfere with sleep.

Tea:

- To make Rhodiola tea, steep 1-2 grams of dried Rhodiola root in hot water for about 10-15 minutes. Strain the tea and drink it once or twice daily.

Capsules/Tablets:

- Follow the dosage instructions on the product label, typically taking 200-400 mg of Rhodiola extract once or twice daily.

Tincture:

- Add 20-30 drops of Rhodiola tincture to a small amount of water or juice, taken 2-3 times daily.

Safety and Precautions

Rhodiola rosea is generally considered safe for most people when used appropriately. However, it is important to consult with a healthcare provider before starting Rhodiola, especially if you are pregnant, breastfeeding, or taking other medications. Some individuals may experience mild side effects such as dizziness, dry mouth, or gastrointestinal discomfort. It is also advisable to avoid taking Rhodiola late in the day to prevent potential interference with sleep.

Rhodiola rosea is a potent adaptogen that can significantly enhance energy levels and reduce fatigue, making it an invaluable herb for managing stress and improving overall vitality. Its ability to optimize cellular energy production, regulate cortisol levels, and enhance mood and cognitive function makes Rhodiola an excellent natural remedy for those seeking to boost their resilience to stress and maintain peak physical and mental performance. Always consult with a healthcare provider to ensure its safe and effective use and enjoy the revitalizing benefits of this remarkable herb.

Holy Basil (Tulsi): Promoting Mental Clarity and Emotional Balance

Holy basil, also known as Tulsi (Ocimum sanctum or Ocimum tenuiflorum), is a revered herb in Ayurvedic medicine, often referred to as the "Queen of Herbs" due to its extensive range of therapeutic benefits. Tulsi is considered an adaptogen, a natural substance that helps the body adapt to stress and restore balance. With its rich history and numerous health benefits, holy basil is particularly valued for its ability to promote mental clarity and emotional balance.

Promoting Mental Clarity

Holy basil is renowned for its ability to enhance cognitive function and promote mental clarity. The herb contains several bioactive compounds, including eugenol, rosmarinic acid, apigenin, and ursolic acid, which contribute to its neuroprotective effects. These compounds help protect the brain from oxidative stress and support overall brain health.

Mechanisms of Action:

- **Antioxidant Properties:** Tulsi's antioxidant compounds protect brain cells from oxidative damage, which is crucial for maintaining cognitive function and preventing neurodegenerative diseases.

- **Enhancing Neurotransmitter Activity:** Holy basil helps regulate the levels of neurotransmitters such as dopamine and serotonin, which play key roles in mood regulation, motivation, and cognitive performance.

- **Reducing Cortisol Levels:** By modulating the stress response and lowering cortisol levels, Tulsi helps prevent the cognitive decline associated with chronic stress. Lower cortisol levels also contribute to improved focus and mental clarity.

Research has shown that holy basil can improve cognitive functions such as memory, attention, and decision-making. A study published in the "Journal of Ayurveda and Integrative Medicine" demonstrated that Tulsi extracts significantly enhanced cognitive functions and reduced symptoms of mild cognitive impairment in elderly participants.

Promoting Emotional Balance

Holy basil is also highly effective in promoting emotional balance and reducing symptoms of anxiety and depression. Its adaptogenic properties help the body and mind cope with stress more effectively, leading to a more balanced emotional state.

Mechanisms of Action:

- **Modulating Neurotransmitters:** Tulsi influences the levels of neurotransmitters associated with mood, such as serotonin, dopamine, and norepinephrine. By balancing these chemicals, holy basil helps alleviate symptoms of anxiety and depression.

- **Anti-inflammatory Effects:** Chronic inflammation is linked to mood disorders. Holy basil's anti-inflammatory properties help reduce inflammation in the body and brain, which can improve mood and emotional well-being.

- **Improving Sleep Quality:** Better sleep is crucial for emotional balance. Tulsi promotes relaxation and enhances sleep quality, which in turn supports emotional stability and resilience.

A study published in the "Journal of Ethnopharmacology" found that participants who took holy basil extract experienced significant reductions in anxiety, stress, and depression symptoms. The study highlighted Tulsi's potential as a natural remedy for managing mood disorders and promoting overall emotional health.

Usage and Dosage

Holy basil can be consumed in various forms, including teas, capsules, tinctures, and fresh leaves. Each form offers unique benefits and can be chosen based on personal preference and convenience.

Tea:

- To make holy basil tea, steep 1-2 teaspoons of dried Tulsi leaves or a handful of fresh leaves in a cup of hot water for about 10-15 minutes. Strain the tea and drink it 2-3 times daily. The tea has a pleasant, slightly spicy flavor, which can be enhanced with honey or lemon.

Capsules:

- Holy basil capsules are a convenient option for those who prefer a standardized dosage. The typical dosage is 300-600 mg of Tulsi extract, taken 1-2 times daily. Follow the dosage instructions on the product label.

Tincture:

- Holy basil tinctures are concentrated liquid extracts that can be taken by adding a few drops to a small amount of water or juice. The typical dosage is 30-40 drops, 2-3 times daily.

Fresh Leaves:

- Fresh Tulsi leaves can be chewed directly or added to salads and other dishes for a fresh, herbal flavor. Incorporating fresh leaves into your diet can provide additional nutritional benefits.

Safety and Precautions

Holy basil is generally considered safe for most people when used appropriately. However, it is important to consult with a healthcare provider before starting Tulsi, especially if you are pregnant, breastfeeding, or taking other medications. Some individuals may experience mild side effects such as nausea or diarrhea. It is advisable to start with a lower dose and gradually increase it to assess your tolerance.

Holy basil (Tulsi) is a powerful adaptogen that promotes mental clarity and emotional balance. Its neuroprotective, antioxidant, and anti-inflammatory properties support cognitive function and mood regulation, making it a valuable herb for managing stress and enhancing overall well-being. Whether consumed as a tea, capsule, tincture, or fresh leaves, holy basil can be a beneficial addition to your wellness routine. Always consult with a healthcare provider to ensure its safe and effective use, and enjoy the calming and balancing benefits of this remarkable herb.

Herbal Remedies for Depression

Depression is a complex and multifaceted mental health condition that affects millions of people worldwide. Characterized by persistent feelings of sadness, hopelessness, and a lack of interest in daily activities, depression can significantly impact a person's quality of life. While conventional treatments such as antidepressant medications and psychotherapy are commonly used, many individuals seek natural alternatives to complement or replace these approaches. Herbal remedies offer a promising solution, providing a holistic and gentle way to alleviate depressive symptoms and promote emotional well-being. This chapter explores various herbs known for their antidepressant properties, delving into their mechanisms of action, benefits, and practical applications. By understanding and utilizing these natural remedies, individuals can take proactive steps towards managing depression and improving their mental health.

Recognizing the Symptoms of Depression and When to Seek Help

Depression is a serious mental health condition that goes beyond temporary feelings of sadness or "the blues." It can affect every aspect of a person's life, from their emotional well-being to their physical health and daily functioning. Recognizing the symptoms of depression early on is crucial for seeking appropriate help and managing the condition effectively. Here are some of the key symptoms to watch for and guidelines on when to seek professional assistance.

Symptoms of Depression

Emotional Symptoms:

- **Persistent Sadness:** Feeling sad, empty, or tearful most of the day, nearly every day.

- **Hopelessness:** A pervasive sense of hopelessness or pessimism about the future.

- **Guilt and Worthlessness:** Excessive feelings of guilt, worthlessness, or self-blame.

- **Loss of Interest:** A marked loss of interest or pleasure in activities once enjoyed, including hobbies, socializing, and sexual activity.

- **Irritability:** Increased irritability, frustration, or anger over small matters.

Cognitive Symptoms:

- **Difficulty Concentrating:** Trouble focusing, making decisions, or remembering details.

- **Indecisiveness:** Difficulty making even simple decisions.

- **Negative Thinking:** Persistent thoughts of death, suicide, or self-harm.

Physical Symptoms:

- **Fatigue:** Persistent fatigue or loss of energy, even with adequate rest.

- **Sleep Disturbances:** Insomnia, waking up too early, or oversleeping.

- **Changes in Appetite:** Significant weight loss or gain, or changes in appetite.

- **Physical Aches and Pains:** Unexplained aches, pains, or digestive problems that do not respond to treatment.

- **Decreased Energy:** Feeling physically slowed down or restless.

Behavioral Symptoms:

- **Social Withdrawal:** Avoiding social interactions and activities.

- **Neglecting Responsibilities:** Difficulty fulfilling responsibilities at work, school, or home.

- **Substance Abuse:** Increased use of alcohol or drugs as a coping mechanism.

When to Seek Help

It is essential to seek help if you or someone you know is experiencing symptoms of depression that persist for more than two weeks and interfere with daily functioning. Here are some specific situations that warrant professional assistance:

Persistent Symptoms:

- If the emotional, cognitive, physical, and behavioral symptoms of depression persist for more than two weeks, it is important to seek help. Depression is a treatable condition, and early intervention can prevent it from worsening.

Impact on Daily Life:

- When depression significantly impacts your ability to function at work, school, or in social settings, it is time to seek professional support. Difficulty performing daily tasks and responsibilities is a clear sign that help is needed.

Suicidal Thoughts:

- If you or someone you know is experiencing thoughts of suicide, self-harm, or death, it is crucial to seek immediate help. Contact a mental health professional, call a crisis hotline, or go to the nearest emergency room.

Substance Abuse:

- If depression leads to increased use of alcohol or drugs, professional help is necessary. Substance abuse can worsen depression and complicate the recovery process.

Lack of Improvement:

- If self-help strategies and support from friends and family do not lead to improvement, seeking professional help is important. A mental health professional can provide a comprehensive evaluation and recommend appropriate treatments.

Recognizing the symptoms of depression and knowing when to seek help are critical steps in managing this condition effectively. Depression affects many aspects of life, and early intervention can lead to better outcomes and improved quality of life. If you or someone you know is experiencing persistent symptoms of depression, reaching out to a mental health professional can provide the necessary support and treatment to begin the journey towards recovery.

Lavender: Calming Effects and Its Role in Mental Health

Lavender (Lavandula angustifolia) is a fragrant herb well-known for its calming and soothing properties. Widely used in aromatherapy and traditional medicine, lavender has been revered for centuries for its ability to promote relaxation and alleviate stress. Its gentle and pleasant scent, along with its versatility in various forms such as essential oils, teas, and extracts, makes lavender a popular choice for improving mental health and well-being.

Calming Effects of Lavender

Lavender is particularly effective in reducing symptoms of anxiety and promoting relaxation. The herb contains several bioactive compounds, including linalool and linalyl acetate, which are primarily responsible for its calming effects. These compounds interact with the brain's neurotransmitter systems, specifically by modulating gamma-aminobutyric acid (GABA) activity, which helps to reduce neuronal excitability and induce a state of calm.

Mechanisms of Action:

- **GABA Modulation:** By enhancing GABA activity, lavender helps to calm the nervous system, reduce anxiety, and promote relaxation.

- **Antioxidant Properties:** Lavender's antioxidant compounds help protect brain cells from oxidative stress, which is crucial for maintaining cognitive function and mental health.

- **Neuroprotective Effects:** The herb's neuroprotective properties support overall brain health, potentially preventing neurodegenerative conditions linked to chronic stress and anxiety.

Research has demonstrated that inhaling lavender essential oil or using it in aromatherapy can significantly reduce anxiety levels. A study published in the "Journal of Alternative and Complementary Medicine" found that participants who inhaled lavender oil reported lower levels of anxiety and better mood compared to those who did not use lavender. Another study published in "Phytomedicine" highlighted that lavender oil capsules were as effective as some anti-anxiety medications in reducing symptoms of generalized anxiety disorder (GAD) without causing sedative side effects.

Role in Mental Health

Beyond its calming effects, lavender plays a significant role in improving overall mental health. Its ability to alleviate anxiety and stress contributes to a more balanced emotional state, which can be beneficial for managing conditions like depression and insomnia. Lavender's soothing properties also make it an effective natural remedy for improving sleep quality, which is essential for maintaining mental health.

Improving Sleep:

- Lavender is widely used to promote better sleep due to its sedative effects. A study published in "The Journal of Sleep Medicine & Disorders" showed that participants who used lavender essential oil experienced improved sleep quality and duration. The herb's ability to reduce anxiety and promote relaxation makes it easier to fall asleep and stay asleep.

Alleviating Depression:

- While lavender is primarily known for its anti-anxiety effects, it also shows promise in alleviating symptoms of depression. The herb's mood-enhancing properties help elevate emotional well-being and reduce feelings of sadness. A study in "International Journal of Psychiatry in Clinical Practice" found that lavender oil capsules significantly improved depressive symptoms in patients with mild to moderate depression.

Stress Reduction:

- Chronic stress is a major contributor to mental health disorders. Lavender's ability to lower cortisol levels, the body's primary stress hormone, helps mitigate the effects of chronic stress. Using lavender in aromatherapy, baths, or as a supplement can create a sense of calm and reduce the overall impact of stress on the body and mind.

Usage and Dosage

Lavender can be used in various forms, each offering its own benefits and applications:

Essential Oil:

- Lavender essential oil is commonly used in aromatherapy. Add a few drops to a diffuser, inhale directly, or apply diluted oil to the skin. For sleep and relaxation, add a few drops to a warm bath or sprinkle on your pillow before bedtime.

Tea:

- Lavender tea can be made by steeping 1-2 teaspoons of dried lavender flowers in hot water for about 10 minutes. Drinking lavender tea 1-2 times daily can promote relaxation and improve sleep quality.

Capsules:

- Lavender oil capsules are available for oral consumption. The typical dosage is 80 mg of lavender oil per day, but it is important to follow the specific dosage instructions provided by the product manufacturer.

Topical Applications:

- Lavender can be applied topically as an oil, cream, or lotion to relieve tension and promote relaxation. Always dilute lavender essential oil with a carrier oil before applying it to the skin.

Lavender is a versatile and effective herb for promoting mental health through its calming effects. Its ability to reduce anxiety, improve sleep, and alleviate symptoms of depression makes it a valuable natural remedy for managing mental health conditions. Whether used in aromatherapy, as a tea, in capsules, or topically, lavender offers a gentle and pleasant way to enhance emotional well-being and support overall mental health. Always consult with a healthcare provider to ensure its safe and effective use and enjoy the soothing benefits of this remarkable herb.

Cognitive Enhancers and Memory Support

Maintaining cognitive health and memory function is essential for overall well-being, particularly as we age. Cognitive enhancers, also known as nootropics, are natural substances that can improve brain function, enhance memory, and support mental clarity. These substances work through various mechanisms, such as boosting blood flow to the brain, protecting neurons from damage, and modulating neurotransmitter levels. Incorporating cognitive enhancers into your daily routine can help sharpen focus, improve recall, and sustain mental performance. This chapter explores a range of herbs and natural remedies known for their cognitive-enhancing and memory-supporting properties, providing insights into their benefits and practical applications. By understanding and utilizing these powerful natural aids, individuals can optimize their cognitive health and enhance their overall mental capabilities.

The Importance of Cognitive Health and Memory Support

Cognitive health and memory function are critical components of overall well-being, affecting how we think, learn, remember, and interact with the world. Maintaining cognitive health is essential not only for daily functioning but also for long-term mental resilience and quality of life. As we age, the natural decline in cognitive abilities can impact various aspects of life, from professional performance to personal relationships. Therefore, supporting cognitive health and memory is crucial for ensuring a healthy, fulfilling life.

Enhancing Daily Functioning

Cognitive abilities such as attention, problem-solving, and decision-making are fundamental for managing everyday tasks and responsibilities. Strong cognitive function enables individuals to process information efficiently, stay organized, and perform complex tasks with ease. Memory support, in particular, plays a vital role in learning new skills, retaining important information, and recalling past experiences. Enhancing these cognitive functions can lead to improved productivity, better academic and professional performance, and a more structured approach to daily activities.

Promoting Mental Health

Cognitive health is closely linked to mental health. Cognitive impairments can lead to frustration, stress, and a sense of helplessness, contributing to mental health issues such as anxiety and depression. Conversely, maintaining good cognitive health can boost confidence, reduce stress, and promote a positive outlook on life. By supporting cognitive functions and memory, individuals can better manage mental health challenges and enhance their emotional well-being.

Preventing Age-Related Decline

As people age, they naturally experience a decline in cognitive abilities, including memory, attention, and processing speed. Conditions such as mild cognitive impairment (MCI) and dementia, including Alzheimer's disease, are common in older adults. Supporting cognitive health through lifestyle choices, diet, and natural remedies can help slow down the progression of cognitive decline and improve the quality of life for aging individuals. Regular mental stimulation, physical activity, and a healthy diet rich in brain-boosting nutrients are crucial for preserving cognitive function.

Enhancing Quality of Life

Good cognitive health and memory are essential for maintaining independence and a high quality of life. They enable individuals to stay engaged in their communities, maintain meaningful relationships, and enjoy hobbies and activities that bring joy and fulfillment. Cognitive health supports not only personal well-being but also social and professional interactions, contributing to a well-rounded and satisfying life.

Supporting Overall Brain Health

Cognitive enhancers and memory support are part of a holistic approach to brain health. These natural remedies often provide neuroprotective benefits, reducing oxidative stress and inflammation, and supporting overall brain function. By protecting neurons and promoting healthy brain activity, these substances can help maintain cognitive vitality and prevent neurodegenerative diseases.

Maintaining cognitive health and memory support is vital for overall well-being, daily functioning, and long-term mental resilience. The decline in cognitive abilities with age underscores the importance of proactive measures to enhance and preserve brain function. By incorporating cognitive enhancers and memory-supporting natural remedies into daily routines, individuals can improve their mental performance, prevent age-related decline, and enhance their quality of life. The following sections will explore specific herbs and natural substances that offer significant benefits for cognitive health and memory support, providing practical guidance on their use and applications.

Ginkgo Biloba: Improving Blood Flow and Cognitive Function

Ginkgo biloba, derived from one of the oldest living tree species, has been used for thousands of years in traditional medicine to treat various ailments. Today, it is widely recognized for its ability to enhance cognitive function and improve blood flow, making it a popular natural remedy for maintaining brain health and preventing cognitive decline.

Enhancing Blood Flow

One of the primary ways Ginkgo biloba supports cognitive health is by improving blood flow to the brain. The herb contains potent antioxidants called flavonoids and terpenoids, which help to dilate blood vessels, reduce blood viscosity, and increase circulation. Enhanced blood flow ensures that the brain receives an adequate supply of oxygen and essential nutrients, which are critical for optimal brain function.

Mechanisms of Action:

- **Vasodilation:** Ginkgo biloba promotes the widening of blood vessels, which enhances circulation and reduces the risk of vascular-related cognitive issues.

- **Anti-Platelet Effects:** The herb has anti-platelet properties that help prevent blood clot formation, further ensuring smooth blood flow to the brain.

- **Neuroprotection:** By improving blood flow, Ginkgo biloba helps protect brain cells from ischemic damage and supports overall brain health.

Research has demonstrated that Ginkgo biloba can significantly improve blood flow to the brain, which is particularly beneficial for older adults who may experience reduced circulation due to aging. A study published in "Psychopharmacology" found that Ginkgo biloba extract improved cerebral blood flow and cognitive performance in healthy elderly individuals.

Improving Cognitive Function

In addition to enhancing blood flow, Ginkgo biloba is well-known for its cognitive-enhancing properties. The herb's ability to support neurotransmitter function and protect neurons from oxidative stress makes it an effective natural remedy for boosting memory, attention, and mental clarity.

Mechanisms of Action:

- **Neurotransmitter Modulation:** Ginkgo biloba influences the levels of key neurotransmitters such as dopamine, norepinephrine, and serotonin, which are involved in mood regulation, memory, and cognitive processing.

- **Antioxidant Effects:** The herb's rich antioxidant content helps neutralize free radicals, reducing oxidative stress and protecting neurons from damage. This neuroprotective effect is crucial for maintaining cognitive function and preventing neurodegenerative diseases.

- **Anti-Inflammatory Properties:** Ginkgo biloba's anti-inflammatory effects help reduce inflammation in the brain, which is linked to cognitive decline and disorders such as Alzheimer's disease.

Several studies have supported the cognitive benefits of Ginkgo biloba. For instance, a meta-analysis published in the "Journal of Alzheimer's Disease" reviewed numerous clinical trials and concluded that Ginkgo biloba extract significantly improved cognitive function in individuals with mild cognitive impairment and dementia. Another study published in "Phytomedicine" found that Ginkgo biloba improved memory and executive function in healthy adults, highlighting its potential as a cognitive enhancer.

Usage and Dosage

Ginkgo biloba is available in various forms, including capsules, tablets, liquid extracts, and teas. Standardized extracts are commonly used in clinical studies and provide a reliable dosage of the herb's active compounds.

Capsules/Tablets:

- The recommended dosage for Ginkgo biloba extract is typically 120-240 mg per day, divided into two or three doses. It is important to follow the dosage instructions provided by the product manufacturer.

Liquid Extracts:

- Ginkgo biloba liquid extracts can be taken by adding a specified number of drops to water or juice. The typical dosage is 30-40 drops, taken 2-3 times daily.

Tea:

- To make Ginkgo biloba tea, steep 1-2 teaspoons of dried Ginkgo leaves in hot water for about 10-15 minutes. Strain and drink the tea 1-2 times daily.

Safety and Precautions

Ginkgo biloba is generally considered safe for most people when used appropriately. However, it is important to consult with a healthcare provider before starting Ginkgo biloba, especially if you are taking medications such as blood thinners, anti-platelet drugs, or anti-inflammatory medications, as the herb may interact with these drugs. Some individuals may experience mild side effects such as gastrointestinal discomfort, headache, or dizziness.

Ginkgo biloba is a powerful herb that supports cognitive function and improves blood flow to the brain. Its ability to enhance circulation, modulate neurotransmitters, and protect neurons from oxidative stress makes it an effective natural remedy for maintaining brain health and preventing cognitive decline. Whether consumed as a capsule, liquid extract, or tea, Ginkgo biloba offers significant benefits for those seeking to boost their mental performance and support long-term cognitive health. Always consult with a healthcare provider to ensure its safe and effective use and enjoy the cognitive-enhancing properties of this remarkable herb.

Bacopa Monnieri: Enhancing Memory and Learning

Bacopa monnieri, commonly known as Brahmi, is a traditional herb that has been used for centuries in Ayurvedic medicine to enhance cognitive function, particularly memory and learning. Native to the wetlands of India, Bacopa monnieri is highly regarded for its neuroprotective and cognitive-enhancing properties. Modern scientific research has confirmed many of the traditional uses of this herb, making it a popular natural supplement for improving mental performance.

Enhancing Memory

Bacopa monnieri is renowned for its ability to improve memory retention and recall. The herb contains active compounds called bacosides, which have been shown to enhance synaptic communication in the brain. This improved communication helps to strengthen the connections between neurons, which is essential for forming and retaining memories.

Mechanisms of Action:

- **Synaptic Plasticity:** Bacosides in Bacopa monnieri enhance synaptic plasticity, the ability of synapses to strengthen or weaken over time. This plasticity is crucial for learning and memory formation.

- **Neurotransmitter Modulation:** Bacopa monnieri influences the levels of key neurotransmitters such as acetylcholine, serotonin, and dopamine, which play vital roles in memory, mood regulation, and cognitive processing.

- **Antioxidant Protection:** The herb's antioxidant properties help protect brain cells from oxidative stress and free radical damage, which can impair memory and cognitive function.

Studies have shown that Bacopa monnieri can significantly improve memory performance. In a double-blind, placebo-controlled trial published in the journal "Psychopharmacology," participants who took Bacopa monnieri extract for 12 weeks demonstrated significant improvements in memory retention and recall compared to the placebo group. Another study published in the "Journal of Alternative and Complementary Medicine" found that elderly participants experienced enhanced memory and cognitive function after taking Bacopa monnieri.

Enhancing Learning

In addition to its memory-boosting effects, Bacopa monnieri is also known for enhancing learning abilities. The herb helps improve cognitive processing speed and information retention, making it easier to learn new skills and concepts.

Mechanisms of Action:

- **Cognitive Processing:** Bacopa monnieri improves cognitive processing speed, allowing for faster and more efficient learning. This is particularly beneficial in tasks that require quick thinking and problem-solving.

- **Attention and Focus:** The herb helps increase attention span and focus, which are critical for effective learning. By reducing distractions and enhancing concentration, Bacopa monnieri supports sustained cognitive effort.

- **Reducing Anxiety:** Bacopa monnieri has anxiolytic properties that help reduce anxiety and stress, which can interfere with learning. By promoting a calm and focused mind, the herb creates an optimal environment for acquiring new information.

Research supports the cognitive benefits of Bacopa monnieri in enhancing learning. A study published in the journal "Neuropsychopharmacology" demonstrated that participants who took Bacopa monnieri showed improvements in learning rate, visual information processing, and working memory. These findings highlight the herb's potential as a natural cognitive enhancer for both students and professionals.

Usage and Dosage

Bacopa monnieri is available in various forms, including capsules, tablets, liquid extracts, and powders. Standardized extracts are commonly used in clinical studies and provide a consistent dosage of the herb's active compounds.

Capsules/Tablets:

- The recommended dosage for Bacopa monnieri extract is typically 300-600 mg per day, standardized to contain 50% bacosides. It is important to follow the dosage instructions provided by the product manufacturer.

Liquid Extracts:

- Bacopa monnieri liquid extracts can be taken by adding a specified number of drops to water or juice. The typical dosage is 30-40 drops, taken 2-3 times daily.

Powder:

- Bacopa monnieri powder can be mixed into smoothies, yogurt, or other foods. The recommended dosage is 1/2 to 1 teaspoon per day.

Tea:

- To make Bacopa monnieri tea, steep 1-2 teaspoons of dried Bacopa leaves in hot water for about 10-15 minutes. Strain and drink the tea 1-2 times daily.

Safety and Precautions

Bacopa monnieri is generally considered safe for most people when used appropriately. However, it is important to consult with a healthcare provider before starting Bacopa monnieri, especially if you are pregnant, breastfeeding, or taking other medications. Some individuals may experience mild side effects such as gastrointestinal discomfort, nausea, or dry mouth. Starting with a lower dose and gradually increasing it can help minimize potential side effects.

Bacopa monnieri is a powerful herb that enhances memory and learning, making it a valuable natural remedy for improving cognitive function. Its ability to boost synaptic communication, modulate neurotransmitters, and protect neurons from oxidative stress supports overall brain health and mental performance. Whether consumed as a capsule, liquid extract, powder, or tea, Bacopa monnieri offers significant benefits for those seeking to enhance their cognitive abilities and support long-term brain health. Always consult with a healthcare provider to ensure its safe and effective use, and enjoy the cognitive-enhancing properties of this remarkable herb.

Gotu Kola: Supporting Brain Health and Reducing Anxiety

Gotu kola (Centella asiatica), often referred to as the "herb of longevity," is a staple in traditional Ayurvedic and Chinese medicine. Known for its wide range of therapeutic benefits, Gotu kola is highly valued for its ability to support brain health, enhance cognitive function, and reduce anxiety. This versatile herb has been used for centuries to promote mental clarity, improve memory, and treat various mental health conditions.

Supporting Brain Health

Gotu kola is renowned for its neuroprotective properties, which help maintain and enhance brain health. The herb contains several active compounds, including triterpenoids, asiaticoside, and madecassoside, which contribute to its cognitive-enhancing effects. These compounds support brain health through various mechanisms.

Mechanisms of Action:

- **Neurogenesis:** Gotu kola promotes the growth of new neurons and dendrites, a process known as neurogenesis. This is crucial for learning, memory, and overall cognitive function.

- **Synaptic Plasticity:** The herb enhances synaptic plasticity, which is the ability of synapses to strengthen or weaken over time, influencing learning and memory.

- **Antioxidant Protection:** Gotu kola's antioxidant properties protect brain cells from oxidative stress and free radical damage, which are linked to cognitive decline and neurodegenerative diseases.

- **Blood Flow:** Gotu kola improves cerebral blood flow, ensuring that the brain receives adequate oxygen and nutrients essential for optimal functioning.

Several studies have demonstrated Gotu kola's effectiveness in enhancing cognitive function. A study published in the "Journal of Ethnopharmacology" showed that Gotu kola extract improved memory and cognitive performance in elderly participants. Another study in "Evidence-Based Complementary and Alternative Medicine" found that Gotu kola enhanced cognitive function and reduced oxidative stress in rats, suggesting its potential for preventing cognitive decline.

Reducing Anxiety

In addition to its cognitive benefits, Gotu kola is also highly effective in reducing anxiety and promoting relaxation. The herb's calming effects are attributed to its ability to modulate neurotransmitters and reduce stress hormone levels.

Mechanisms of Action:

- **GABA Modulation:** Gotu kola enhances the activity of gamma-aminobutyric acid (GABA), an inhibitory neurotransmitter that promotes relaxation and reduces neuronal excitability. Increased GABA activity helps alleviate anxiety and stress.

- **Cortisol Regulation:** The herb helps regulate cortisol levels, the body's primary stress hormone. By reducing cortisol production, Gotu kola mitigates the physiological impact of stress and promotes a sense of calm.

- **Serotonin Modulation:** Gotu kola influences serotonin levels, a neurotransmitter associated with mood regulation and anxiety. Enhanced serotonin activity contributes to improved mood and reduced anxiety symptoms.

Clinical studies support Gotu kola's anxiolytic properties. A study published in the "Journal of Clinical Psychopharmacology" found that participants who took Gotu kola extract experienced significant reductions in anxiety and stress levels compared to the placebo group. Another study in the "Indian Journal of Psychiatry" showed that Gotu kola effectively reduced symptoms of generalized anxiety disorder (GAD) without causing sedation.

Usage and Dosage

Gotu kola can be consumed in various forms, including capsules, tablets, liquid extracts, and teas. Standardized extracts provide a consistent dosage of the herb's active compounds.

Capsules/Tablets:

- The recommended dosage for Gotu kola extract is typically 300-500 mg per day, standardized to contain 10% asiaticosides. It is important to follow the dosage instructions provided by the product manufacturer.

Liquid Extracts:

- Gotu kola liquid extracts can be taken by adding a specified number of drops to water or juice. The typical dosage is 30-40 drops, taken 2-3 times daily.

Powder:

- Gotu kola powder can be mixed into smoothies, yogurt, or other foods. The recommended dosage is 1/2 to 1 teaspoon per day.

Tea:

- To make Gotu kola tea, steep 1-2 teaspoons of dried Gotu kola leaves in hot water for about 10-15 minutes. Strain and drink the tea 1-2 times daily.

Safety and Precautions

Gotu kola is generally considered safe for most people when used appropriately. However, it is important to consult with a healthcare provider before starting Gotu kola, especially if you are pregnant, breastfeeding, or taking other medications. Some individuals may experience mild side effects such as gastrointestinal discomfort, headache, or dizziness. Starting with a lower dose and gradually increasing it can help minimize potential side effects.

Gotu kola is a powerful herb that supports brain health and reduces anxiety, making it a valuable natural remedy for enhancing cognitive function and promoting mental well-being. Its ability to stimulate neurogenesis, improve blood flow, and modulate neurotransmitters underscores its potential as a cognitive enhancer and anxiolytic agent. Whether consumed as a capsule, liquid extract, powder, or tea, Gotu kola offers significant benefits for those seeking to maintain brain health and manage anxiety. Always consult with a healthcare provider to ensure its safe and effective use, and enjoy the cognitive and calming properties of this remarkable herb.

Rosemary: Stimulating Memory and Mental Clarity

Rosemary (Rosmarinus officinalis) is a fragrant herb commonly used in culinary dishes, but it also boasts a rich history in traditional medicine for its cognitive-enhancing properties. Known as the "herb of remembrance," rosemary has been associated with memory and mental clarity for centuries. Modern scientific research has begun to validate these traditional uses, highlighting rosemary's potential as a natural remedy for boosting cognitive function.

Rosemary contains a variety of active compounds, including rosmarinic acid, caffeic acid, and essential oils like cineole and camphor. These compounds contribute to its neuroprotective and cognitive-enhancing effects. One of the primary ways rosemary stimulates memory and mental clarity is by improving blood circulation to the brain. Enhanced blood flow ensures that the brain receives adequate oxygen and nutrients, which are essential for optimal cognitive function.

The herb's ability to modulate neurotransmitters is another key factor in its cognitive benefits. Rosemary influences the levels of acetylcholine, a neurotransmitter crucial for memory and learning. By inhibiting the breakdown of acetylcholine, rosemary helps maintain higher levels of this neurotransmitter in the brain, thereby supporting memory retention and recall. This mechanism is similar to how certain medications for Alzheimer's disease work, making rosemary a valuable natural alternative for cognitive support.

Rosemary also has potent antioxidant properties that protect brain cells from oxidative stress and free radical damage. Oxidative stress is a significant contributor to cognitive decline and neurodegenerative diseases. The antioxidants in rosemary neutralize free radicals, reducing inflammation and preventing cellular damage. This neuroprotective effect helps maintain cognitive health and can slow down the progression of age-related cognitive decline.

Aromatherapy with rosemary essential oil is a popular method for reaping its cognitive benefits. Inhalation of rosemary aroma has been shown to enhance cognitive performance and mood. A study published in the journal "Therapeutic Advances in Psychopharmacology" found that participants exposed to rosemary aroma demonstrated improved performance in cognitive tasks, including memory speed and accuracy. The stimulating effects of rosemary aroma can be attributed to its ability to increase brain wave activity and boost alertness.

In addition to its memory-boosting properties, rosemary also enhances mental clarity and focus. The herb's stimulating effects help reduce mental fatigue and improve concentration. This makes rosemary particularly beneficial for individuals who need to stay mentally sharp and alert, whether for academic purposes, professional tasks, or daily activities.

Incorporating rosemary into your daily routine can be done in various ways, including using fresh or dried rosemary in cooking, drinking rosemary tea, or using rosemary essential oil for aromatherapy. For a simple cognitive boost, adding a few drops of rosemary essential oil to a diffuser or inhaling it directly from the bottle can provide immediate mental clarity and focus.

Overall, rosemary is a versatile and powerful herb that supports cognitive health. Its ability to stimulate memory, enhance mental clarity, and protect brain cells from oxidative damage makes it an excellent natural remedy for maintaining and improving cognitive function. By incorporating rosemary into your wellness routine, you can enjoy the mental sharpness and clarity that this remarkable herb offers.

Creating Herbal Blends for Cognitive Enhancement

Combining various herbs known for their cognitive-enhancing properties can create powerful synergies that amplify their individual benefits. By carefully selecting and blending herbs, you can formulate an effective natural remedy to boost memory, focus, and overall mental clarity. Here are some popular herbs for cognitive enhancement and how to blend them:

Key Herbs for Cognitive Enhancement

1. **Ginkgo Biloba**:
    - **Benefits**: Improves blood flow to the brain, enhances memory, and protects neurons.
    - **Form**: Capsules, tablets, liquid extracts, or dried leaves for tea.

2. **Bacopa Monnieri**:
    - **Benefits**: Enhances memory retention, supports learning, and protects brain cells from oxidative stress.
    - **Form**: Capsules, tablets, liquid extracts, or powder.

3. **Gotu Kola**:
    - **Benefits**: Supports brain health, improves cognitive function, and reduces anxiety.
    - **Form**: Capsules, tablets, liquid extracts, or dried leaves for tea.

4. **Rosemary**:

- **Benefits**: Stimulates memory, enhances mental clarity, and provides antioxidant protection.
- **Form**: Fresh or dried leaves for cooking, tea, or essential oil for aromatherapy.

5. **Rhodiola Rosea**:
  - **Benefits**: Enhances energy, reduces fatigue, and improves cognitive function under stress.
  - **Form**: Capsules, tablets, liquid extracts, or dried root for tea.

Sample Herbal Blends

Memory Boosting Blend:

- **Ingredients**:
  - 1 part Ginkgo Biloba
  - 1 part Bacopa Monnieri
  - 1 part Gotu Kola

- **Preparation**:
  - Combine equal parts of Ginkgo biloba, Bacopa monnieri, and Gotu kola in a jar.
  - Use 1-2 teaspoons of the blend to make a tea by steeping in hot water for 10-15 minutes.
  - Drink 1-2 cups daily to support memory and cognitive function.

Focus and Clarity Blend:

- **Ingredients**:
  - 1 part Rosemary
  - 1-part Rhodiola Rosea
  - 1-part Gotu Kola

- **Preparation**:
  - Mix equal parts of dried rosemary, Rhodiola rosea, and Gotu kola.
  - Brew 1-2 teaspoons of the blend in hot water for 10-15 minutes to make a tea.
  - Enjoy a cup in the morning or early afternoon to enhance mental clarity and focus.

Stress-Relief Cognitive Blend:

- **Ingredients**:
  - 1-part Ashwagandha (an adaptogen for stress relief)

- 1-part Bacopa Monnieri
    - 1-part Gotu Kola
- **Preparation**:
    - Combine the herbs in equal proportions.
    - Use the blend to prepare a tea or take in capsule form as directed.
    - This blend helps manage stress while enhancing cognitive function.

Tips for Creating Herbal Blends

1. **Quality of Ingredients**: Always use high-quality, organic herbs to ensure the best results and avoid contaminants.

2. **Proportions**: Adjust the proportions based on your specific needs and preferences. Some herbs may need to be in higher quantities than others depending on their potency and your goals.

3. **Form of Herbs**: Decide whether you prefer teas, tinctures, or capsules. Teas are great for hydration and slower absorption, while tinctures and capsules offer more concentrated doses.

4. **Consultation**: Before starting any new herbal regimen, consult with a healthcare provider, especially if you have any existing health conditions or are taking other medications.

5. **Experimentation**: Feel free to experiment with different combinations and proportions to find what works best for you. Herbal blends can be personalized to suit your unique needs and lifestyle.

Creating herbal blends for cognitive enhancement is an effective way to harness the combined benefits of various herbs. By selecting herbs that support memory, focus, and mental clarity, you can formulate potent blends that cater to your specific cognitive needs. Whether you prefer teas, tinctures, or capsules, these blends offer a natural and holistic approach to boosting brain health and cognitive function. Always prioritize quality and consult with a healthcare provider to ensure safe and effective use.

BOOK 13:

Herbs for Women's Health: Natural Remedies for Every Stage of Life

Natural Treatment for Menstrual Disorders

Menstrual disorders are common issues that many women face at some point in their lives, affecting both physical and emotional well-being. Conditions such as premenstrual syndrome (PMS), dysmenorrhea (painful periods), menorrhagia (heavy menstrual bleeding), and irregular cycles can significantly impact daily life. While conventional treatments are available, many women seek natural alternatives to manage their symptoms effectively and safely. Herbal remedies offer a holistic approach to menstrual health, addressing the root causes of these disorders and providing relief through nature's bounty. This chapter explores various herbs known for their efficacy in treating menstrual disorders, providing insights into their benefits, mechanisms of action, and practical applications. By understanding and utilizing these natural treatments, women can achieve better menstrual health and overall well-being.

Overview of Common Menstrual Disorders

Menstrual disorders encompass a range of conditions that affect the regularity, flow, and pain associated with the menstrual cycle. These disorders can significantly impact a woman's quality of life, causing physical discomfort and emotional distress. Understanding the various types of menstrual disorders is crucial for identifying appropriate treatments and managing symptoms effectively.

Premenstrual Syndrome (PMS)

Premenstrual Syndrome (PMS) is a common condition that affects many women in the days leading up to their menstrual period. PMS encompasses a wide array of symptoms, including mood swings, irritability, anxiety, depression, bloating, breast tenderness, headaches, and fatigue. The exact cause of PMS is not fully understood, but it is believed to be related to hormonal fluctuations during the menstrual cycle. While PMS is not typically debilitating, its symptoms can significantly impact daily activities and overall well-being.

Dysmenorrhea

Dysmenorrhea refers to painful menstruation, which can be classified into primary and secondary dysmenorrhea. Primary dysmenorrhea is characterized by cramping pain in the lower abdomen that occurs just before or during menstruation, without any underlying pelvic pathology. This type of dysmenorrhea is commonly experienced by adolescents and young women and is usually linked to the production of prostaglandins, which cause uterine contractions. Secondary dysmenorrhea, on the other hand, is caused by underlying reproductive health issues such as endometriosis, fibroids, or pelvic inflammatory disease. The pain associated with secondary dysmenorrhea tends to be more severe and prolonged than primary dysmenorrhea.

Menorrhagia

Menorrhagia is defined as abnormally heavy or prolonged menstrual bleeding. Women with menorrhagia may experience periods lasting longer than seven days or lose more blood than is typical during their menstrual cycle, which can lead to anemia and severe fatigue. The causes of menorrhagia can vary, including hormonal imbalances, uterine fibroids, polyps, and blood clotting disorders. In some cases, the condition may also be linked to the use of certain medications or intrauterine devices (IUDs).

Irregular Menstrual Cycles

Irregular menstrual cycles refer to variations in the length and regularity of the menstrual cycle. While some variability is normal, significantly irregular cycles can indicate underlying health issues. Causes of irregular menstrual cycles can include hormonal imbalances, polycystic ovary syndrome (PCOS), thyroid disorders, stress, excessive exercise, and significant weight loss or gain. Irregular cycles can complicate family planning and may be accompanied by other symptoms such as acne, hirsutism, and metabolic issues, particularly in the case of PCOS.

Amenorrhea

Amenorrhea is the absence of menstruation. Primary amenorrhea refers to the absence of menstruation by the age of 15 in girls who have not shown other signs of puberty. Secondary amenorrhea occurs when a woman who has previously had regular periods stops menstruating for three months or longer. Amenorrhea can result from a variety of factors, including hormonal imbalances, extreme weight loss or gain, excessive exercise, stress, and underlying medical conditions such as PCOS or thyroid dysfunction.

Premenstrual Dysphoric Disorder (PMDD)

Premenstrual Dysphoric Disorder (PMDD) is a severe form of PMS that affects a smaller percentage of women but can be debilitating. PMDD is characterized by extreme mood swings, severe irritability, depression, and anxiety in the week or two before menstruation begins. The symptoms are more intense than those of PMS and can interfere significantly with daily life, relationships, and work.

Understanding the various types of menstrual disorders is essential for managing symptoms and seeking appropriate treatment. While these conditions can vary in severity and impact, they all share the potential to disrupt a woman's daily life and overall well-being. In the following sections, we will explore natural remedies and herbal treatments that can help alleviate the symptoms of these common menstrual disorders, offering women a holistic and effective approach to menstrual health.

Herbs for Regulating Menstrual Cycles

Regulating menstrual cycles is essential for maintaining reproductive health and overall well-being. Irregular menstrual cycles can be caused by a variety of factors, including hormonal imbalances, stress, poor diet, and underlying health conditions such as polycystic ovary syndrome (PCOS) and thyroid disorders. Herbal remedies offer a natural and gentle approach to regulating menstrual cycles, promoting hormonal balance, and addressing the root causes of irregular periods. Here are some herbs commonly used for this purpose:

Vitex (Chasteberry)

Vitex agnus-castus, commonly known as chasteberry, is one of the most well-known herbs for regulating menstrual cycles. Vitex works by influencing the pituitary gland to balance the production of hormones such as estrogen and progesterone. It is particularly effective for conditions like PMS, amenorrhea, and PCOS, where hormonal imbalances play a significant role. By normalizing hormone levels, Vitex can help regulate the menstrual cycle, reduce PMS symptoms, and improve fertility. It is typically taken as a tincture or in capsule form, with recommended doses varying based on individual needs.

Dong Quai

Dong Quai (Angelica sinensis) is a traditional Chinese herb known as the "female ginseng." It is highly regarded for its ability to regulate the menstrual cycle and alleviate menstrual pain. Dong Quai acts as a phytoestrogen, helping to balance estrogen levels in the body. It also improves blood flow to the pelvic area, which can help normalize menstrual cycles and reduce symptoms of menstrual irregularities. Dong Quai is often used in combination with other herbs in formulations for women's health. It can be consumed as a tea, tincture, or in capsule form.

Black Cohosh

Black Cohosh (Cimicifuga racemosa) is an herb commonly used to treat menopausal symptoms, but it is also effective in regulating menstrual cycles. Black Cohosh has estrogenic properties, which help balance hormone levels and promote regular ovulation. It is particularly beneficial for women experiencing irregular periods due to hormonal imbalances or approaching menopause. Black Cohosh can help reduce the severity of PMS symptoms, including mood swings and menstrual cramps. It is available in various forms, including tinctures, capsules, and teas.

Red Raspberry Leaf

Red Raspberry Leaf (Rubus idaeus) is a popular herb for women's reproductive health. It is rich in vitamins and minerals, including iron, calcium, and magnesium, which support overall reproductive health. Red Raspberry Leaf is known for its ability to tone the uterine muscles, promote regular menstrual cycles, and alleviate menstrual cramps. It also helps balance hormone levels, making it beneficial for women with irregular cycles. Red Raspberry Leaf is most commonly consumed as a tea, which can be taken daily to support menstrual health.

Cinnamon

Cinnamon (Cinnamomum verum) is not only a popular spice but also a valuable herb for regulating menstrual cycles. Cinnamon has been shown to improve insulin resistance and lower blood sugar levels, which can help regulate menstrual cycles, especially in women with PCOS. Cinnamon also has anti-inflammatory properties that can reduce menstrual pain and promote regular ovulation. It can be incorporated into the diet as a spice or taken as a supplement in capsule form.

Maca Root

Maca Root (Lepidium meyenii) is an adaptogenic herb known for its ability to balance hormones and support reproductive health. Maca helps regulate the endocrine system, which controls hormone production, and can improve symptoms of hormonal imbalances such as irregular menstrual cycles and PMS. It is also known to enhance fertility and increase energy levels. Maca Root is typically available in powder form, which can be added to smoothies, or as capsules and tinctures.

Herbal remedies provide a natural and effective way to regulate menstrual cycles and address the underlying causes of irregular periods. Herbs such as Vitex, Dong Quai, Black Cohosh, Red Raspberry Leaf, Cinnamon, and Maca Root offer numerous benefits for hormonal balance and menstrual health. Incorporating these herbs into your daily routine can help promote regular menstrual cycles, reduce symptoms of PMS, and support overall reproductive health. As with any herbal treatment, it is important to consult with a healthcare provider to ensure safe and appropriate use based on your individual health needs.

Pain Relief and Symptom Management with Herbal Remedies

Managing menstrual pain and symptoms can be challenging for many women. Common issues such as cramps, headaches, bloating, and mood swings can significantly impact daily life. While over-the-counter medications are often used to alleviate these symptoms, herbal remedies offer a natural alternative that can provide effective relief with fewer side effects. Here are some herbs commonly used for pain relief and symptom management during menstruation:

Cramp Bark

Cramp Bark (Viburnum opulus) is an herb renowned for its ability to relieve menstrual cramps. It works as a muscle relaxant, specifically targeting the smooth muscles of the uterus, which helps to ease the painful contractions that cause cramps. Cramp Bark can also alleviate other menstrual-related pain, such as backaches and leg pain. It is typically consumed as a tea or tincture, providing quick relief from discomfort. Regular use of Cramp Bark during the menstrual period can significantly reduce the severity of cramps and improve overall comfort.

Ginger

Ginger (Zingiber officinale) is a versatile herb with powerful anti-inflammatory and analgesic properties, making it highly effective for managing menstrual pain. Studies have shown that ginger can reduce the production of prostaglandins, chemicals in the body that trigger inflammation and pain. Consuming ginger tea or supplements can help alleviate cramps, headaches, and nausea associated with menstruation. Ginger is also beneficial for reducing bloating and improving digestion, which can be particularly helpful during the menstrual cycle.

Turmeric

Turmeric (Curcuma longa) is another potent anti-inflammatory herb that can help manage menstrual symptoms. The active compound in turmeric, curcumin, has been shown to reduce inflammation and pain. Turmeric can be particularly effective for alleviating menstrual cramps and joint pain that some women experience during their periods. Adding turmeric to your diet, drinking turmeric tea, or taking turmeric supplements can provide significant relief from menstrual discomfort. Its anti-inflammatory properties also help improve overall well-being and reduce the severity of PMS symptoms.

Chamomile

Chamomile (Matricaria chamomilla) is a gentle herb known for its calming and anti-inflammatory properties. Chamomile tea is commonly used to relieve menstrual cramps and promote relaxation. The herb works by reducing muscle spasms and inflammation, which helps to alleviate pain. Additionally, chamomile can help ease anxiety, irritability, and insomnia, which are common symptoms of PMS. Drinking chamomile tea regularly before and during menstruation can provide both physical and emotional relief.

Peppermint

Peppermint (Mentha piperita) is a soothing herb that can help manage menstrual pain and digestive issues. Peppermint has muscle-relaxing properties that can ease cramps and reduce bloating. The menthol in peppermint also acts as an analgesic, providing pain relief. Drinking peppermint tea or using peppermint essential oil in aromatherapy can help alleviate headaches, nausea, and abdominal discomfort associated with menstruation. Peppermint is a refreshing and effective option for symptom management during the menstrual cycle.

Evening Primrose Oil

Evening Primrose Oil (Oenothera biennis) is a natural supplement that can help reduce PMS symptoms and menstrual pain. It contains gamma-linolenic acid (GLA), an omega-6 fatty acid that has anti-inflammatory properties. Evening Primrose Oil can help alleviate breast tenderness, bloating, and mood swings associated with PMS. It is typically taken in capsule form, with a recommended dose based on individual needs. Regular use of Evening Primrose Oil can improve menstrual health and reduce discomfort during periods.

Red Raspberry Leaf

Red Raspberry Leaf (Rubus idaeus) is a well-known herb for women's health, particularly for its ability to tone the uterine muscles and reduce menstrual cramps. It contains fragarine, a compound that helps relax the muscles of the uterus, reducing the severity of cramps. Red Raspberry Leaf also supports overall reproductive health and can help regulate menstrual cycles. Drinking Red Raspberry Leaf tea daily, especially in the weeks leading up to menstruation, can provide significant relief from menstrual pain and discomfort.

Conclusion

Herbal remedies offer a natural and effective approach to managing menstrual pain and symptoms. Herbs such as Cramp Bark, Ginger, Turmeric, Chamomile, Peppermint, Evening Primrose Oil, and Red Raspberry Leaf provide relief from cramps, inflammation, headaches, bloating, and mood swings. Incorporating these herbs into your routine can help you achieve a more comfortable and manageable menstrual cycle. As with any herbal treatment, it is important to consult with a healthcare provider to ensure safe and appropriate use based on your individual health needs.

Herbal Teas and Supplements for Menstrual Health

Herbal teas and supplements provide a natural and effective way to support menstrual health. They offer various benefits, from regulating menstrual cycles and reducing cramps to alleviating PMS symptoms and promoting overall reproductive health. Incorporating these herbal remedies into your daily routine can lead to a more balanced and comfortable menstrual experience. Here are some of the most beneficial herbal teas and supplements for menstrual health:

Red Raspberry Leaf Tea

Red Raspberry Leaf (Rubus idaeus) tea is a popular herbal remedy for women's reproductive health. Known for its high content of vitamins and minerals, including iron, calcium, and magnesium, Red Raspberry Leaf helps to strengthen the uterine muscles and promote a regular menstrual cycle. The tea contains fragarine, a compound that tones and relaxes the muscles of the pelvic region, reducing cramps and easing menstrual pain. Drinking Red Raspberry Leaf tea daily, particularly in the weeks leading up to your period, can help create a smoother and less painful menstrual experience. This tea is not only beneficial for menstruation but also supports overall reproductive health.

Ginger Tea

Ginger (Zingiber officinale) tea is renowned for its potent anti-inflammatory and analgesic properties, making it an excellent choice for managing menstrual cramps and pain. Ginger helps reduce the production of prostaglandins, which are responsible for inflammation and pain during menstruation. Consuming ginger tea during your menstrual period can provide quick relief from cramps, headaches, and nausea. Additionally, ginger aids digestion and can help alleviate bloating and digestive discomfort associated with PMS. For maximum benefits, drink ginger tea two to three times a day during your menstrual cycle.

Chamomile Tea

Chamomile (Matricaria chamomilla) tea is well-known for its calming effects and ability to reduce muscle spasms. The anti-inflammatory and antispasmodic properties of chamomile make it an effective remedy for menstrual cramps and discomfort. Drinking chamomile tea can help relax the muscles of the uterus, alleviating pain and reducing the severity of cramps. Chamomile also promotes relaxation and helps relieve anxiety and irritability associated with PMS. Enjoying a cup of chamomile tea before bed can improve sleep quality and help manage insomnia related to menstrual cycles.

Peppermint Tea

Peppermint (Mentha piperita) tea is a refreshing and soothing herbal remedy for menstrual health. The muscle-relaxing properties of peppermint help ease menstrual cramps and reduce bloating. The menthol in peppermint acts as an analgesic, providing pain relief and alleviating headaches and digestive discomfort. Drinking peppermint tea can help reduce nausea and improve overall digestive health, which is particularly beneficial during menstruation. Incorporating peppermint tea into your daily routine can provide both physical and mental relief during your menstrual period.

Evening Primrose Oil Supplements

Evening Primrose Oil (Oenothera biennis) is a natural supplement rich in gamma-linolenic acid (GLA), an omega-6 fatty acid with anti-inflammatory properties. This supplement is highly effective in reducing PMS symptoms such as breast tenderness, bloating, mood swings, and irritability. Taking Evening Primrose Oil supplements regularly can help balance hormones and improve menstrual health. The recommended dosage varies based on individual needs, so it is important to follow the instructions on the supplement label or consult with a healthcare provider.

Vitex (Chasteberry) Supplements

Vitex agnus-castus, commonly known as chasteberry, is a powerful herb for regulating menstrual cycles and balancing hormones. Vitex works by influencing the pituitary gland to normalize the production of hormones such as estrogen and progesterone. This herb is particularly beneficial for women with irregular menstrual cycles, PMS, or hormonal imbalances. Vitex supplements are available in capsule or tincture form, and the typical dosage varies depending on the product and individual needs. Consistent use of Vitex can help promote regular menstrual cycles and reduce PMS symptoms.

Turmeric Supplements

Turmeric (Curcuma longa) is a potent anti-inflammatory herb that can help manage menstrual pain and symptoms. The active compound in turmeric, curcumin, reduces inflammation and alleviates pain associated with menstrual cramps. Taking turmeric supplements during your menstrual period can help reduce the severity of cramps and improve overall well-being. Turmeric supplements are available in capsule form, and the recommended dosage should be followed as per the product instructions. Additionally, incorporating turmeric into your diet can provide ongoing benefits for menstrual health.

Herbal teas and supplements offer a natural and effective way to support menstrual health and manage symptoms associated with menstruation. Red Raspberry Leaf, Ginger, Chamomile, and Peppermint teas provide relief from cramps, pain, and digestive discomfort, while Evening Primrose Oil, Vitex, and Turmeric supplements help balance hormones and reduce PMS symptoms. Incorporating these herbal remedies into your daily routine can lead to a more comfortable and balanced menstrual experience. As always, it is important to consult with a healthcare provider to ensure safe and appropriate use based on your individual health needs.

Case Studies and Success Stories

Case Study 1: Regulating Irregular Cycles with Vitex and Red Raspberry Leaf

Background: Sarah, a 28-year-old woman, had struggled with irregular menstrual cycles since her teenage years. Her cycles ranged from 35 to 60 days, making it difficult for her to predict her periods and plan her activities. Sarah also experienced severe PMS symptoms, including mood swings, bloating, and breast tenderness.

Intervention: Sarah consulted with a naturopathic doctor who recommended a regimen of Vitex (chasteberry) supplements and Red Raspberry Leaf tea. She was advised to take 400 mg of Vitex extract each morning and drink two cups of Red Raspberry Leaf tea daily.

Results: After three months of consistent use, Sarah noticed a significant improvement in her menstrual regularity. Her cycles became more predictable, averaging 30 to 32 days. Additionally, her PMS symptoms were markedly reduced, with less bloating and breast tenderness. Sarah reported feeling more in control of her menstrual health and appreciated the natural approach to managing her symptoms.

Case Study 2: Managing Menstrual Pain with Ginger and Turmeric

Background: Emma, a 34-year-old woman, experienced debilitating menstrual cramps that often caused her to miss work and social engagements. She relied heavily on over-the-counter pain medications but was interested in finding a natural solution to manage her pain.

Intervention: Emma began incorporating ginger and turmeric into her daily routine. She drank ginger tea three times a day and took 500 mg of turmeric supplements twice daily. She also added fresh ginger and turmeric to her meals whenever possible.

Results: Within two menstrual cycles, Emma noticed a significant reduction in the intensity of her cramps. The combination of ginger and turmeric not only alleviated her pain but also reduced inflammation. Emma found that she no longer needed to rely on pain medications and felt more energetic and positive during her menstrual periods. She appreciated the holistic approach to pain management and continued using the herbs regularly.

Case Study 3: Alleviating PMS Symptoms with Evening Primrose Oil and Chamomile Tea

Background: Laura, a 42-year-old woman, suffered from severe PMS symptoms, including irritability, anxiety, insomnia, and breast tenderness. These symptoms disrupted her daily life and affected her relationships and work performance.

Intervention: Laura's healthcare provider recommended Evening Primrose Oil supplements and Chamomile tea. She started taking 1000 mg of Evening Primrose Oil daily and drank a cup of Chamomile tea every evening before bed.

Results: After two months, Laura experienced significant relief from her PMS symptoms. Her mood swings and anxiety levels were much lower, and she reported improved sleep quality. The breast tenderness she previously experienced was also considerably reduced. Laura felt more balanced and emotionally stable throughout her cycle and continued using Evening Primrose Oil and Chamomile tea as part of her routine.

Success Story 1: Enhancing Menstrual Health with Peppermint Tea

Background: Rachel, a 30-year-old woman, struggled with bloating and digestive discomfort during her menstrual periods. These symptoms made her feel sluggish and uncomfortable, affecting her daily activities.

Intervention: Rachel started drinking two cups of Peppermint tea daily, particularly during the week leading up to her period and throughout her menstrual cycle.

Results: Rachel noticed a significant improvement in her bloating and digestive issues. The Peppermint tea helped relax her digestive muscles, reducing bloating and discomfort. Rachel felt lighter and more energetic during her menstrual periods and was pleased with the natural approach to managing her symptoms.

Success Story 2: Balancing Hormones with Maca Root

Background: Sophie, a 25-year-old woman, experienced hormonal imbalances that led to irregular periods and acne. She was looking for a natural solution to balance her hormones and improve her menstrual health.

Intervention: Sophie began taking Maca Root powder, adding one teaspoon to her morning smoothie each day. She continued this regimen consistently for several months.

Results: Sophie's menstrual cycles became more regular, averaging 28 to 30 days. Her hormonal acne also cleared up, and she noticed an overall improvement in her skin health. Sophie felt more balanced and energetic, attributing these positive changes to the regular use of Maca Root. She was delighted with the natural solution to her hormonal issues and continued using Maca Root as part of her daily routine.

Conclusion

These case studies and success stories highlight the effectiveness of herbal remedies in managing menstrual health. Herbs such as Vitex, Red Raspberry Leaf, Ginger, Turmeric, Evening Primrose Oil, Chamomile, Peppermint, and Maca Root have provided significant relief and improvements for women dealing with irregular cycles, menstrual pain, PMS symptoms, and hormonal imbalances. These natural approaches offer safe and holistic solutions, allowing women to take control of their menstrual health and improve their overall well-being. Always consult with a healthcare provider before starting any new herbal regimen to ensure it is appropriate for your individual health needs.

Menopause: Support and Relief

Menopause is a natural phase in a woman's life that marks the end of her reproductive years, typically occurring between the ages of 45 and 55. This transition, while normal, often comes with a variety of physical and emotional symptoms that can significantly impact a woman's quality of life. Common symptoms include hot flashes, night sweats, mood swings, vaginal dryness, and sleep disturbances. These changes are primarily due to fluctuating and declining hormone levels, particularly estrogen and progesterone. While conventional treatments like hormone replacement therapy (HRT) are available, many women seek natural alternatives to manage their symptoms. Herbal remedies offer a holistic approach to supporting the body through menopause, helping to alleviate symptoms and promote overall well-being. This chapter explores various herbs known for their effectiveness in providing support and relief during menopause, offering practical guidance on how to incorporate these natural solutions into daily life.

Understanding Menopause and Its Symptoms

Menopause is a significant biological transition in a woman's life, marking the end of her menstrual cycles and reproductive years. It is officially diagnosed after a woman has gone 12 consecutive months without a menstrual period. Menopause typically occurs between the ages of 45 and 55, although the timing can vary widely. The process leading up to menopause, known as perimenopause, can begin several years before the final menstrual period and is characterized by gradual changes in hormone levels. During this time, the ovaries produce less estrogen and progesterone, leading to various physical and emotional symptoms.

One of the most well-known symptoms of menopause is hot flashes, sudden feelings of intense heat that can cause sweating and discomfort. Hot flashes can vary in frequency and intensity and are often accompanied by night sweats, which can disrupt sleep and contribute to fatigue. The exact cause of hot flashes is not fully understood, but they are believed to be related to changes in the body's temperature regulation mechanisms due to fluctuating estrogen levels.

Mood swings and emotional changes are also common during menopause. Women may experience increased irritability, anxiety, and feelings of sadness or depression. These mood changes can be attributed to hormonal fluctuations, as well as the stress and life changes that often occur during this stage of life. Additionally, menopause can affect memory and cognitive function, sometimes leading to difficulties with concentration and recall.

Another significant symptom of menopause is vaginal dryness, which can cause discomfort and pain during intercourse. This is due to decreased estrogen levels, which lead to thinning and drying of the vaginal tissues. Women may also experience urinary symptoms such as increased frequency, urgency, and a higher risk of urinary tract infections. These changes can affect sexual health and overall quality of life.

Sleep disturbances are prevalent during menopause, often resulting from night sweats or hormonal changes that disrupt the sleep cycle. Insomnia and restless sleep can exacerbate other menopausal symptoms, such as fatigue, mood swings, and cognitive difficulties. Proper management of sleep issues is crucial for maintaining overall health and well-being during this transition.

Bone health is another important consideration during menopause. The decline in estrogen levels can lead to decreased bone density, increasing the risk of osteoporosis and fractures. Women in menopause need to focus on maintaining bone health through diet, exercise, and, in some cases, supplementation.

Menopause can also affect cardiovascular health. Estrogen is known to have a protective effect on the heart and blood vessels, and its decline can increase the risk of cardiovascular diseases such as heart disease and stroke. Women should be mindful of their cardiovascular health and adopt lifestyle changes that support heart health during and after menopause.

Understanding the range of symptoms associated with menopause is essential for managing this transition effectively. By recognizing these symptoms and their underlying causes, women can seek appropriate treatments and support to alleviate discomfort and maintain their quality of life. While conventional treatments like hormone replacement therapy (HRT) are available, many women prefer natural alternatives. Herbal remedies offer a holistic approach to managing menopausal symptoms, providing relief and promoting overall well-being. The following sections will explore various herbs known for their effectiveness in supporting women through menopause and offer practical guidance on incorporating these natural solutions into daily life.

Herbs for Hormone Balance and Symptom Relief

Managing menopause through natural remedies can provide effective relief from the various symptoms associated with this transition. Several herbs are known for their ability to balance hormones and alleviate menopausal symptoms such as hot flashes, night sweats, mood swings, and vaginal dryness. Here are some of the most effective herbs for hormone balance and symptom relief during menopause:

Black Cohosh

Black Cohosh (Cimicifuga racemosa) is one of the most well-researched herbs for menopause. It has been traditionally used to treat a variety of menopausal symptoms, particularly hot flashes and night sweats. Black Cohosh works by influencing the serotonin receptors in the brain, which helps regulate body temperature and reduce the frequency and intensity of hot flashes. Additionally, it may have a mild estrogenic effect, which can help balance hormone levels and alleviate symptoms such as vaginal dryness and mood swings. Black Cohosh is typically taken in capsule or tincture form, with a standard dosage of 20-40 mg twice daily.

Red Clover

Red Clover (Trifolium pratense) contains isoflavones, which are plant-based compounds that mimic estrogen in the body. These phytoestrogens can help alleviate menopausal symptoms by compensating for the decline in natural estrogen levels. Red Clover is particularly effective in reducing hot flashes, night sweats, and improving bone density, which is crucial for preventing osteoporosis. It can also support cardiovascular health, which is important as the risk of heart disease increases after menopause. Red Clover is available in various forms, including capsules, tinctures, and teas.

Dong Quai

Dong Quai (Angelica sinensis), often referred to as "female ginseng," is a traditional Chinese herb known for its ability to balance hormones and support reproductive health. Dong Quai helps alleviate menopausal symptoms by regulating estrogen levels and improving blood circulation. It is particularly beneficial for reducing hot flashes, night sweats, and menstrual irregularities that can occur during perimenopause. Dong Quai is commonly used in combination with other herbs in formulations for women's health. It is available in capsules, tinctures, and teas.

Maca Root

Maca Root (Lepidium meyenii) is an adaptogenic herb that helps balance hormone levels and improve overall energy and vitality. Maca does not contain hormones but works by supporting the endocrine system, which regulates hormone production. It is particularly effective in alleviating symptoms such as hot flashes, night sweats, mood swings, and fatigue. Maca is also known to enhance libido and sexual function, which can be affected during menopause. Maca Root is available in powder form, which can be added to smoothies, or in capsules and tinctures.

Evening Primrose Oil

Evening Primrose Oil (Oenothera biennis) is rich in gamma-linolenic acid (GLA), an omega-6 fatty acid with anti-inflammatory properties. This oil is highly effective in reducing PMS and menopausal symptoms, including breast tenderness, mood swings, and hot flashes. Evening Primrose Oil helps balance hormones and supports overall reproductive health. It is typically taken in capsule form, with a recommended dosage based on individual needs. Regular use of Evening Primrose Oil can significantly improve menopausal symptoms and enhance well-being.

Sage

Sage (Salvia officinalis) is a herb well-known for its ability to reduce excessive sweating and hot flashes during menopause. Sage contains compounds that have estrogenic effects, which help balance hormone levels and alleviate symptoms. Drinking sage tea or taking sage supplements can provide quick relief from hot flashes and night sweats. Sage also has antioxidant properties that support overall health. For sage tea, steep one to two teaspoons of dried sage leaves in hot water for 10-15 minutes and drink 1-2 cups daily.

Licorice Root

Licorice Root (Glycyrrhiza glabra) is another effective herb for balancing hormones and reducing menopausal symptoms. It contains phytoestrogens that help compensate for declining estrogen levels. Licorice Root can help alleviate hot flashes, mood swings, and vaginal dryness. However, it should be used with caution, as excessive use can lead to elevated blood pressure. It is best to use Licorice Root under the guidance of a healthcare provider. It is available in capsules, tinctures, and teas.

Conclusion

Herbal remedies offer a natural and effective approach to managing menopausal symptoms and balancing hormones. Herbs such as Black Cohosh, Red Clover, Dong Quai, Maca Root, Evening Primrose Oil, Sage, and Licorice Root provide significant relief from hot flashes, night sweats, mood swings, and other menopausal symptoms. Incorporating these herbs into your daily routine can help you navigate menopause more comfortably and maintain overall well-being. As with any herbal treatment, it is important to consult with a healthcare provider to ensure safe and appropriate use based on your individual health needs.

Managing Hot Flashes and Night Sweats Naturally

Hot flashes and night sweats are among the most common and distressing symptoms experienced during menopause. Characterized by sudden feelings of intense heat, sweating, and often accompanied by a flushed face and rapid heartbeat, these symptoms can disrupt daily activities and sleep. Fortunately, several natural remedies can help manage hot flashes and night sweats effectively, providing relief without the side effects associated with conventional treatments.

Black Cohosh

Black Cohosh (Cimicifuga racemosa) is one of the most well-known herbal remedies for managing hot flashes and night sweats. It works by influencing serotonin receptors in the brain, which helps regulate body temperature. Studies have shown that Black Cohosh can significantly reduce the frequency and severity of hot flashes. It is typically taken in capsule or tincture form, with a standard dosage of 20-40 mg twice daily. Consistent use over several weeks is often required to achieve the best results.

Red Clover

Red Clover (Trifolium pratense) contains isoflavones, which are plant-based compounds that act like estrogen in the body. These phytoestrogens help alleviate menopausal symptoms by balancing hormone levels. Red Clover has been shown to reduce the frequency and intensity of hot flashes and night sweats. It can be taken as a tea, capsule, or tincture. Drinking Red Clover tea 1-2 times daily or following the dosage instructions for capsules or tinctures can provide effective symptom relief.

Sage

Sage (Salvia officinalis) is a traditional remedy for excessive sweating and hot flashes. It contains compounds with estrogenic properties that help balance hormone levels. Sage also has cooling and astringent properties that help reduce sweating. Drinking sage tea or taking sage supplements can provide quick relief from hot flashes and night sweats. To make sage tea, steep one to two teaspoons of dried sage leaves in hot water for 10-15 minutes and drink 1-2 cups daily.

Flaxseed

Flaxseed (Linum usitatissimum) is rich in lignans, which are plant compounds that have estrogen-like effects. These lignans help balance hormone levels and can reduce the frequency and severity of hot flashes. Flaxseed also provides omega-3 fatty acids, which have anti-inflammatory properties and support overall health. Adding ground flaxseed to your diet by sprinkling it on cereal, yogurt, or smoothies can help manage menopausal symptoms. The recommended intake is about one to two tablespoons daily.

Dong Quai

Dong Quai (Angelica sinensis) is a traditional Chinese herb known for its hormone-balancing effects. It helps alleviate menopausal symptoms such as hot flashes and night sweats by regulating estrogen levels. Dong Quai improves blood circulation, which can also help manage temperature regulation in the body. It is often used in combination with other herbs in formulations for women's health. Dong Quai can be taken in capsule, tincture, or tea form, following the recommended dosage instructions.

Evening Primrose Oil

Evening Primrose Oil (Oenothera biennis) is rich in gamma-linolenic acid (GLA), an omega-6 fatty acid with anti-inflammatory properties. This oil helps balance hormones and can reduce hot flashes and night sweats. Evening Primrose Oil is typically taken in capsule form, with a recommended dosage of 500-1000 mg daily. Consistent use over several weeks may be necessary to achieve noticeable results.

Lifestyle Modifications

In addition to herbal remedies, certain lifestyle changes can help manage hot flashes and night sweats:

- **Dress in Layers:** Wear lightweight, breathable clothing and dress in layers to adjust to temperature changes easily.

- **Stay Cool:** Use fans, air conditioning, or cool showers to lower body temperature. Keep your sleeping environment cool by using lightweight bedding and keeping windows open or using a fan.

- **Hydrate:** Drink plenty of water throughout the day to stay hydrated and help regulate body temperature.

- **Avoid Triggers:** Identify and avoid triggers that may exacerbate hot flashes, such as spicy foods, caffeine, alcohol, and stress.

- **Exercise Regularly:** Engage in regular physical activity to improve overall health and reduce stress, which can help manage hot flashes.

- **Practice Relaxation Techniques:** Techniques such as deep breathing, meditation, and yoga can help reduce stress and improve symptom management.

Managing hot flashes and night sweats naturally involves a combination of herbal remedies and lifestyle modifications. Herbs such as Black Cohosh, Red Clover, Sage, Flaxseed, Dong Quai, and Evening Primrose Oil provide effective relief by balancing hormones and reducing the severity of symptoms. Incorporating these natural remedies into your daily routine, along with making lifestyle adjustments, can help you navigate menopause more comfortably. As with any treatment, it is important to consult with a healthcare provider to ensure safe and appropriate use based on your individual health needs.

Supporting Bone Health and Preventing Osteoporosis

As women age and transition through menopause, the decline in estrogen levels can significantly impact bone density, increasing the risk of osteoporosis. Osteoporosis is a condition characterized by weak and brittle bones, making them more susceptible to fractures. Supporting bone health during and after menopause is crucial to maintaining overall well-being and mobility. Several natural strategies, including diet, lifestyle changes, and herbal remedies, can help strengthen bones and prevent osteoporosis.

Calcium and Vitamin D

Adequate intake of calcium and vitamin D is essential for bone health. Calcium is a key building block of bone tissue, while vitamin D helps the body absorb calcium effectively. Women should aim to consume 1,000 to 1,200 mg of calcium daily, which can be obtained from dietary sources such as dairy products, leafy green vegetables, and fortified foods. Vitamin D can be synthesized through exposure to sunlight and is also found in foods like fatty fish, fortified milk, and eggs. A daily supplement may be necessary for those with limited sun exposure or dietary intake, with a recommended dosage of 600 to 800 IU of vitamin D.

Weight-Bearing Exercise

Regular weight-bearing exercise is crucial for maintaining bone density and strength. Activities such as walking, jogging, dancing, and resistance training stimulate bone formation and slow down bone loss. Weight-bearing exercises apply stress to the bones, encouraging them to rebuild and become stronger. Aim for at least 30 minutes of moderate exercise most days of the week to support bone health and overall fitness.

Magnesium

Magnesium plays a vital role in bone health by helping to regulate calcium levels and contributing to bone structure. Many people do not get enough magnesium through their diet. Foods rich in magnesium include nuts, seeds, whole grains, and leafy green vegetables. A daily intake of 320 mg of magnesium is recommended for adult women. If dietary intake is insufficient, a magnesium supplement can help meet the body's needs and support bone health.

Herbal Remedies

Several herbs are known for their bone-strengthening properties and can be incorporated into a daily regimen to support bone health and prevent osteoporosis.

Red Clover:

- Red Clover (Trifolium pratense) contains isoflavones, which are phytoestrogens that mimic estrogen in the body. These compounds can help maintain bone density and reduce the risk of osteoporosis. Red Clover can be taken as a tea, capsule, or tincture. Drinking Red Clover tea daily can provide ongoing support for bone health.

Horsetail:

- Horsetail (Equisetum arvense) is rich in silica, a mineral essential for bone formation and strength. Silica helps the body utilize calcium more effectively and supports collagen production in bone tissue. Horsetail can be consumed as a tea or taken in capsule form. Regular use of horsetail can help maintain bone density and prevent fractures.

Nettle:

- Nettle (Urtica dioica) is a nutrient-dense herb that contains calcium, magnesium, and other minerals important for bone health. Nettle tea or capsules can provide a natural source of these essential nutrients, supporting bone density and strength. Drinking nettle tea daily or taking nettle supplements can help fortify bones and prevent osteoporosis.

Black Cohosh:

- Black Cohosh (Cimicifuga racemosa) is known for its hormone-balancing effects and can help support bone health during menopause. By mimicking the effects of estrogen, Black Cohosh can help reduce bone loss and maintain bone density. It is typically taken in capsule or tincture form.

Omega-3 Fatty Acids

Omega-3 fatty acids, found in fish oil and flaxseed, have anti-inflammatory properties and may help support bone health. Omega-3s can reduce bone loss and increase bone formation by promoting the activity of bone-forming cells. Including fatty fish such as salmon, mackerel, and sardines in your diet, or taking an omega-3 supplement, can contribute to stronger bones and overall health.

Lifestyle Modifications

In addition to diet and exercise, certain lifestyle changes can help support bone health and prevent osteoporosis:

- **Avoid Smoking:** Smoking can reduce bone density and increase the risk of fractures. Quitting smoking is essential for maintaining healthy bones.

- **Limit Alcohol Intake:** Excessive alcohol consumption can interfere with the body's ability to absorb calcium and other nutrients essential for bone health. Limit alcohol intake to moderate levels to protect your bones.

- **Maintain a Healthy Weight:** Being underweight increases the risk of bone loss and fractures, while being overweight can put extra stress on bones. Maintaining a healthy weight through a balanced diet and regular exercise is important for bone health.

Supporting bone health and preventing osteoporosis during and after menopause requires a multifaceted approach that includes adequate intake of calcium and vitamin D, regular weight-bearing exercise, and the use of bone-strengthening herbs and supplements. Incorporating Red Clover, Horsetail, Nettle, and Black Cohosh into your daily regimen, along with omega-3 fatty acids, can provide natural support for maintaining bone density and strength. Lifestyle modifications such as avoiding smoking, limiting alcohol intake, and maintaining a healthy weight further contribute to bone health. By adopting these strategies, women can reduce the risk of osteoporosis and enjoy better overall well-being. As always, it is important to consult with a healthcare provider before starting any new supplement or herbal regimen to ensure safe and appropriate use.

Emotional Well-Being and Mood Support with Herbs

Navigating the emotional ups and downs during menopause can be challenging for many women. Hormonal fluctuations can lead to mood swings, anxiety, depression, and irritability. While lifestyle changes and conventional treatments can help, herbal remedies offer a natural and effective way to support emotional well-being and stabilize mood. Here are some herbs known for their mood-enhancing and calming properties:

St. John's Wort

St. John's Wort (Hypericum perforatum) is one of the most well-known herbs for managing mild to moderate depression. It works by increasing levels of serotonin, dopamine, and norepinephrine in the brain, which are neurotransmitters associated with mood regulation. Studies have shown that St. John's Wort can be as effective as some conventional antidepressants with fewer side effects. It is typically taken in capsule, tablet, or tincture form.

The standard dosage is usually 300 mg of standardized extract taken three times daily. It is important to note that St. John's Wort can interact with various medications, so consulting with a healthcare provider before use is crucial.

Ashwagandha

Ashwagandha (Withania somnifera) is an adaptogenic herb known for its ability to reduce stress and anxiety. It helps the body adapt to stress by regulating cortisol levels and supporting the adrenal glands. Ashwagandha also enhances mood and promotes emotional balance. Regular use of Ashwagandha can improve sleep quality, reduce anxiety, and enhance overall well-being. It is available in various forms, including capsules, powders, and tinctures. A common dosage is 300-500 mg of standardized extract taken twice daily.

Lavender

Lavender (Lavandula angustifolia) is widely recognized for its calming and soothing properties. It is often used in aromatherapy to reduce stress, anxiety, and promote relaxation. Inhaling lavender essential oil or using it in a diffuser can help create a sense of calm and improve mood. Lavender tea is another effective way to harness its calming effects. Drinking a cup of lavender tea before bed can promote restful sleep and reduce nighttime anxiety. For aromatherapy, a few drops of lavender essential oil can be added to a diffuser or a warm bath.

Lemon Balm

Lemon Balm (Melissa officinalis) is a member of the mint family known for its calming effects and ability to reduce anxiety and stress. It works by increasing GABA (gamma-aminobutyric acid) levels in the brain, which helps promote relaxation and reduce excitability. Lemon Balm can be consumed as a tea, tincture, or capsule. Drinking Lemon Balm tea 2-3 times daily can help alleviate anxiety and improve mood. The tea has a pleasant, lemony flavor, making it a soothing choice for emotional support.

Rhodiola Rosea

Rhodiola Rosea is an adaptogenic herb that helps the body cope with stress and fatigue. It enhances mental resilience and supports emotional well-being by balancing neurotransmitter levels and reducing cortisol production. Rhodiola is particularly effective for reducing symptoms of anxiety and depression. It is commonly taken in capsule or tincture form. The recommended dosage is typically 200-600 mg per day of standardized extract. Rhodiola should be taken earlier in the day as it can be stimulating for some people.

Passionflower

Passionflower (Passiflora incarnata) is a calming herb traditionally used to treat anxiety and insomnia. It works by increasing GABA levels in the brain, promoting relaxation and reducing stress. Passionflower can be particularly helpful for managing anxiety-related sleep disturbances. It is available in various forms, including tea, tincture, and capsules. Drinking Passionflower tea before bed can help improve sleep quality and reduce nighttime anxiety. For tinctures and capsules, following the dosage instructions on the product label is recommended.

Valerian Root

Valerian Root (Valeriana officinalis) is well-known for its sedative properties and ability to promote restful sleep. It helps reduce anxiety and stress by increasing GABA levels in the brain. Valerian Root is often used to manage insomnia and anxiety-related sleep disturbances. It can be consumed as a tea, tincture, or capsule. Drinking Valerian Root tea or taking a tincture 30 minutes before bed can help promote relaxation and improve sleep quality. Valerian Root should be used with caution during the day as it can cause drowsiness.

Herbal remedies offer a natural and effective way to support emotional well-being and stabilize mood during menopause. Herbs such as St. John's Wort, Ashwagandha, Lavender, Lemon Balm, Rhodiola Rosea, Passionflower, and Valerian Root provide significant relief from stress, anxiety, depression, and mood swings. Incorporating these herbs into your daily routine can enhance overall emotional health and improve quality of life. As with any herbal treatment, it is important to consult with a healthcare provider to ensure safe and appropriate use based on your individual health needs.

Personal Stories and Experiences

Sarah's Journey with St. John's Wort

Sarah, a 52-year-old woman, began experiencing significant mood swings and bouts of depression during her menopausal transition. These emotional changes impacted her daily life, making it difficult to maintain her usual level of productivity and positivity. After consulting with her healthcare provider, Sarah decided to try St. John's Wort as a natural remedy for her symptoms.

Sarah started taking 300 mg of standardized St. John's Wort extract three times a day. Within a few weeks, she noticed a marked improvement in her mood. The depressive episodes became less frequent and less intense, allowing her to feel more like herself. Sarah also found that her anxiety levels decreased, and she was able to manage stress more effectively. She continued using St. John's Wort, finding it a vital part of her emotional well-being regimen.

Emily's Experience with Ashwagandha

Emily, a 48-year-old woman, was struggling with heightened anxiety and stress as she entered menopause. The increased responsibilities at work and home only added to her stress, leading to sleepless nights and constant worry. After researching natural remedies, Emily decided to incorporate Ashwagandha into her daily routine.

Emily began taking 500 mg of standardized Ashwagandha extract twice a day. Over the next month, she experienced a significant reduction in her anxiety levels. The adaptogenic properties of Ashwagandha helped her better manage stress and improved her resilience. Emily also noticed that her sleep quality improved, and she felt more rested and energized each morning. Ashwagandha became a staple in her efforts to maintain emotional balance and overall health during menopause.

Claire's Relief with Lavender

Claire, a 50-year-old woman, found herself dealing with intense stress and frequent bouts of irritability during her menopausal years. The stress also affected her sleep, leading to restless nights. Claire decided to try lavender for its reputed calming effects.

She started by using lavender essential oil in a diffuser at night and drinking lavender tea before bed. The calming aroma of the lavender oil helped Claire relax and created a soothing environment conducive to sleep. Drinking lavender tea also promoted relaxation and eased her transition into sleep. Within a few weeks, Claire noticed a significant reduction in her stress levels and improved sleep quality. Lavender became a key component in her nightly routine, providing the emotional support she needed.

Rachel's Calm with Lemon Balm

Rachel, a 47-year-old woman, struggled with anxiety and occasional panic attacks as she navigated menopause. These episodes were disruptive and impacted her ability to focus on her work and family. Seeking a natural solution, Rachel turned to Lemon Balm.

Rachel began drinking Lemon Balm tea three times a day. The pleasant, lemony flavor made it easy to incorporate into her routine. She soon noticed that her anxiety levels began to diminish, and the frequency of her panic attacks decreased. Lemon Balm's calming effect helped Rachel manage her anxiety more effectively, allowing her to feel more in control and focused. The herb became an integral part of her strategy to maintain emotional stability.

Laura's Balance with Rhodiola Rosea

Laura, a 49-year-old woman, experienced extreme fatigue and emotional exhaustion during her menopausal transition. She found it challenging to keep up with her daily responsibilities and felt overwhelmed. After learning about the benefits of Rhodiola Rosea, Laura decided to give it a try.

Laura started taking 400 mg of standardized Rhodiola Rosea extract each morning. Within a few weeks, she felt a noticeable increase in her energy levels and a significant improvement in her mood. Rhodiola helped her feel more balanced and resilient, reducing the emotional exhaustion she had been experiencing. The adaptogenic properties of Rhodiola supported her mental clarity and overall well-being, making it an essential part of her daily routine.

Megan's Serenity with Passionflower

Megan, a 46-year-old woman, was dealing with severe anxiety and insomnia during menopause. The lack of sleep exacerbated her anxiety, creating a vicious cycle. Megan decided to try Passionflower, known for its calming and sleep-promoting properties.

Megan began drinking Passionflower tea every evening before bed. The soothing effects of Passionflower helped her relax and prepare for sleep. Over time, Megan noticed that her anxiety levels decreased, and her sleep quality improved significantly. The regular use of Passionflower allowed her to break the cycle of anxiety and insomnia, leading to better emotional well-being and restful nights.

These personal stories highlight the positive impact of herbal remedies on managing emotional well-being and mood during menopause. Herbs like St. John's Wort, Ashwagandha, Lavender, Lemon Balm, Rhodiola Rosea, and Passionflower have provided significant relief and support for women navigating this life transition. These natural solutions offer a safe and effective way to enhance emotional health and improve overall quality of life during menopause. As always, it is important to consult with a healthcare provider before starting any new herbal regimen to ensure it is appropriate for your individual needs.

BOOK 14:

Fertility and Pregnancy: Precautions and Benefits

Fertility and pregnancy are critical stages in a woman's life that require careful attention to health and well-being. During these times, many women seek natural remedies to support reproductive health and manage pregnancy-related symptoms. While certain herbs can offer significant benefits, it is crucial to use them with caution due to the sensitive nature of these stages. Understanding which herbs are safe and effective, as well as those that should be avoided, is essential for promoting a healthy pregnancy and optimizing fertility. This chapter explores the benefits and precautions associated with herbal remedies during fertility and pregnancy, providing guidance on their appropriate use to ensure the best outcomes for both mother and baby.

Herbs to Support Reproductive Health and Boost Fertility

Maintaining reproductive health and enhancing fertility naturally can be effectively supported by incorporating specific herbs known for their beneficial properties. These herbs can help balance hormones, support the reproductive organs, and improve overall well-being, thereby increasing the chances of conception. Here are some herbs commonly used to support reproductive health and boost fertility:

Vitex (Chasteberry)

Vitex agnus-castus, commonly known as chasteberry, is one of the most well-known herbs for supporting reproductive health and boosting fertility. Vitex works by regulating the pituitary gland, which controls the production of hormones such as estrogen and progesterone. By balancing these hormones, Vitex can help normalize menstrual cycles, improve ovulation, and enhance overall reproductive health. It is particularly beneficial for women with irregular cycles or conditions like polycystic ovary syndrome (PCOS). Vitex is typically taken in capsule, tablet, or tincture form, with a recommended dosage of 400-1000 mg daily.

Maca Root

Maca Root (Lepidium meyenii) is an adaptogenic herb that has been used for centuries to boost fertility and enhance reproductive health. Maca supports the endocrine system, helping to balance hormones and improve energy levels. It is rich in vitamins, minerals, and amino acids that promote overall health. Maca is beneficial for both men and women, as it can improve sperm quality and motility in men and regulate menstrual cycles and ovulation in women. Maca Root is available in powder form, which can be added to smoothies, or in capsules and tinctures. A common dosage is 1,500-3,000 mg daily.

Red Clover

Red Clover (Trifolium pratense) contains isoflavones, which are phytoestrogens that mimic estrogen in the body. These compounds help balance hormone levels and improve overall reproductive health. Red Clover is known for its ability to detoxify the body, improve blood circulation to the reproductive organs, and promote hormonal balance. It can also enhance the health of the uterine lining, which is crucial for implantation. Red Clover is typically consumed as a tea, but it is also available in capsule and tincture forms. Drinking 1-2 cups of Red Clover tea daily can provide significant benefits.

Dong Quai

Dong Quai (Angelica sinensis) is a traditional Chinese herb often referred to as "female ginseng." It is highly regarded for its ability to support reproductive health and boost fertility. Dong Quai helps regulate the menstrual cycle, improve blood flow to the reproductive organs, and balance estrogen levels. It is particularly beneficial for women experiencing menstrual irregularities or hormonal imbalances. Dong Quai can be taken in capsule, tincture, or tea form. A common dosage is 1-2 grams of dried root per day, or as directed on supplement packaging.

Tribulus

Tribulus terrestris is an herb known for its ability to enhance fertility and improve reproductive health. Tribulus works by regulating hormone levels and supporting ovarian function, which can improve ovulation and increase the chances of conception. It is also beneficial for men, as it can improve sperm quality and libido. Tribulus is typically taken in capsule or tablet form, with a recommended dosage of 500-1500 mg daily.

Nettle

Nettle (Urtica dioica) is a nutrient-dense herb that supports overall reproductive health. It is rich in vitamins and minerals, including iron, calcium, and magnesium, which are essential for hormonal balance and reproductive function. Nettle helps detoxify the body, support the adrenal glands, and improve the health of the reproductive organs. Nettle tea is a popular way to consume this herb, but it is also available in capsules and tinctures. Drinking 1-2 cups of Nettle tea daily can provide excellent support for reproductive health.

Ashwagandha

Ashwagandha (Withania somnifera) is an adaptogenic herb that helps balance hormones, reduce stress, and improve overall reproductive health. By supporting the adrenal glands and reducing cortisol levels, Ashwagandha helps create a more conducive environment for conception. It is beneficial for both men and women, improving sperm quality in men and regulating menstrual cycles and ovulation in women. Ashwagandha is available in various forms, including capsules, powders, and tinctures. A common dosage is 300-500 mg of standardized extract taken twice daily.

Herbs such as Vitex, Maca Root, Red Clover, Dong Quai, Tribulus, Nettle, and Ashwagandha offer significant benefits for supporting reproductive health and boosting fertility. These herbs help balance hormones, improve menstrual regularity, enhance the health of reproductive organs, and increase the chances of conception. Incorporating these natural remedies into your daily routine can promote overall well-being and reproductive success. As with any herbal treatment, it is important to consult with a healthcare provider to ensure safe and appropriate use based on your individual health needs.

Safe Herbal Remedies During Pregnancy

During pregnancy, it is essential to prioritize safety when considering herbal remedies. While some herbs can provide valuable support for common pregnancy-related issues such as nausea, anxiety, and sleep disturbances, others should be avoided due to potential risks to the mother and baby. Here are some safe herbal remedies that can help manage pregnancy symptoms and promote overall well-being.

Ginger

Ginger (Zingiber officinale) is widely recognized for its effectiveness in alleviating nausea and vomiting, which are common during the first trimester of pregnancy. Ginger can be consumed in various forms, including ginger tea, ginger candies, or fresh ginger added to foods. Studies have shown that ginger can significantly reduce the severity of morning sickness without harmful side effects. Drinking ginger tea or taking ginger capsules (250 mg up to four times daily) can provide relief from nausea and improve digestive health.

Peppermint

Peppermint (Mentha piperita) is known for its calming and digestive properties. It can help relieve nausea, indigestion, and headaches, which are common during pregnancy. Peppermint tea is a soothing option that can be safely consumed during pregnancy. However, it is important to use peppermint in moderation, as excessive amounts may cause heartburn in some individuals. Drinking 1-2 cups of peppermint tea daily can help alleviate digestive discomfort and promote relaxation.

Chamomile

Chamomile (Matricaria chamomilla) is a gentle herb that promotes relaxation and can help with insomnia and anxiety during pregnancy. Chamomile tea is a popular way to enjoy its calming effects. It is important to use chamomile in moderation and choose high-quality, organic sources to avoid contamination. Drinking a cup of chamomile tea before bedtime can improve sleep quality and reduce stress. However, chamomile should be avoided in large quantities due to potential uterine stimulant effects.

Raspberry Leaf

Red Raspberry Leaf (Rubus idaeus) is a well-known herb for supporting reproductive health and preparing the body for labor. It is rich in vitamins and minerals, including iron, calcium, and magnesium. Red Raspberry Leaf helps tone the uterine muscles, which can lead to more efficient contractions during labor. It is generally recommended to start using Red Raspberry Leaf tea in the second or third trimester, as it can help strengthen the uterus and support a healthy pregnancy. Drinking 1-2 cups of Red Raspberry Leaf tea daily is considered safe and beneficial.

Lemon Balm

Lemon Balm (Melissa officinalis) is a calming herb that can help reduce anxiety and improve sleep during pregnancy. It has mild sedative properties and can be consumed as a tea to promote relaxation. Lemon Balm tea is safe for use during pregnancy and can help manage stress and insomnia. Drinking 1-2 cups of Lemon Balm tea daily can provide gentle support for emotional well-being.

Oat Straw

Oat Straw (Avena sativa) is a nourishing herb rich in vitamins and minerals, including calcium and magnesium, which support overall health during pregnancy. Oat Straw can help reduce stress, improve sleep, and support the nervous system. It is commonly consumed as an infusion or tea. Drinking 1-2 cups of Oat Straw tea daily can provide nutritional support and promote relaxation.

Nettle

Nettle (Urtica dioica) is a nutrient-dense herb that provides essential vitamins and minerals, such as iron, calcium, and magnesium. Nettle supports overall health and can help prevent anemia during pregnancy. It is also known for its ability to support the kidneys and reduce water retention. Nettle tea is a safe and beneficial option for pregnant women. Drinking 1-2 cups of Nettle tea daily can provide valuable nutritional support.

Conclusion

Herbal remedies such as Ginger, Peppermint, Chamomile, Red Raspberry Leaf, Lemon Balm, Oat Straw, and Nettle can safely support health and alleviate common pregnancy-related symptoms. These herbs offer gentle and effective solutions for nausea, anxiety, insomnia, digestive issues, and overall well-being. As with any treatment during pregnancy, it is crucial to consult with a healthcare provider before starting any new herbal regimen to ensure safety and appropriateness for your individual needs.

Precautions and Contraindications for Pregnant Women

During pregnancy, the use of herbal remedies should be approached with caution. While many herbs can offer safe and effective relief from pregnancy-related symptoms, others may pose risks to the mother and developing baby. It is crucial to be aware of which herbs are safe and which should be avoided. Here are some general precautions and a list of herbs that are contraindicated during pregnancy.

General Precautions

1. **Consult with a Healthcare Provider**: Before taking any herbal remedies, pregnant women should consult with their healthcare provider. This ensures that any chosen herb is safe for their specific health conditions and circumstances.

2. **Use High-Quality Products**: Choose high-quality, organic herbs from reputable sources to avoid contamination with pesticides, heavy metals, or other harmful substances.

3. **Avoid High Doses**: Even safe herbs should be used in moderation. High doses of certain herbs can lead to adverse effects.

4. **Be Aware of Potential Allergies**: Like any substance, herbs can cause allergic reactions in some individuals. Start with a small amount to ensure there are no adverse reactions.

5. **Avoid Combining Multiple Herbs Without Guidance**: Combining herbs can sometimes lead to unexpected interactions. It is best to use one herb at a time unless advised otherwise by a healthcare provider.

6. **Monitor for Side Effects**: Pay attention to any side effects or unusual symptoms that arise after starting an herbal remedy. If any adverse effects occur, discontinue use and consult a healthcare provider.

Herbs to Avoid During Pregnancy

1. **Pennyroyal (Mentha pulegium)**: Known to induce uterine contractions and has been associated with miscarriages.

2. **Blue Cohosh (Caulophyllum thalictroides)**: Can stimulate uterine contractions and is associated with adverse effects on the cardiovascular system of the fetus.

3. **Dong Quai (Angelica sinensis)**: While beneficial for reproductive health, it is contraindicated during pregnancy due to its potential to stimulate uterine contractions.

4. **Goldenseal (Hydrastis canadensis)**: Contains berberine, which can cross the placenta and potentially cause brain damage in the developing fetus.

5. **Black Cohosh (Cimicifuga racemosa)**: While often used for menopausal symptoms, it should be avoided during pregnancy as it can induce labor.

6. **Aloe Vera (internal use)**: Can stimulate uterine contractions and cause electrolyte imbalances.

7. **Mugwort (Artemisia vulgaris)**: Known to stimulate the uterus and is associated with miscarriages.

8. **Sage (Salvia officinalis)**: High doses can stimulate uterine contractions and is linked to increased risk of miscarriage.

9. **Parsley (Petroselinum crispum) (in large amounts)**: Can stimulate uterine contractions and should be used cautiously.

10. **Tansy (Tanacetum vulgare)**: Known for its abortifacient properties and should be strictly avoided during pregnancy.

11. **Fennel (Foeniculum vulgare) (in high doses)**: While small amounts are generally safe, high doses can stimulate the uterus.

12. **Licorice Root (Glycyrrhiza glabra)**: Can lead to hypertension and preterm labor due to its effects on hormone levels and blood pressure.

While many herbs can offer safe and beneficial support during pregnancy, it is essential to approach their use with caution. Consulting with a healthcare provider, using high-quality products, and being aware of potential risks are crucial steps for ensuring the health and safety of both the mother and the developing baby. Avoiding certain herbs that are known to pose risks during pregnancy is equally important. By following these guidelines, pregnant women can safely benefit from herbal remedies to alleviate symptoms and support their overall well-being.

Herbal Support for Common Pregnancy Issues

Pregnancy can bring a variety of physical and emotional challenges, including nausea, fatigue, digestive issues, and anxiety. While many women prefer natural remedies to manage these symptoms, it's essential to choose herbs that are safe for both the mother and the developing baby. Here are some herbal remedies that can provide effective relief for common pregnancy issues.

Nausea and Morning Sickness

Ginger (Zingiber officinale): Ginger is one of the most effective herbs for relieving nausea and morning sickness. It works by stimulating digestive function and reducing inflammation in the gastrointestinal tract. Ginger can be consumed as tea, in capsule form, or as ginger candies.

- **Ginger Tea:** Steep 1-2 grams of fresh grated ginger in hot water for 10 minutes. Drink 1-2 cups per day.
- **Ginger Capsules:** 250 mg up to four times daily.

Peppermint (Mentha piperita): Peppermint can help relieve nausea and improve digestion. It has a soothing effect on the stomach and can reduce feelings of queasiness.

- **Peppermint Tea:** Steep 1 teaspoon of dried peppermint leaves in hot water for 10 minutes. Drink 1-2 cups per day.

Fatigue

Maca Root (Lepidium meyenii): Maca root is an adaptogen that helps balance hormones and increase energy levels. It can combat fatigue and improve overall stamina.

- **Maca Powder:** Add 1-2 teaspoons to smoothies or juice daily.

- **Maca Capsules:** Follow the recommended dosage on the product label, usually 1,500-3,000 mg daily.

Nettle (Urtica dioica): Nettle is rich in vitamins and minerals, including iron, which is essential for combating fatigue. It helps support overall energy levels and replenishes vital nutrients.

- **Nettle Tea:** Steep 1-2 teaspoons of dried nettle leaves in hot water for 10-15 minutes. Drink 1-2 cups per day.

Digestive Issues

Fennel (Foeniculum vulgare): Fennel can help relieve bloating, gas, and indigestion. It has carminative properties that soothe the digestive tract.

- **Fennel Tea:** Steep 1 teaspoon of crushed fennel seeds in hot water for 10 minutes. Drink 1-2 cups per day.

Chamomile (Matricaria chamomilla): Chamomile is gentle and effective for soothing digestive issues, reducing gas, and relieving indigestion. It also promotes relaxation and better sleep.

- **Chamomile Tea:** Steep 1-2 teaspoons of dried chamomile flowers in hot water for 10 minutes. Drink 1-2 cups per day, especially before bedtime.

Anxiety and Stress

Lavender (Lavandula angustifolia): Lavender is well-known for its calming properties. It can help reduce anxiety and promote relaxation.

- **Lavender Tea:** Steep 1 teaspoon of dried lavender flowers in hot water for 10 minutes. Drink 1-2 cups per day.

- **Lavender Aromatherapy:** Use a few drops of lavender essential oil in a diffuser or add to a warm bath.

Lemon Balm (Melissa officinalis): Lemon Balm is a soothing herb that helps reduce anxiety and promote a sense of calm. It can also improve sleep quality.

- **Lemon Balm Tea:** Steep 1-2 teaspoons of dried lemon balm leaves in hot water for 10 minutes. Drink 1-2 cups per day.

Sleep Disturbances

Oat Straw (Avena sativa): Oat Straw is nourishing and supports the nervous system, promoting relaxation and better sleep.

- **Oat Straw Tea:** Steep 1-2 teaspoons of dried oat straw in hot water for 10-15 minutes. Drink 1-2 cups per day.

Passionflower (Passiflora incarnata): Passionflower is effective in promoting restful sleep and reducing anxiety-related sleep disturbances.

- **Passionflower Tea:** Steep 1-2 teaspoons of dried passionflower in hot water for 10-15 minutes. Drink a cup before bedtime.

Herbal remedies can provide safe and effective relief for common pregnancy issues such as nausea, fatigue, digestive problems, anxiety, and sleep disturbances. Herbs like ginger, peppermint, maca root, nettle, fennel, chamomile, lavender, lemon balm, oat straw, and passionflower offer natural solutions to support overall well-being during pregnancy. Always consult with a healthcare provider before starting any new herbal regimen to ensure it is appropriate for your individual health needs and circumstances.

Promoting a Healthy Pregnancy with Herbal Nutrition

Maintaining a healthy pregnancy requires a balanced diet rich in essential nutrients, and certain herbs can play a supportive role by providing additional vitamins, minerals, and other beneficial compounds. Herbal nutrition can help ensure both the mother and developing baby receive the necessary nutrients for optimal health. Here are some herbs known for their nutritional benefits during pregnancy:

Red Raspberry Leaf

Red Raspberry Leaf (Rubus idaeus): Red Raspberry Leaf is renowned for its ability to tone the uterine muscles, which can help prepare the body for labor and delivery. It is rich in vitamins and minerals, including vitamins C, E, and A, as well as iron, calcium, and magnesium. These nutrients support overall health and can help reduce the risk of complications during pregnancy.

- **Red Raspberry Leaf Tea:** Steep 1-2 teaspoons of dried Red Raspberry Leaf in hot water for 10-15 minutes. Drink 1-2 cups daily, increasing to 3 cups in the third trimester.

Nettle

Nettle (Urtica dioica): Nettle is a powerhouse of nutrients, providing high levels of vitamins A, C, D, and K, as well as iron, calcium, potassium, and magnesium. These nutrients are essential for supporting the increased nutritional demands during pregnancy. Nettle can help prevent anemia, support kidney function, and promote overall energy and well-being.

- **Nettle Tea:** Steep 1-2 teaspoons of dried nettle leaves in hot water for 10-15 minutes. Drink 1-2 cups daily.

Oat Straw

Oat Straw (Avena sativa): Oat Straw is highly nutritious, offering a good source of calcium, magnesium, and silica, which are important for bone health and overall strength. It also supports the nervous system, helping to reduce stress and improve sleep.

- **Oat Straw Tea:** Steep 1-2 teaspoons of dried oat straw in hot water for 10-15 minutes. Drink 1-2 cups daily.

Alfalfa

Alfalfa (Medicago sativa): Alfalfa is rich in vitamins A, D, E, and K, as well as calcium, magnesium, and iron. It can help boost overall nutritional intake and is especially beneficial in the later stages of pregnancy to support blood clotting due to its high vitamin K content.

- **Alfalfa Tea:** Steep 1-2 teaspoons of dried alfalfa leaves in hot water for 10-15 minutes. Drink 1-2 cups daily.

- **Alfalfa Capsules:** Follow the dosage instructions on the product label.

Dandelion

Dandelion (Taraxacum officinale): Dandelion is a great source of vitamins A, C, and K, as well as iron and calcium. It supports liver function, helps manage fluid retention, and provides gentle diuretic effects, which can be helpful in reducing pregnancy-related swelling.

- **Dandelion Tea:** Steep 1-2 teaspoons of dried dandelion leaves or roots in hot water for 10-15 minutes. Drink 1-2 cups daily.

- **Dandelion Greens:** Can be added to salads or smoothies.

Ginger

Ginger (Zingiber officinale): Ginger is not only effective for reducing nausea but also provides anti-inflammatory and digestive benefits. It can help improve overall digestion and nutrient absorption, which is crucial during pregnancy.

- **Ginger Tea:** Steep 1-2 grams of fresh grated ginger in hot water for 10 minutes. Drink 1-2 cups daily.

- **Ginger Capsules:** Follow the dosage instructions on the product label.

Lemon Balm

Lemon Balm (Melissa officinalis): Lemon Balm supports emotional well-being by reducing anxiety and promoting relaxation. It is also rich in antioxidants, which help protect cells from damage.

- **Lemon Balm Tea:** Steep 1-2 teaspoons of dried lemon balm leaves in hot water for 10 minutes. Drink 1-2 cups daily.

Tips for Incorporating Herbal Nutrition

1. **Start Slowly:** If you are new to using herbal teas and supplements, start with small amounts and gradually increase to the recommended dosage to ensure there are no adverse reactions.

2. **Combine Herbs:** Creating a blend of these herbs can provide a broad spectrum of nutrients. For example, combining Red Raspberry Leaf, Nettle, and Oat Straw into a single tea blend can enhance overall nutritional benefits.

3. **Consistency is Key:** Consistent daily use of these herbs can help maintain optimal health throughout pregnancy. Incorporate them into your daily routine to ensure regular intake.

4. **Hydration:** Drinking herbal teas not only provides nutritional benefits but also helps maintain hydration, which is essential during pregnancy.

5. **Consult Your Healthcare Provider:** Always discuss any new herbal regimen with your healthcare provider to ensure it is safe and appropriate for your specific health needs.

Herbs like Red Raspberry Leaf, Nettle, Oat Straw, Alfalfa, Dandelion, Ginger, and Lemon Balm offer valuable nutritional support during pregnancy. These herbs provide essential vitamins and minerals, support overall health, and help manage common pregnancy-related symptoms. Incorporating these herbal remedies into your daily routine can promote a healthy pregnancy and ensure both the mother and developing baby receive the necessary nutrients for optimal health. Always consult with a healthcare provider before starting any new herbal regimen to ensure safety and appropriateness for your individual circumstances.

Testimonials and Real-Life Experiences

Testimonial 1: Sarah's Journey with Red Raspberry Leaf and Nettle

Background: Sarah, a 32-year-old expectant mother, was looking for natural ways to support her pregnancy. She wanted to ensure she was getting enough nutrients and managing common pregnancy symptoms naturally.

Experience: Sarah started drinking Red Raspberry Leaf and Nettle tea during her second trimester after hearing about their benefits from a friend. She began with one cup of tea daily, gradually increasing to two cups as she approached her third trimester. Sarah noticed that her energy levels improved, and she felt more balanced and less fatigued. The iron content in Nettle helped her maintain healthy iron levels, preventing anemia. She also experienced fewer leg cramps and less swelling as a result of these herbal teas.

Testimonial: "Drinking Red Raspberry Leaf and Nettle tea was a game-changer for me during my pregnancy. I felt more energized, and my iron levels were great throughout. Plus, it was a relaxing routine that I looked forward to every day."

Testimonial 2: Emily's Success with Ginger for Morning Sickness

Background: Emily, a 28-year-old woman in her first trimester, struggled with severe morning sickness. She was wary of taking medications and wanted a natural remedy to alleviate her nausea.

Experience: Emily started drinking ginger tea as soon as she woke up and found it significantly reduced her morning sickness. She also carried ginger candies with her to help manage nausea throughout the day. The ginger tea not only helped with her nausea but also improved her overall digestion, making her feel more comfortable.

Testimonial: "Ginger tea was my lifesaver during those tough early weeks of pregnancy. It made my mornings much more bearable, and I could finally enjoy my meals again without feeling queasy."

Testimonial 3: Rachel's Relief with Lemon Balm and Chamomile

Background: Rachel, a 35-year-old pregnant woman, experienced high levels of anxiety and had trouble sleeping as her due date approached. She wanted a safe and natural way to calm her nerves and get better sleep.

Experience: Rachel started drinking a blend of Lemon Balm and Chamomile tea in the evenings. This nightly ritual helped her relax and unwind. Over a few weeks, she noticed a significant reduction in her anxiety levels and was able to fall asleep more easily. The combination of these calming herbs provided the emotional support she needed during this stressful time.

Testimonial: "The Lemon Balm and Chamomile tea blend was wonderful. It helped me relax and get much-needed sleep. I felt more at ease and better prepared for my baby's arrival."

Testimonial 4: Laura's Balanced Nutrition with Alfalfa and Oat Straw

Background: Laura, a 30-year-old expectant mother, wanted to ensure she was getting all the necessary nutrients for a healthy pregnancy. She sought natural supplements to complement her diet.

Experience: Laura incorporated Alfalfa and Oat Straw tea into her daily routine. She found that these teas provided a rich source of vitamins and minerals that supported her overall health. Alfalfa helped boost her vitamin K levels, which are important for blood clotting, while Oat Straw provided calcium and magnesium, promoting strong bones and reducing muscle cramps.

Testimonial: "Alfalfa and Oat Straw teas were fantastic additions to my pregnancy diet. They gave me peace of mind knowing I was getting extra nutrients naturally. Plus, they tasted great and were easy to include in my daily routine."

Testimonial 5: Megan's Enhanced Well-Being with Nettle and Dandelion

Background: Megan, a 33-year-old pregnant woman, was dealing with swelling and water retention during her second trimester. She looked for natural diuretic options to manage these symptoms.

Experience: Megan started drinking Nettle and Dandelion tea daily. These herbs helped reduce her swelling and water retention, making her feel more comfortable and less bloated. Nettle provided additional nutrients that supported her overall health, while Dandelion's gentle diuretic effect helped manage fluid retention.

Testimonial: "Using Nettle and Dandelion tea made a huge difference in my pregnancy. I had less swelling, and I felt more at ease knowing I was supporting my body with natural, nutrient-rich herbs."

Conclusion

These testimonials highlight the positive impact of herbal remedies on various aspects of pregnancy, from managing morning sickness and anxiety to ensuring adequate nutrition and reducing swelling. Real-life experiences from women like Sarah, Emily, Rachel, Laura, and Megan demonstrate how incorporating herbs such as Red Raspberry Leaf, Nettle, Ginger, Lemon Balm, Chamomile, Alfalfa, Oat Straw, and Dandelion into their daily routines can provide effective and natural support during pregnancy. As always, it is essential to consult with a healthcare provider before starting any new herbal regimen to ensure it is safe and appropriate for individual health needs.

Herbal Remedies for Postpartum Care

The postpartum period, also known as the fourth trimester, is a critical time for new mothers as they recover from childbirth and adjust to the demands of caring for a newborn. This period can bring a range of physical and emotional challenges, including hormonal imbalances, fatigue, pain, and emotional upheaval. Herbal remedies offer a natural and supportive way to promote healing, boost energy, and enhance emotional well-being during this time. By incorporating specific herbs into postpartum care, new mothers can aid their recovery, improve lactation, and support their overall health. This chapter explores various herbal remedies that are safe and effective for postpartum care, providing practical guidance on their use to help new mothers navigate this transformative period with greater ease and comfort.

Postpartum Recovery and Healing with Herbs

The postpartum period is a time of significant physical and emotional adjustment for new mothers. During this phase, the body undergoes numerous changes as it heals from childbirth and adapts to the demands of caring for a newborn. Herbal remedies can provide valuable support, promoting recovery, enhancing energy levels, and alleviating common postpartum discomforts. Here are some herbs that are particularly beneficial for postpartum recovery and healing:

Red Raspberry Leaf

Red Raspberry Leaf (Rubus idaeus): Red Raspberry Leaf is highly regarded for its ability to tone the uterine muscles and support uterine health. It helps reduce postpartum bleeding and promotes faster recovery of the uterus to its pre-pregnancy size. Additionally, Red Raspberry Leaf is rich in vitamins and minerals, which can help replenish nutrients lost during childbirth.

- **Red Raspberry Leaf Tea:** Steep 1-2 teaspoons of dried Red Raspberry Leaf in hot water for 10-15 minutes. Drink 1-2 cups daily to support uterine recovery and overall health.

Nettle

Nettle (Urtica dioica): Nettle is a nutrient-dense herb that provides essential vitamins and minerals, including iron, calcium, and magnesium. These nutrients are crucial for replenishing the body's stores and supporting overall recovery. Nettle also helps increase milk supply, making it beneficial for breastfeeding mothers.

- **Nettle Tea:** Steep 1-2 teaspoons of dried nettle leaves in hot water for 10-15 minutes. Drink 1-2 cups daily to boost nutrient intake and support lactation.

Calendula

Calendula (Calendula officinalis): Calendula is known for its healing and anti-inflammatory properties. It can be used topically to soothe and heal perineal tears, hemorrhoids, and cesarean section scars. Calendula helps reduce inflammation, promote tissue regeneration, and prevent infection.

- **Calendula Sitz Bath:** Add a handful of dried calendula flowers to a warm sitz bath. Soak for 15-20 minutes to promote healing of perineal tears and reduce inflammation.

Witch Hazel

Witch Hazel (Hamamelis virginiana): Witch Hazel is an astringent herb that can help reduce swelling, soothe hemorrhoids, and promote healing of the perineal area. It provides relief from discomfort and supports tissue repair.

- **Witch Hazel Pads:** Soak cotton pads in witch hazel and apply them to the perineal area or hemorrhoids for soothing relief.

Motherwort

Motherwort (Leonurus cardiaca): Motherwort is known for its calming and uterine-toning properties. It can help reduce postpartum anxiety, promote emotional well-being, and support uterine recovery. Motherwort is also beneficial for alleviating afterbirth pains.

- **Motherwort Tincture:** Take 10-20 drops of motherwort tincture in water 2-3 times daily to support emotional health and uterine recovery.

Fenugreek

Fenugreek (Trigonella foenum-graecum): Fenugreek is well-known for its ability to enhance milk production in breastfeeding mothers. It can help establish and maintain a healthy milk supply.

- **Fenugreek Capsules:** Follow the recommended dosage on the product label, usually 1-2 capsules 2-3 times daily.
- **Fenugreek Tea:** Steep 1 teaspoon of fenugreek seeds in hot water for 10-15 minutes. Drink 1-2 cups daily to support lactation.

Lemon Balm

Lemon Balm (Melissa officinalis): Lemon Balm is a calming herb that can help reduce postpartum anxiety and promote relaxation. It supports emotional well-being and can improve sleep quality.

- **Lemon Balm Tea:** Steep 1-2 teaspoons of dried lemon balm leaves in hot water for 10 minutes. Drink 1-2 cups daily to promote relaxation and emotional balance.

Herbs like Red Raspberry Leaf, Nettle, Calendula, Witch Hazel, Motherwort, Fenugreek, and Lemon Balm offer valuable support for postpartum recovery and healing. These herbs help tone the uterus, replenish essential nutrients, soothe perineal tears and hemorrhoids, enhance milk production, and promote emotional well-being. Incorporating these herbal remedies into your postpartum care routine can facilitate a smoother recovery and improve overall health during this transformative period. As always, it is important to consult with a healthcare provider before starting any new herbal regimen to ensure it is safe and appropriate for your individual needs.

Enhancing Lactation and Milk Production Naturally

Breastfeeding provides essential nutrients and antibodies to newborns, promoting their health and development. However, some mothers may experience challenges with lactation and milk production. Fortunately, several natural remedies can help enhance lactation and ensure an adequate milk supply. Here are some effective herbs and practices to support breastfeeding:

Fenugreek

Fenugreek (Trigonella foenum-graecum): Fenugreek is one of the most well-known herbs for increasing milk production. It contains phytoestrogens that help stimulate the mammary glands, thereby enhancing milk supply.

- **Fenugreek Capsules:** The usual recommended dosage is 1-2 capsules (580-610 mg each) taken 2-3 times daily. Results are typically seen within 24-72 hours.
- **Fenugreek Tea:** Steep 1 teaspoon of fenugreek seeds in hot water for 10-15 minutes. Drink 1-2 cups daily.

Blessed Thistle

Blessed Thistle (Cnicus benedictus): Blessed Thistle is often used in combination with fenugreek to boost milk supply. It works by stimulating the flow of milk and supporting the overall health of the mother.

- **Blessed Thistle Capsules:** The recommended dosage is usually 1-2 capsules (390-450 mg each) taken 2-3 times daily.
- **Blessed Thistle Tea:** Steep 1 teaspoon of dried blessed thistle in hot water for 10-15 minutes. Drink 1-2 cups daily.

Fennel

Fennel (Foeniculum vulgare): Fennel contains phytoestrogens that can help increase milk production. It also aids in digestion, which can be beneficial for both the mother and the baby.

- **Fennel Tea:** Steep 1 teaspoon of crushed fennel seeds in hot water for 10-15 minutes. Drink 1-2 cups daily.
- **Fennel Seeds:** Chew on a teaspoon of fennel seeds or add them to meals.

Milk Thistle

Milk Thistle (Silybum marianum): Milk Thistle is known for its liver-supporting properties, but it can also help enhance milk production. It is believed to work by promoting overall health and hormonal balance.

- **Milk Thistle Capsules:** The typical dosage is 1-2 capsules (200-400 mg each) taken 2-3 times daily.

- **Milk Thistle Tea:** Steep 1 teaspoon of dried milk thistle seeds in hot water for 10-15 minutes. Drink 1-2 cups daily.

Alfalfa

Alfalfa (Medicago sativa): Alfalfa is rich in vitamins and minerals that support overall health and lactation. It helps increase milk production and provides essential nutrients to the mother.

- **Alfalfa Capsules:** The recommended dosage is usually 2-3 capsules (500 mg each) taken 3 times daily.

- **Alfalfa Tea:** Steep 1-2 teaspoons of dried alfalfa leaves in hot water for 10-15 minutes. Drink 1-2 cups daily.

Goat's Rue

Goat's Rue (Galega officinalis): Goat's Rue is an herb that can help increase the development of mammary tissue, making it particularly useful for adoptive mothers or those with low milk supply.

- **Goat's Rue Capsules:** Follow the dosage instructions on the product label, typically 1-2 capsules (300-500 mg each) taken 2-3 times daily.

- **Goat's Rue Tea:** Steep 1 teaspoon of dried goat's rue in hot water for 10-15 minutes. Drink 1-2 cups daily.

Additional Tips for Enhancing Lactation

1. **Frequent Nursing:** Nursing frequently and on demand helps stimulate milk production. Aim to breastfeed every 2-3 hours.

2. **Stay Hydrated:** Drink plenty of fluids throughout the day to stay hydrated, which is essential for maintaining milk supply.

3. **Balanced Diet:** Eat a balanced diet rich in fruits, vegetables, whole grains, and lean proteins to provide the necessary nutrients for milk production.

4. **Rest and Relaxation:** Ensure you get adequate rest and manage stress, as these factors can impact milk supply.

5. **Breast Massage:** Gently massaging the breasts before and during nursing can help stimulate milk flow.

6. **Pumping:** Using a breast pump after nursing sessions can help increase milk production by emptying the breasts more completely.

Herbs such as Fenugreek, Blessed Thistle, Fennel, Milk Thistle, Alfalfa, and Goat's Rue offer natural and effective ways to enhance lactation and increase milk production. Incorporating these herbs into your daily routine, along with following additional lactation tips, can support successful breastfeeding and ensure your baby receives the necessary nutrition. Always consult with a healthcare provider before starting any new herbal regimen to ensure it is safe and appropriate for your individual needs.

Managing Postpartum Depression and Mood Swings

Postpartum depression (PPD) and mood swings are common challenges many new mothers face. These emotional difficulties can impact a mother's ability to care for herself and her baby, making it essential to find effective ways to manage and alleviate symptoms. Herbal remedies, along with lifestyle changes and support, can provide significant relief and support emotional well-being during the postpartum period. Here are some herbs and strategies that can help manage postpartum depression and mood swings:

St. John's Wort

St. John's Wort (Hypericum perforatum): St. John's Wort is one of the most researched herbs for managing mild to moderate depression. It works by increasing levels of serotonin, dopamine, and norepinephrine in the brain, which are neurotransmitters associated with mood regulation.

- **St. John's Wort Capsules or Tablets:** The recommended dosage is typically 300 mg of standardized extract taken three times daily. However, it is important to consult with a healthcare provider before using St. John's Wort, especially if you are breastfeeding, as it can interact with certain medications.

Ashwagandha

Ashwagandha (Withania somnifera): Ashwagandha is an adaptogenic herb that helps the body manage stress and reduce anxiety. It supports the adrenal glands, balances cortisol levels, and promotes overall emotional well-being.

- **Ashwagandha Capsules or Powder:** The typical dosage is 300-500 mg of standardized extract taken twice daily. Ashwagandha can be taken in capsule form or added to smoothies or teas as a powder.

Lemon Balm

Lemon Balm (Melissa officinalis): Lemon Balm is known for its calming and mood-enhancing properties. It helps reduce anxiety, improve sleep quality, and promote relaxation.

- **Lemon Balm Tea:** Steep 1-2 teaspoons of dried lemon balm leaves in hot water for 10-15 minutes. Drink 1-2 cups daily.

- **Lemon Balm Capsules or Tincture:** Follow the dosage instructions on the product label.

Lavender

Lavender (Lavandula angustifolia): Lavender is widely recognized for its calming effects. It can help reduce anxiety, improve mood, and promote restful sleep.

- **Lavender Aromatherapy:** Use a few drops of lavender essential oil in a diffuser or add to a warm bath.

- **Lavender Tea:** Steep 1 teaspoon of dried lavender flowers in hot water for 10 minutes. Drink 1-2 cups daily.

Motherwort

Motherwort (Leonurus cardiaca): Motherwort is known for its ability to calm anxiety and support emotional well-being. It is particularly helpful for postpartum women experiencing mood swings and emotional instability.

- **Motherwort Tincture:** Take 10-20 drops in water 2-3 times daily. Consult with a healthcare provider for appropriate use during breastfeeding.

Lifestyle Changes and Support

1. **Adequate Rest:** Ensure you get as much rest as possible. Nap when your baby naps and ask for help from family and friends to manage household tasks.

2. **Healthy Diet:** Eat a balanced diet rich in fruits, vegetables, whole grains, and lean proteins. Avoid excessive caffeine and sugar, which can contribute to mood swings.

3. **Hydration:** Stay hydrated by drinking plenty of water throughout the day.

4. **Physical Activity:** Engage in gentle physical activities such as walking, yoga, or postpartum exercise classes to boost endorphins and improve mood.

5. **Social Support:** Connect with other new mothers, join a support group, or talk to a trusted friend or family member about your feelings.

6. **Professional Help:** If symptoms of postpartum depression persist or worsen, seek help from a mental health professional. Therapy, counseling, or medication may be necessary to manage severe depression.

Herbal remedies such as St. John's Wort, Ashwagandha, Lemon Balm, Lavender, and Motherwort can provide natural support for managing postpartum depression and mood swings. These herbs, combined with healthy lifestyle changes and social support, can help improve emotional well-being and enhance the postpartum experience. It is crucial to consult with a healthcare provider before starting any new herbal regimen, especially if you are breastfeeding, to ensure safety and appropriateness for your individual needs. If symptoms of postpartum depression are severe, seeking professional help is essential for effective management and recovery.

Strengthening the Body After Childbirth with Herbal Tonics

The postpartum period is a time for recovery and rejuvenation as the body heals from childbirth. Herbal tonics can play a significant role in strengthening the body, replenishing nutrients, and supporting overall well-being. Here are some beneficial herbal tonics that can help new mothers regain strength and vitality after childbirth:

Red Raspberry Leaf

Red Raspberry Leaf (Rubus idaeus): Red Raspberry Leaf is renowned for its ability to tone the uterine muscles and promote uterine health. It is also rich in vitamins and minerals, such as iron, calcium, and magnesium, which are essential for recovery and overall health.

- **Red Raspberry Leaf Tea:** Steep 1-2 teaspoons of dried Red Raspberry Leaf in hot water for 10-15 minutes. Drink 1-2 cups daily to support uterine recovery and replenish nutrients.

Nettle

Nettle (Urtica dioica): Nettle is a nutrient-dense herb that provides high levels of vitamins A, C, D, and K, as well as iron, calcium, and potassium. It helps combat fatigue, supports the adrenal glands, and boosts overall energy and vitality.

- **Nettle Tea:** Steep 1-2 teaspoons of dried nettle leaves in hot water for 10-15 minutes. Drink 1-2 cups daily to boost nutrient intake and enhance energy levels.

Oat Straw

Oat Straw (Avena sativa): Oat Straw is highly nutritious, offering a good source of calcium, magnesium, and silica, which are important for bone health and overall strength. It also supports the nervous system, helping to reduce stress and improve sleep.

- **Oat Straw Tea:** Steep 1-2 teaspoons of dried oat straw in hot water for 10-15 minutes. Drink 1-2 cups daily to support recovery and relaxation.

Alfalfa

Alfalfa (Medicago sativa): Alfalfa is rich in vitamins A, D, E, and K, as well as calcium, magnesium, and iron. It can help boost overall nutritional intake and support recovery.

- **Alfalfa Tea:** Steep 1-2 teaspoons of dried alfalfa leaves in hot water for 10-15 minutes. Drink 1-2 cups daily to replenish nutrients.
- **Alfalfa Capsules:** Follow the dosage instructions on the product label.

Dandelion

Dandelion (Taraxacum officinale): Dandelion is a great source of vitamins A, C, and K, as well as iron and calcium. It supports liver function, helps manage fluid retention, and provides gentle diuretic effects, which can be helpful in reducing postpartum swelling.

- **Dandelion Tea:** Steep 1-2 teaspoons of dried dandelion leaves or roots in hot water for 10-15 minutes. Drink 1-2 cups daily to support liver health and reduce swelling.
- **Dandelion Greens:** Can be added to salads or smoothies for additional nutritional benefits.

Dong Quai

Dong Quai (Angelica sinensis): Dong Quai is a traditional Chinese herb that supports blood health and circulation. It is often used to rebuild strength and vitality after childbirth, promoting overall recovery and hormonal balance.

- **Dong Quai Capsules:** Follow the dosage instructions on the product label.

- **Dong Quai Tea:** Steep 1 teaspoon of dried Dong Quai root in hot water for 10-15 minutes. Drink 1 cup daily to support recovery.

Ashwagandha

Ashwagandha (Withania somnifera): Ashwagandha is an adaptogenic herb that helps the body cope with stress and fatigue. It supports the adrenal glands, balances cortisol levels, and promotes overall strength and vitality.

- **Ashwagandha Capsules or Powder:** The typical dosage is 300-500 mg of standardized extract taken twice daily. Ashwagandha can be taken in capsule form or added to smoothies or teas as a powder.

Additional Tips for Postpartum Recovery

1. **Balanced Diet:** Ensure you are eating a balanced diet rich in fruits, vegetables, whole grains, and lean proteins to provide the necessary nutrients for recovery.

2. **Hydration:** Stay hydrated by drinking plenty of water and herbal teas throughout the day.

3. **Rest and Sleep:** Prioritize rest and sleep whenever possible to allow your body to heal and rejuvenate.

4. **Gentle Exercise:** Engage in gentle exercises, such as walking or postpartum yoga, to promote circulation and overall well-being.

5. **Social Support:** Seek support from family and friends to help with household tasks and care for the baby, allowing you more time to rest and recover.

Herbal tonics such as Red Raspberry Leaf, Nettle, Oat Straw, Alfalfa, Dandelion, Dong Quai, and Ashwagandha can provide valuable support for postpartum recovery. These herbs help replenish nutrients, boost energy levels, and promote overall strength and vitality. Incorporating these herbal remedies into your daily routine, along with maintaining a balanced diet, staying hydrated, and getting adequate rest, can facilitate a smoother and more effective postpartum recovery. Always consult with a healthcare provider before starting any new herbal regimen to ensure it is safe and appropriate for your individual needs.

Herbal Care for Newborns and Infants

Caring for newborns and infants requires gentle, safe, and effective remedies. Herbal care can provide natural solutions to common infant issues such as colic, teething discomfort, and skin irritations. Here are some carefully selected herbs that are safe for newborns and infants, along with guidelines for their use:

Chamomile

Chamomile (Matricaria chamomilla): Chamomile is well-known for its calming and soothing properties. It can help alleviate colic, promote better sleep, and reduce fussiness in infants. Chamomile is also gentle on the stomach and can relieve digestive discomfort.

- **Chamomile Tea for Infants:** Prepare a weak chamomile tea by steeping 1 teaspoon of dried chamomile flowers in 8 ounces of hot water for 5 minutes. Strain and cool the tea. Give 1-2 teaspoons of the cooled tea to your baby before feeding or bedtime.
- **Chamomile Bath:** Add a few chamomile tea bags to your baby's bathwater to soothe skin irritations and promote relaxation.

Fennel

Fennel (Foeniculum vulgare): Fennel is effective in relieving gas and colic in infants. It helps to relax the gastrointestinal tract and reduce bloating.

- **Fennel Water:** Steep 1/2 teaspoon of crushed fennel seeds in 8 ounces of hot water for 10 minutes. Strain and cool the tea. Give 1 teaspoon of the cooled fennel water to your baby before feedings.

Ginger

Ginger (Zingiber officinale): Ginger can help with digestive issues and soothe an upset stomach. It is particularly useful for relieving nausea and colic.

- **Ginger Tea:** Prepare a very diluted ginger tea by steeping a small piece of fresh ginger (about the size of a pea) in 8 ounces of hot water for 5 minutes. Strain and cool the tea. Give 1 teaspoon of the cooled tea to your baby as needed for digestive discomfort.

Lavender

Lavender (Lavandula angustifolia): Lavender has calming and soothing properties that can help promote sleep and reduce fussiness in infants. It is also beneficial for soothing skin irritations.

- **Lavender Oil:** Dilute a few drops of lavender essential oil in a carrier oil (such as coconut oil) and use it for a gentle massage. Avoid using essential oils directly on the skin without dilution.
- **Lavender Bath:** Add a few drops of lavender essential oil to your baby's bathwater to promote relaxation and calmness.

Calendula

Calendula (Calendula officinalis): Calendula is excellent for treating diaper rash, minor cuts, and other skin irritations. It has anti-inflammatory and healing properties.

- **Calendula Salve:** Use a natural calendula salve on diaper rashes or minor skin irritations. Ensure the salve is free of any harsh chemicals and additives.

- **Calendula Bath:** Add calendula tea bags or a few drops of calendula extract to your baby's bathwater to soothe irritated skin.

Catnip

Catnip (Nepeta cataria): Catnip can help alleviate colic and promote relaxation in infants. It has mild sedative properties and can soothe digestive issues.

- **Catnip Tea:** Prepare a weak catnip tea by steeping 1/2 teaspoon of dried catnip leaves in 8 ounces of hot water for 5 minutes. Strain and cool the tea. Give 1-2 teaspoons of the cooled tea to your baby before feedings.

Tips for Using Herbs with Newborns and Infants

1. **Consult with a Pediatrician:** Always consult with your pediatrician before introducing any herbal remedies to ensure they are safe and appropriate for your baby's specific needs.

2. **Use Small Amounts:** Start with very small amounts of any herbal remedy to ensure there are no adverse reactions.

3. **Monitor for Allergies:** Watch for any signs of allergic reactions, such as rash, hives, or difficulty breathing. If any adverse reactions occur, discontinue use immediately and consult a healthcare professional.

4. **Avoid Essential Oils Internally:** Never give essential oils internally to infants. Use only properly diluted essential oils externally and with caution.

5. **High-Quality Products:** Use high-quality, organic herbs to avoid exposure to pesticides and contaminants.

Herbal care can provide gentle and effective solutions for common issues in newborns and infants, such as colic, digestive discomfort, teething pain, and skin irritations. Chamomile, fennel, ginger, lavender, calendula, and catnip are some of the safe herbs that can support your baby's well-being. Always consult with a pediatrician before using any herbal remedies and monitor your baby for any signs of allergies or adverse reactions. By using these herbs thoughtfully and carefully, you can help ensure a healthy and comfortable start for your little one.

Stories from New Mothers

Sarah's Experience with Chamomile for Colic

Background: Sarah, a first-time mother, was overwhelmed when her newborn, Jack, started experiencing severe colic at just two weeks old. The endless crying episodes were distressing for both Jack and Sarah, making it difficult for her to rest or feel at ease.

Experience: After consulting with her pediatrician and exploring various remedies, Sarah decided to try chamomile tea, known for its gentle and calming properties. She prepared a weak chamomile tea and gave Jack 1-2 teaspoons before his feedings. Within a few days, Sarah noticed a significant improvement. Jack seemed more at ease, and his crying episodes reduced dramatically. The chamomile tea helped soothe his digestive system, allowing him to sleep better and reducing the overall stress in their household.

Testimonial: "Chamomile tea was a lifesaver for us. Seeing Jack in pain was heartbreaking, but the chamomile tea provided the relief he needed. It not only helped with his colic but also made our lives much more peaceful. I'm grateful for this natural remedy."

Emily's Success with Fennel for Digestive Issues

Background: Emily's daughter, Lily, struggled with gas and bloating from the first month of her life. These issues often led to long nights filled with crying and discomfort. Emily was determined to find a natural solution that would ease Lily's digestive troubles without any side effects.

Experience: Emily learned about fennel's benefits for digestive health and decided to give it a try. She prepared a fennel tea by steeping crushed fennel seeds and gave Lily a teaspoon of the cooled tea before feedings. The results were remarkable. Lily's gas and bloating issues started to subside, and she became much calmer and happier. Emily was relieved to see her daughter more comfortable and sleeping better at night.

Testimonial: "Fennel tea made a huge difference for Lily. It was heartbreaking to see her in so much discomfort, but the fennel tea provided gentle relief that worked wonders. It's amazing how such a simple, natural remedy can have such a profound effect."

Rachel's Relief with Lavender for Sleep

Background: Rachel, a mother of two, found herself struggling with her newborn, Ethan's, sleep patterns. Ethan had difficulty settling down and would wake up frequently during the night, leaving both exhausted.

Experience: Rachel decided to use lavender to help improve Ethan's sleep. She started adding a few drops of lavender essential oil to a diffuser in Ethan's room and included a few drops in his evening bath. The calming aroma of lavender helped create a soothing bedtime routine. Within a week, Rachel noticed that Ethan was more relaxed at bedtime and began sleeping for longer stretches. The lavender not only helped Ethan but also made Rachel feel more relaxed and less stressed.

Testimonial: "Lavender became an essential part of our bedtime routine. The calming scent helped Ethan settle down and sleep better, and it made our evenings much more peaceful. I'm so thankful for the calm and rest it brought to our home."

Laura's Journey with Calendula for Diaper Rash

Background: Laura's baby, Mia, developed a persistent diaper rash that over-the-counter creams failed to alleviate. Concerned about using too many chemical-based products on Mia's sensitive skin, Laura sought a natural alternative.

Experience: Laura discovered calendula's healing properties and decided to try a natural calendula salve. She applied the salve to Mia's diaper area during each change. Within a few days, the redness and irritation began to diminish, and Mia's skin started to heal. The calendula salve not only soothed the rash but also prevented future occurrences.

Testimonial: "Calendula salve was a miracle for Mia's diaper rash. It healed her skin quickly and gently, without any harsh chemicals. Seeing her comfortable and rash-free was such a relief. I'm glad we found this natural remedy."

Megan's Solution with Ginger for Upset Stomach

Background: Megan's son, Noah, frequently experienced an upset stomach, causing him to be fussy and uncomfortable. Megan wanted a natural solution that would help soothe Noah's digestive system without causing any harm.

Experience: After researching, Megan decided to use a very diluted ginger tea. She prepared the tea and gave Noah a teaspoon whenever he seemed uncomfortable. The ginger tea worked effectively, calming Noah's stomach and reducing his fussiness. Megan was pleased to see Noah more content and less distressed.

Testimonial: "The ginger tea was incredibly effective for Noah's upset stomach. It was gentle yet powerful, and it gave him the relief he needed. Knowing I could use a natural remedy to help him feel better was very reassuring."

Conclusion

These stories from new mothers like Sarah, Emily, Rachel, Laura, and Megan highlight the positive impact of herbal remedies on common infant issues. From soothing colic with chamomile tea to easing digestive discomfort with fennel, improving sleep with lavender, healing diaper rash with calendula, and calming an upset stomach with ginger, these natural solutions have provided significant relief for both babies and their mothers. The experiences shared demonstrate the effectiveness and gentle nature of herbal remedies in supporting the health and well-being of newborns and infants. Always consult with a pediatrician before introducing any new herbal remedy to ensure it is safe and appropriate for your baby.

Enhancing Women's Sexual Health Naturally

Sexual health is a vital component of overall well-being, encompassing physical, emotional, and relational aspects. For women, maintaining a healthy sexual life can significantly impact self-esteem, intimate relationships, and quality of life. However, various factors, including hormonal imbalances, stress, and lifestyle changes, can affect sexual health and function. Fortunately, natural remedies and lifestyle adjustments can offer effective support. This chapter explores how herbs, nutrition, and holistic practices can naturally enhance women's sexual health, addressing common issues such as low libido, vaginal dryness, and hormonal imbalances. By integrating these natural approaches, women can foster a more fulfilling and vibrant sexual life.

Herbs for Boosting Libido and Sexual Vitality

Enhancing sexual health and vitality naturally can be achieved through the use of specific herbs known for their aphrodisiac properties and ability to balance hormones. These herbs can help increase libido, improve sexual function, and enhance overall well-being. Here are some of the most effective herbs for boosting libido and sexual vitality in women:

Maca Root

Maca Root (Lepidium meyenii): Maca root, also known as Peruvian ginseng, is a powerful adaptogen that supports hormonal balance, increases energy levels, and enhances sexual desire. It is rich in vitamins, minerals, and amino acids that boost overall vitality and stamina.

- **Maca Powder:** Add 1-2 teaspoons of maca powder to smoothies, oatmeal, or yogurt daily.
- **Maca Capsules:** Follow the dosage instructions on the product label, typically 1,500-3,000 mg per day.

Tribulus

Tribulus (Tribulus terrestris): Tribulus is known for its ability to enhance libido and improve sexual function. It works by increasing the levels of certain hormones, such as testosterone, which play a crucial role in sexual desire.

- **Tribulus Capsules:** The recommended dosage is usually 250-500 mg taken twice daily.
- **Tribulus Tincture:** Follow the dosage instructions on the product label.

Damiana

Damiana (Turnera diffusa): Damiana has been traditionally used as an aphrodisiac and tonic for the nervous system. It helps reduce anxiety, elevate mood, and increase sexual desire.

- **Damiana Tea:** Steep 1-2 teaspoons of dried damiana leaves in hot water for 10-15 minutes. Drink 1-2 cups daily.
- **Damiana Capsules:** Follow the dosage instructions on the product label.

Ashwagandha

Ashwagandha (Withania somnifera): Ashwagandha is an adaptogen that helps reduce stress and anxiety, which are common contributors to low libido. It supports hormonal balance and improves overall vitality and energy levels.

- **Ashwagandha Capsules:** The typical dosage is 300-500 mg of standardized extract taken twice daily.
- **Ashwagandha Powder:** Add 1 teaspoon of ashwagandha powder to smoothies, milk, or warm water daily.

Ginkgo Biloba

Ginkgo Biloba: Ginkgo biloba improves blood flow and circulation, which can enhance sexual function and arousal. It also supports cognitive function and reduces anxiety, contributing to an improved sexual experience.

- **Ginkgo Biloba Capsules:** The recommended dosage is typically 120-240 mg taken daily.
- **Ginkgo Biloba Extract:** Follow the dosage instructions on the product label.

Muira Puama

Muira Puama (Ptychopetalum olacoides): Muira puama, also known as "potency wood," is a traditional aphrodisiac that enhances sexual desire and function. It supports overall energy levels and reduces stress.

- **Muira Puama Tea:** Steep 1 teaspoon of dried muira puama bark in hot water for 10-15 minutes. Drink 1-2 cups daily.
- **Muira Puama Capsules:** Follow the dosage instructions on the product label.

Shatavari

Shatavari (Asparagus racemosus): Shatavari is an adaptogenic herb known for its ability to balance female hormones and support reproductive health. It enhances libido, supports fertility, and alleviates symptoms of menopause.

- **Shatavari Powder:** Add 1 teaspoon of shatavari powder to milk or smoothies daily.
- **Shatavari Capsules:** Follow the dosage instructions on the product label.

Herbs such as Maca Root, Tribulus, Damiana, Ashwagandha, Ginkgo Biloba, Muira Puama, and Shatavari offer natural and effective ways to boost libido and enhance sexual vitality. These herbs work by balancing hormones, reducing stress and anxiety, and improving blood flow and energy levels. Incorporating these herbs into your daily routine can lead to improved sexual health and overall well-being. As always, it is important to consult with a healthcare provider before starting any new herbal regimen to ensure it is safe and appropriate for your individual needs.

Natural Solutions for Vaginal Health and Lubrication

Maintaining vaginal health and adequate lubrication is essential for comfort, sexual satisfaction, and overall well-being. Various factors, including hormonal changes, stress, and aging, can affect vaginal moisture and health. Natural solutions, including herbs, oils, and lifestyle adjustments, can help address these issues effectively. Here are some natural remedies for enhancing vaginal health and lubrication:

Aloe Vera

Aloe Vera (Aloe barbadensis): Aloe vera is known for its soothing and hydrating properties. It can help alleviate vaginal dryness and irritation. Ensure you use pure aloe vera gel without any additives or preservatives.

- **Aloe Vera Gel:** Apply a small amount of pure aloe vera gel to the vaginal area as needed to relieve dryness.

Coconut Oil

Coconut Oil: Coconut oil is an excellent natural lubricant that can help maintain vaginal moisture. It has antifungal and antibacterial properties, which can help prevent infections.

- **Coconut Oil:** Apply a small amount of organic, unrefined coconut oil to the vaginal area as needed for lubrication and moisture.

Vitamin E

Vitamin E: Vitamin E is beneficial for skin health and can help improve vaginal moisture. It can be used topically to alleviate dryness.

- **Vitamin E Oil:** Apply a small amount of vitamin E oil to the vaginal area as needed. You can also puncture a vitamin E capsule and use the oil inside.

Olive Oil

Olive Oil: Olive oil is a natural moisturizer that can help relieve vaginal dryness. It is safe to use and can provide long-lasting moisture.

- **Olive Oil:** Apply a small amount of extra virgin olive oil to the vaginal area as needed for lubrication.

Calendula

Calendula (Calendula officinalis): Calendula has anti-inflammatory and healing properties that can help soothe irritated vaginal tissues and promote moisture.

- **Calendula Oil:** Apply a small amount of calendula-infused oil to the vaginal area as needed to relieve dryness and irritation.

Sea Buckthorn Oil

Sea Buckthorn Oil: Sea buckthorn oil is rich in omega-7 fatty acids, which are beneficial for mucous membrane health, including the vaginal lining. It can help improve vaginal elasticity and moisture.

- **Sea Buckthorn Oil:** Take sea buckthorn oil supplements as directed on the product label. You can also apply a small amount of sea buckthorn oil topically to the vaginal area.

Fenugreek

Fenugreek (Trigonella foenum-graecum): Fenugreek can help balance hormones and improve vaginal lubrication by increasing natural estrogen levels.

- **Fenugreek Tea:** Steep 1 teaspoon of fenugreek seeds in hot water for 10-15 minutes. Drink 1-2 cups daily.

- **Fenugreek Capsules:** Follow the dosage instructions on the product label.

Lifestyle Adjustments for Vaginal Health

1. **Stay Hydrated:** Drink plenty of water throughout the day to maintain overall hydration, which is crucial for vaginal moisture.

2. **Balanced Diet:** Eat a diet rich in fruits, vegetables, whole grains, and lean proteins. Foods high in phytoestrogens, such as soy products, flaxseeds, and whole grains, can help maintain hormonal balance.

3. **Avoid Harsh Products:** Avoid using harsh soaps, douches, and scented products in the vaginal area, as they can disrupt the natural pH balance and cause dryness.

4. **Practice Safe Sex:** Use protection during sexual activity to prevent infections and maintain vaginal health.

5. **Manage Stress:** Practice stress-reducing activities such as yoga, meditation, and deep breathing exercises, as stress can impact hormonal balance and vaginal health.

6. **Wear Breathable Clothing:** Wear cotton underwear and loose-fitting clothes to allow air circulation and reduce moisture buildup, which can lead to infections.

Natural remedies such as aloe vera, coconut oil, vitamin E, olive oil, calendula, sea buckthorn oil, and fenugreek can provide effective solutions for maintaining vaginal health and improving lubrication. Incorporating these remedies into your routine, along with making lifestyle adjustments, can help enhance vaginal moisture, prevent infections, and promote overall well-being. Always consult with a healthcare provider before starting any new treatment to ensure it is safe and appropriate for your individual needs.

Managing Sexual Dysfunction and Enhancing Pleasure Naturally

Sexual dysfunction can affect women at various stages of life and can be caused by physical, emotional, or psychological factors. Managing these issues and enhancing pleasure naturally can involve using specific herbs, lifestyle changes, and holistic practices. Here are some natural solutions to help manage sexual dysfunction and enhance pleasure:

Herbs for Sexual Health

Maca Root (Lepidium meyenii): Maca root is an adaptogen that supports hormonal balance and increases energy and libido. It has been shown to improve sexual desire and function in women.

- **Maca Powder:** Add 1-2 teaspoons to smoothies, oatmeal, or yogurt daily.

- **Maca Capsules:** Follow the dosage instructions on the product label, typically 1,500-3,000 mg per day.

Ginkgo Biloba: Ginkgo biloba improves blood flow and circulation, which can enhance sexual arousal and function. It also supports cognitive function and reduces anxiety, contributing to improved sexual experiences.

- **Ginkgo Biloba Capsules:** The recommended dosage is typically 120-240 mg taken daily.

- **Ginkgo Biloba Extract:** Follow the dosage instructions on the product label.

Damiana (Turnera diffusa): Damiana has been traditionally used as an aphrodisiac and tonic for the nervous system. It helps reduce anxiety, elevate mood, and increase sexual desire.

- **Damiana Tea:** Steep 1-2 teaspoons of dried damiana leaves in hot water for 10-15 minutes. Drink 1-2 cups daily.

- **Damiana Capsules:** Follow the dosage instructions on the product label.

Ashwagandha (Withania somnifera): Ashwagandha is an adaptogen that helps reduce stress and anxiety, which are common contributors to sexual dysfunction. It supports hormonal balance and improves overall vitality and energy levels.

- **Ashwagandha Capsules:** The typical dosage is 300-500 mg of standardized extract taken twice daily.

- **Ashwagandha Powder:** Add 1 teaspoon of ashwagandha powder to smoothies, milk, or warm water daily.

Tribulus (Tribulus terrestris): Tribulus is known for its ability to enhance libido and improve sexual function by increasing hormone levels.

- **Tribulus Capsules:** The recommended dosage is usually 250-500 mg taken twice daily.

- **Tribulus Tincture:** Follow the dosage instructions on the product label.

Lifestyle and Holistic Practices

1. **Healthy Diet:**

   o Eat a balanced diet rich in fruits, vegetables, whole grains, and lean proteins to support overall health and hormonal balance.

   o Include foods high in phytoestrogens, such as soy products, flaxseeds, and whole grains, to help maintain hormonal balance.

2. **Regular Exercise:**

   o Engage in regular physical activity to improve blood flow, reduce stress, and enhance overall well-being.

   o Include pelvic floor exercises (Kegels) to strengthen pelvic muscles and improve sexual function.

3. **Stress Management:**

   o Practice stress-reducing activities such as yoga, meditation, deep breathing exercises, and mindfulness to reduce anxiety and improve mental health.

- Ensure adequate rest and sleep to support overall health and reduce stress.

4. **Communication and Intimacy:**

   - Openly communicate with your partner about your needs, desires, and concerns to build intimacy and improve sexual satisfaction.

   - Spend quality time together to strengthen emotional bonds and enhance sexual connection.

5. **Arousal and Lubrication:**

   - Use natural lubricants such as aloe vera, coconut oil, or olive oil to reduce discomfort and enhance pleasure during sexual activity.

   - Explore different forms of sexual expression and foreplay to enhance arousal and intimacy.

6. **Pelvic Floor Therapy:**

   - Consider pelvic floor therapy or physical therapy to address any pelvic floor dysfunction that may be contributing to sexual dysfunction.

   - Perform regular pelvic floor exercises to strengthen the muscles and improve sexual function.

Natural Supplements for Sexual Health

L-Arginine: L-Arginine is an amino acid that helps increase blood flow by converting to nitric oxide in the body. Improved blood flow can enhance sexual arousal and function.

- **L-Arginine Supplements:** Follow the dosage instructions on the product label, typically 1,000-2,000 mg daily.

Omega-3 Fatty Acids: Omega-3 fatty acids support cardiovascular health, which can improve blood flow and sexual function. They also help reduce inflammation and support overall health.

- **Omega-3 Supplements:** Take fish oil or flaxseed oil supplements as directed on the product label.

Managing sexual dysfunction and enhancing pleasure naturally involves a holistic approach that includes the use of specific herbs, lifestyle changes, and natural supplements. Herbs such as Maca Root, Ginkgo Biloba, Damiana, Ashwagandha, and Tribulus can help improve libido and sexual function. Adopting a healthy diet, regular exercise, stress management techniques, and open communication with your partner can further enhance sexual health and satisfaction. Always consult with a healthcare provider before starting any new herbal regimen or supplement to ensure it is safe and appropriate for your individual needs.

Supporting Emotional Intimacy and Connection with Herbs

Emotional intimacy and connection are essential components of a healthy and fulfilling relationship. While various factors contribute to building and maintaining intimacy, herbal remedies can provide additional support by promoting relaxation, reducing stress, and enhancing mood. Here are some herbs that can help foster emotional intimacy and connection:

Lavender

Lavender (Lavandula angustifolia): Lavender is renowned for its calming and soothing properties. It helps reduce stress and anxiety, promoting a sense of relaxation and well-being. The calming aroma of lavender can create a peaceful environment conducive to emotional connection. Using lavender essential oil in a diffuser or adding a few drops to a warm bath can help both partners relax and open up emotionally.

- **Lavender Aromatherapy:** Use a diffuser with a few drops of lavender essential oil to create a calming atmosphere in your living space or bedroom.
- **Lavender Bath:** Add a few drops of lavender essential oil to a warm bath and enjoy a relaxing soak together to enhance emotional bonding.

Ashwagandha

Ashwagandha (Withania somnifera): Ashwagandha is an adaptogenic herb that helps reduce stress and anxiety while promoting emotional balance. By supporting the adrenal glands and regulating cortisol levels, ashwagandha helps create a more relaxed state of mind, making it easier to connect emotionally with your partner. Consuming ashwagandha regularly can enhance overall well-being and improve mood, fostering a deeper emotional connection.

- **Ashwagandha Capsules:** Take 300-500 mg of standardized extract twice daily to reduce stress and promote emotional balance.
- **Ashwagandha Powder:** Add 1 teaspoon of ashwagandha powder to smoothies, milk, or warm water daily.

Passionflower

Passionflower (Passiflora incarnata): Passionflower is known for its calming effects and ability to reduce anxiety. It helps promote relaxation and can be particularly beneficial for individuals experiencing stress or nervousness that hinders emotional intimacy. Drinking passionflower tea together can create a calming ritual that enhances emotional connection and opens up pathways for deeper communication.

- **Passionflower Tea:** Steep 1-2 teaspoons of dried passionflower in hot water for 10-15 minutes. Drink a cup of tea together before bed to promote relaxation and emotional closeness.

Damiana

Damiana (Turnera diffusa): Damiana has traditionally been used as an aphrodisiac and mood enhancer. It helps reduce anxiety, elevate mood, and increase feelings of well-being. By enhancing relaxation and emotional openness, damiana can support deeper emotional intimacy and connection between partners. Drinking damiana tea together can create a bonding experience that fosters closeness.

- **Damiana Tea:** Steep 1-2 teaspoons of dried damiana leaves in hot water for 10-15 minutes. Drink a cup of tea together to enhance mood and emotional connection.
- **Damiana Capsules:** Follow the dosage instructions on the product label.

Lemon Balm

Lemon Balm (Melissa officinalis): Lemon Balm is a calming herb that helps reduce anxiety and promote a sense of calm and relaxation. It is particularly effective in soothing nervousness and enhancing emotional well-being. Drinking lemon balm tea together can create a relaxing ritual that encourages open communication and emotional bonding.

- **Lemon Balm Tea:** Steep 1-2 teaspoons of dried lemon balm leaves in hot water for 10-15 minutes. Drink a cup of tea together in the evening to promote relaxation and emotional intimacy.

Rhodiola Rosea

Rhodiola Rosea: Rhodiola Rosea is an adaptogenic herb that helps the body cope with stress and fatigue. By promoting emotional resilience and reducing anxiety, Rhodiola can help create a more balanced and relaxed state of mind, making it easier to connect emotionally with your partner.

- **Rhodiola Capsules:** Take 200-400 mg of standardized extract daily to reduce stress and enhance emotional resilience.
- **Rhodiola Tea:** Steep 1 teaspoon of dried Rhodiola root in hot water for 10-15 minutes. Drink a cup of tea together to support emotional balance and connection.

Conclusion

Herbs such as Lavender, Ashwagandha, Passionflower, Damiana, Lemon Balm, and Rhodiola Rosea offer natural support for reducing stress, promoting relaxation, and enhancing mood. Incorporating these herbs into your daily routine can create a calming and nurturing environment that fosters emotional intimacy and connection with your partner. Whether through aromatherapy, herbal teas, or supplements, these natural remedies can help you and your partner build a deeper emotional bond and improve your overall relationship. Always consult with a healthcare provider before starting any new herbal regimen to ensure it is safe and appropriate for your individual needs.

Creating Herbal Blends for Sexual Health

Combining specific herbs into blends can enhance their individual benefits, providing a comprehensive approach to supporting sexual health. Herbal blends can help address various aspects of sexual function, including libido, hormonal balance, stress reduction, and overall vitality. Here are some effective herbal blends tailored for sexual health:

Libido-Boosting Blend

Ingredients:

- Maca Root (Lepidium meyenii)

- Damiana (Turnera diffusa)

- Tribulus (Tribulus terrestris)

- Ginkgo Biloba

Preparation:

1. **Maca Root Powder:** 2 teaspoons

2. **Damiana Leaves:** 1 teaspoon

3. **Tribulus Powder:** 1 teaspoon

4. **Ginkgo Biloba Leaves:** 1 teaspoon

Instructions:

1. Combine all the dried herbs in a bowl and mix well.

2. Store the blend in an airtight container in a cool, dark place.

3. To make tea, steep 1-2 teaspoons of the herbal blend in a cup of hot water for 10-15 minutes. Strain and drink 1-2 cups daily.

4. Alternatively, you can add Maca Root powder to smoothies or yogurt and take the other herbs in capsule form according to the dosage instructions.

Hormonal Balance Blend

Ingredients:

- Shatavari (Asparagus racemosus)

- Ashwagandha (Withania somnifera)

- Red Clover (Trifolium pratense)

- Nettle (Urtica dioica)

Preparation:

1. **Shatavari Powder:** 2 teaspoons

2. **Ashwagandha Powder:** 1 teaspoon

3. **Red Clover Blossoms:** 1 teaspoon

4. **Nettle Leaves:** 1 teaspoon

Instructions:

1. Combine all the dried herbs in a bowl and mix well.

2. Store the blend in an airtight container in a cool, dark place.

3. To make tea, steep 1-2 teaspoons of the herbal blend in a cup of hot water for 10-15 minutes. Strain and drink 1-2 cups daily.

4. You can also add Shatavari and Ashwagandha powders to your smoothies or yogurt.

Stress Reduction and Relaxation Blend

Ingredients:

- Lavender (Lavandula angustifolia)
- Lemon Balm (Melissa officinalis)
- Passionflower (Passiflora incarnata)
- Chamomile (Matricaria chamomilla)

Preparation:

1. **Lavender Flowers:** 1 teaspoon
2. **Lemon Balm Leaves:** 1 teaspoon
3. **Passionflower Leaves:** 1 teaspoon
4. **Chamomile Flowers:** 1 teaspoon

Instructions:

1. Combine all the dried herbs in a bowl and mix well.

2. Store the blend in an airtight container in a cool, dark place.

3. To make tea, steep 1-2 teaspoons of the herbal blend in a cup of hot water for 10-15 minutes. Strain and drink 1-2 cups daily, especially in the evening to promote relaxation.

Vitality and Energy Blend

Ingredients:

- Rhodiola Rosea
- Eleuthero (Eleutherococcus senticosus)
- Ginseng (Panax ginseng)
- Holy Basil (Ocimum sanctum)

Preparation:

1. **Rhodiola Rosea Root:** 1 teaspoon
2. **Eleuthero Root:** 1 teaspoon

3. **Ginseng Root:** 1 teaspoon

4. **Holy Basil Leaves:** 1 teaspoon

Instructions:

1. Combine all the dried herbs in a bowl and mix well.

2. Store the blend in an airtight container in a cool, dark place.

3. To make tea, steep 1-2 teaspoons of the herbal blend in a cup of hot water for 10-15 minutes. Strain and drink 1-2 cups daily.

4. Alternatively, you can take these herbs in capsule or tincture form according to the dosage instructions.

Tips for Using Herbal Blends

1. **Consistency:** For best results, use the herbal blends consistently over a period of time. It may take several weeks to notice significant effects.

2. **Quality:** Use high-quality, organic herbs to ensure safety and efficacy.

3. **Consultation:** Always consult with a healthcare provider before starting any new herbal regimen, especially if you have underlying health conditions or are taking other medications.

4. **Customization:** Feel free to adjust the blends according to your specific needs and preferences. You can add or remove herbs based on your individual health goals.

Creating herbal blends tailored for sexual health can provide a comprehensive approach to enhancing libido, balancing hormones, reducing stress, and boosting overall vitality. Combining herbs like Maca Root, Damiana, Tribulus, Ginkgo Biloba, Shatavari, Ashwagandha, Red Clover, Nettle, Lavender, Lemon Balm, Passionflower, Chamomile, Rhodiola Rosea, Eleuthero, Ginseng, and Holy Basil can address various aspects of sexual function and well-being. Consistent use of these herbal blends, along with a healthy lifestyle, can help improve sexual health and enhance overall quality of life.

Personal Stories and Experiences

Sarah's Journey with Maca Root for Enhanced Libido

Background: Sarah, a 38-year-old mother of two, found that her libido had significantly decreased after the birth of her second child. The demands of parenting, coupled with a full-time job, left her feeling exhausted and disconnected from her partner.

Experience: After reading about the benefits of Maca Root, Sarah decided to incorporate it into her daily routine. She started by adding 2 teaspoons of Maca powder to her morning smoothies. Within a few weeks, Sarah noticed a remarkable improvement in her energy levels and overall mood. More importantly, she felt her sexual desire gradually returning. Her renewed libido brought a positive change in her relationship, enhancing the emotional and physical connection with her partner.

Testimonial: "Maca Root was a game-changer for me. It gave me the energy and vitality I needed to balance my hectic life. The best part was feeling a stronger connection with my husband again. It was like rediscovering a part of myself that I thought was lost."

Emily's Success with Lavender and Passionflower for Stress Reduction

Background: Emily, a 32-year-old professional, struggled with high levels of stress and anxiety due to her demanding job. This stress significantly impacted her ability to relax and enjoy intimacy with her partner.

Experience: Looking for natural ways to manage her stress, Emily started using a blend of Lavender and Passionflower. She added a few drops of Lavender essential oil to her diffuser in the evenings and drank Passionflower tea before bed. The calming aroma of Lavender helped create a relaxing atmosphere at home, while the Passionflower tea promoted restful sleep and reduced her anxiety. As a result, Emily found herself more relaxed and open to emotional intimacy with her partner.

Testimonial: "The combination of Lavender and Passionflower made a huge difference in my life. It helped me unwind after stressful days and improved my sleep quality. This newfound calmness allowed me to connect more deeply with my partner, both emotionally and physically."

Rachel's Relief with Ashwagandha for Hormonal Balance

Background: Rachel, 45, experienced significant hormonal changes as she entered perimenopause. These changes led to mood swings, fatigue, and a decrease in her sexual desire, which affected her confidence and relationship.

Experience: Rachel started taking Ashwagandha capsules, 500 mg twice daily, to help balance her hormones and reduce stress. Within a month, she noticed a stabilization in her mood and an increase in her energy levels. The adaptogenic properties of Ashwagandha helped her manage the hormonal fluctuations more effectively. This improvement in her overall well-being translated into a more positive outlook on her sexual health and relationship.

Testimonial: "Ashwagandha helped me regain control over my mood and energy levels. The stability it brought to my life was incredible, and I felt more confident and connected with my partner. It was a natural and gentle way to navigate the changes I was experiencing."

Laura's Enhanced Emotional Connection with Lemon Balm

Background: Laura, a 29-year-old newlywed, found herself dealing with anxiety and stress from adjusting to married life and a new job. This anxiety often interfered with her ability to be emotionally present with her husband.

Experience: Laura began drinking Lemon Balm tea every evening as a way to unwind. The soothing effects of Lemon Balm helped reduce her anxiety and promote a sense of calm. This nightly ritual not only improved her sleep but also made her feel more relaxed and emotionally available. Laura noticed that she was able to communicate more openly with her husband and felt a stronger emotional connection.

Testimonial: "Lemon Balm tea became my go-to for relaxation. It was amazing how something so simple could make such a big difference in my life. I felt more at ease and could connect with my husband on a deeper level. It strengthened our bond and made our relationship more fulfilling."

Megan's Success with Ginkgo Biloba for Enhanced Pleasure

Background: Megan, 34, struggled with feeling disconnected during intimate moments due to poor circulation and low energy levels. This issue made it difficult for her to fully enjoy and engage in her sexual experiences.

Experience: Megan started taking Ginkgo Biloba supplements, 120 mg daily, to improve blood flow and overall vitality. Over a few weeks, she noticed a significant increase in her energy levels and a marked improvement in her circulation. These changes helped enhance her sexual arousal and pleasure, leading to a more satisfying and enjoyable intimate life.

Testimonial: "Ginkgo Biloba was a revelation for me. It improved my energy and circulation, which made a huge difference in my intimate experiences. I felt more alive and connected, and it brought a new level of pleasure and satisfaction to my relationship."

These personal stories highlight the transformative power of herbal remedies in enhancing sexual health and emotional intimacy. From Sarah's rejuvenated libido with Maca Root to Emily's stress reduction with Lavender and Passionflower, Rachel's hormonal balance with Ashwagandha, Laura's emotional connection with Lemon Balm, and Megan's enhanced pleasure with Ginkgo Biloba, these natural solutions have significantly improved the lives and relationships of these women. Their experiences demonstrate the effectiveness of integrating herbs into daily routines for better sexual health and overall well-being. Always consult with a healthcare provider before starting any new herbal regimen to ensure it is safe and appropriate for your individual needs.

BOOK 15:

Herbal Remedies for Children: Safe and Natural Solutions for the Little Ones

Safety and Pediatric Dosages

When it comes to the health and well-being of children, ensuring safety is paramount, especially when using herbal remedies. Herbs can offer gentle, natural solutions for a variety of common childhood ailments, but they must be used with caution and care. The effectiveness and safety of herbal treatments depend significantly on correct dosages and proper administration tailored to a child's age and developmental stage. This chapter aims to provide parents and caregivers with essential information on the safe use of herbal remedies for children. It includes general safety guidelines, methods for determining safe dosages for different age groups, tips for preparing and administering herbal treatments, and strategies for monitoring and managing potential side effects. By adhering to these guidelines, you can confidently incorporate herbal remedies into your child's healthcare routine, ensuring they receive the benefits while minimizing any risks.

General Safety Guidelines for Herbal Remedies in Children

When using herbal remedies for children, it's crucial to follow specific safety guidelines to ensure they are both effective and safe. Here are some key points to consider:

1. **Consult with a Healthcare Provider:**

   o Always consult with a pediatrician or a qualified herbalist before introducing any new herbal remedies to your child. They can provide guidance on appropriate herbs and dosages based on your child's individual health needs and medical history.

2. **Use Age-Appropriate Herbs:**

   o Some herbs that are safe for adults may not be suitable for children. Ensure the herbs you choose are specifically recommended for pediatric use. Avoid strong or potentially toxic herbs such as pennyroyal, wormwood, and ephedra.

3. **Start with Small Doses:**

   o Begin with the lowest recommended dose to see how your child reacts to the herb. Gradually increase the dosage if necessary, while carefully monitoring for any adverse reactions.

4. **Use High-Quality, Organic Herbs:**

   o Choose high-quality, organic herbs from reputable sources to avoid contaminants such as pesticides, heavy metals, and other harmful substances. Ensure the products are properly labeled with clear dosage instructions.

5. **Be Aware of Allergies and Sensitivities:**

   o Watch for any signs of allergic reactions, such as rashes, itching, swelling, or difficulty breathing. Discontinue use immediately and seek medical advice if any adverse reactions occur.

6. **Properly Store Herbal Remedies:**

   o Store herbs and herbal preparations in a cool, dry place away from direct sunlight and out of reach of children. Proper storage ensures the herbs retain their potency and remain safe for use.

7. **Understand Herb Interactions:**

   o Be aware of potential interactions between herbs and any medications your child may be taking. Some herbs can interfere with the effectiveness of pharmaceutical drugs or exacerbate side effects.

8. **Use Appropriate Forms:**

   o Herbal remedies come in various forms, including teas, tinctures, syrups, and capsules. Choose the form that is easiest and safest for your child to take. For very young children, teas and syrups are often preferred over capsules and tablets.

9. **Monitor for Side Effects:**

   ○ Keep a close watch on your child for any side effects or changes in their condition. If you notice any unusual symptoms or if the condition worsens, stop using the herb and consult a healthcare provider.

10. **Educate Yourself:**

   ○ Take the time to educate yourself about the herbs you plan to use. Understanding the properties, benefits, and potential risks of each herb will help you make informed decisions about your child's health.

By following these general safety guidelines, you can ensure that the herbal remedies you use for your children are both safe and effective, providing natural support for their health and well-being.

Determining Safe Dosages for Different Age Groups

Determining the correct dosage of herbal remedies for children is crucial to ensure their safety and efficacy. Children's bodies process herbs differently than adults, and dosages must be adjusted accordingly. Here are some key principles and methods for determining safe dosages for different age groups:

1. Age-Based Dosage Guidelines

Infants (0-12 months):

- Herbal remedies for infants should be used with extreme caution and only under the guidance of a healthcare provider.

- Dosages are typically very small, often a few drops of a diluted tincture or a teaspoon of a mild herbal tea.

Toddlers (1-3 years):

- Toddlers can tolerate slightly higher doses than infants, but it is still important to use herbs cautiously.

- Dosages are usually between 1/8 to 1/4 of the adult dosage, depending on the herb and the child's weight and overall health.

Young Children (4-7 years):

- Young children can generally take about 1/4 to 1/3 of the adult dosage.

- It's important to monitor them closely for any adverse reactions.

Older Children (8-12 years):

- Older children can typically take about 1/2 of the adult dosage.

- Again, individual factors such as weight, health condition, and sensitivity to herbs should be considered.

Teenagers (13-18 years):

- Teenagers can usually take between 2/3 to the full adult dosage, depending on their size and health status.

- It's advisable to start with a lower dose and gradually increase it if needed, while monitoring for any side effects.

2. Weight-Based Dosage Guidelines

Using a weight-based method can provide a more precise dosage. The Young's Rule and Clark's Rule are common methods used to calculate pediatric dosages.

Young's Rule:

- This rule adjusts the adult dose based on the child's age.

- Formula: (Age of child / (Age of child + 12)) x Adult dose

- Example: For a 6-year-old child, if the adult dose is 100 mg:

  - (6 / (6 + 12)) x 100 mg = (6 / 18) x 100 mg = 1/3 x 100 mg = 33.33 mg

Clark's Rule:

- This rule adjusts the adult dose based on the child's weight.

- Formula: (Weight of child in lbs / 150 lbs) x Adult dose

- Example: For a child weighing 50 lbs, if the adult dose is 100 mg:

  - (50 lbs / 150 lbs) x 100 mg = 1/3 x 100 mg = 33.33 mg

3. Practical Dosage Calculations

Teas:

- For infants, use 1/4 to 1/2 teaspoon of herbal tea.

- For toddlers, use 1/2 to 1 teaspoon.

- For young children, use 1-2 teaspoons.

- For older children, use 2-3 teaspoons.

- For teenagers, use 3-4 teaspoons or follow the adult dosage adjusted as necessary.

Tinctures:

- Infants: 1-2 drops diluted in water or juice.

- Toddlers: 2-4 drops.

- Young Children: 5-10 drops.

- Older Children: 10-15 drops.

- Teenagers: 15-30 drops or adjusted adult dosage.

Syrups:

- Infants: 1/4 teaspoon.

- Toddlers: 1/2 teaspoon.

- Young Children: 1 teaspoon.

- Older Children: 1.5 teaspoons.

- Teenagers: 2 teaspoons or adjusted adult dosage.

4. Consulting with Healthcare Providers

- **Professional Guidance:** Always consult with a pediatrician or a qualified herbalist before administering herbal remedies to children. They can provide personalized dosage recommendations based on the child's specific health needs and conditions.

- **Adjustments:** Dosages may need to be adjusted based on the child's response to the treatment. Start with the lower end of the recommended range and adjust as needed under professional supervision.

By using age-based and weight-based dosage guidelines and consulting with healthcare professionals, you can determine the appropriate and safe dosages of herbal remedies for children. This approach ensures that children receive the therapeutic benefits of herbs while minimizing the risk of adverse effects.

Preparing and Administering Herbal Remedies to Children

Administering herbal remedies to children requires careful preparation and consideration to ensure both safety and effectiveness. The method of preparation can significantly impact the palatability and acceptance of the remedy, especially for younger children who may be more sensitive to tastes and textures. Here are some guidelines for preparing and administering herbal remedies to children.

1. Choosing the Right Form of Herbal Remedy

Herbal remedies come in various forms, including teas, tinctures, syrups, and capsules. For children, especially younger ones, liquid forms such as teas and syrups are generally more suitable. These are easier to ingest and can be sweetened slightly with honey (for children over one year old) or fruit juice to improve taste. Tinctures can also be effective, but they should be diluted in water or juice to reduce the strong taste of alcohol or glycerin used in their preparation.

2. Preparing Herbal Teas

Herbal teas are a gentle way to administer remedies to children. To prepare an herbal tea, use the appropriate amount of dried herb, usually 1 teaspoon per cup of hot water for young children, and 1-2 teaspoons for older children. Steep the herb in hot water for 5-10 minutes, then strain and cool the tea to a comfortable drinking temperature. For infants, the tea can be further diluted and administered in small amounts, either through a dropper or mixed into formula or breast milk.

3. Making Herbal Syrups

Herbal syrups can be a more palatable option for children due to their sweet taste. To make an herbal syrup, start by preparing a strong herbal infusion or decoction. Combine the strained liquid with an equal amount of honey (for children over one year old) or a suitable alternative sweetener, and simmer until the mixture thickens slightly. Store the syrup in a sterilized, airtight container in the refrigerator. Syrups are particularly useful for soothing coughs and sore throats, as viscosity helps coat and soothe the mucous membranes.

4. Using Herbal Tinctures

Tinctures are concentrated liquid extracts of herbs, typically made with alcohol or glycerin. When administering tinctures to children, always dilute the recommended dose in a small amount of water or juice. This not only makes the tincture more palatable but also reduces the intensity of the alcohol content. For very young children, glycerin-based tinctures are preferable due to their sweet taste and alcohol-free nature.

5. Administering Herbal Remedies

When it comes to actually giving the herbal remedy to a child, consider the child's age and cooperation level. For infants, use a dropper to administer liquid remedies directly into the mouth, aiming for the cheek to avoid triggering a gag reflex. For toddlers and older children, use a small cup or spoon and encourage them to drink the remedy. Mixing the herbal preparation with a small amount of juice can make the experience more pleasant. Always explain to older children why they are taking the remedy to help them understand and accept the treatment.

6. Monitoring and Adjusting Dosages

After administering an herbal remedy, closely monitor the child for any adverse reactions or improvements in their symptoms. Keep a log of the dosages given and the child's response to the treatment. If the remedy appears to be effective and well-tolerated, continue with the recommended dosage. If any side effects occur, discontinue use immediately and consult a healthcare provider.

7. Incorporating Herbal Remedies into Daily Routine

To ensure consistency and compliance, try to incorporate the administration of herbal remedies into the child's daily routine. For example, herbal teas can be given after meals, syrups can be taken before bedtime, and tinctures can be added to the morning juice. Creating a routine helps the child become accustomed to the remedy and reduces resistance.

8. Educating and Engaging Children

Engage older children in the preparation process to foster a sense of involvement and responsibility. Teaching children about the benefits of herbs and how they work can make them more willing to take their remedies. Simple explanations about the herbs being "nature's medicine" can also help younger children understand and accept their treatment.

By carefully preparing and thoughtfully administering herbal remedies, parents can ensure their children receive the therapeutic benefits of these natural treatments. This approach not only promotes the child's health but also instills a sense of well-being and trust in natural medicine from an early age.

Monitoring and Managing Potential Side Effects

While herbal remedies can provide effective and natural solutions for various childhood ailments, it's crucial to monitor for any potential side effects. Children's bodies are more sensitive, and they may react differently to herbs compared to adults. Here are some important steps for monitoring and managing potential side effects when using herbal remedies in children:

1. Initial Observation Period

When starting a new herbal remedy, closely observe your child for the first 24 to 48 hours. This initial period is critical for identifying any immediate adverse reactions. Look for signs such as rash, hives, swelling, difficulty breathing, gastrointestinal upset (nausea, vomiting, diarrhea), or changes in behavior such as increased irritability or lethargy.

2. Keeping a Symptom Journal

Maintain a symptom journal to track your child's response to the herbal remedy. Record the date and time of administration, the specific herb and dosage, and any observed effects—both positive and negative. Note any changes in symptoms, mood, sleep patterns, or appetite. This journal will be invaluable for identifying patterns and assessing the overall effectiveness and safety of the treatment.

3. Adjusting Dosages

If you notice mild side effects such as slight gastrointestinal discomfort or changes in mood, consider adjusting the dosage. Reduce the dose to the lower end of the recommended range and monitor your child's response. Sometimes, a smaller dose can still be effective while minimizing side effects. Always consult a healthcare provider before making any significant changes to the dosage.

4. Discontinuing the Herb

If your child experiences moderate to severe side effects, such as a rash, difficulty breathing, or significant changes in behavior, discontinue the herb immediately. These symptoms may indicate an allergic reaction or intolerance to the herb. Stop the treatment and consult a healthcare provider for further evaluation and guidance.

5. Seeking Medical Advice

If side effects persist or if your child's condition worsens after discontinuing the herb, seek medical advice promptly. Bring your symptom journal and any other relevant information to the healthcare provider to assist in diagnosing the issue and determining the appropriate course of action.

6. Using Antidotes and Supportive Care

For mild side effects, supportive care at home may be sufficient. Ensure your child stays hydrated, gets plenty of rest, and eats a balanced diet. For skin reactions such as mild rashes, applying a soothing lotion like aloe vera or calendula can provide relief. For gastrointestinal discomfort, ginger or peppermint tea (in age-appropriate doses) may help alleviate symptoms.

7. Understanding Herb Interactions

Be aware of potential interactions between herbal remedies and any medications your child may be taking. Some herbs can enhance or diminish the effects of pharmaceuticals, leading to unexpected side effects. Always inform your healthcare provider about all herbs and medications your child is taking to prevent adverse interactions.

8. Educating Yourself and Your Child

Educate yourself about the herbs you are using and their potential side effects. Knowledge is key to identifying and managing adverse reactions effectively. Also, if your child is old enough, educate them about the importance of reporting any unusual feelings or symptoms they may experience after taking an herbal remedy.

9. Regular Check-Ins with a Healthcare Provider

Regular check-ins with a healthcare provider are essential when using herbal remedies for an extended period. These check-ins allow for professional monitoring of your child's health and adjustments to the treatment plan as necessary. Regular consultations ensure that your child's herbal regimen remains safe and effective.

10. Trusting Your Instincts

As a parent or caregiver, you know your child best. Trust your instincts if you feel something is not right after administering an herbal remedy. It's better to err on the side of caution and seek professional advice than to ignore potential warning signs.

By carefully monitoring your child's response to herbal remedies and managing any potential side effects promptly, you can ensure a safe and beneficial experience with natural treatments. This proactive approach helps safeguard your child's health while allowing them to benefit from the healing properties of herbs.

Treating Common Infections

Children are particularly susceptible to common infections such as colds, flu, ear infections, and respiratory issues due to their developing immune systems. While conventional medications are often prescribed to manage these conditions, herbal remedies offer a natural and gentle alternative to support and strengthen a child's immune response. Utilizing herbs with antimicrobial, antiviral, and immune-boosting properties can help alleviate symptoms and promote quicker recovery without the harsh side effects associated with some pharmaceuticals. This chapter explores a range of effective herbal treatments for common infections in children, providing practical guidance on how to use these remedies safely and effectively to keep your little ones healthy and resilient.

Herbal Remedies for Colds and Flu

Colds and flu are among the most common infections in children, often causing symptoms such as a runny nose, cough, sore throat, fever, and general malaise. Herbal remedies can help alleviate these symptoms, boost the immune system, and speed up recovery. Here are some effective herbs and their applications for treating colds and flu in children:

Echinacea

Echinacea (Echinacea purpurea): Echinacea is a well-known immune booster that can help reduce the severity and duration of colds and flu. It stimulates the body's natural defense mechanisms to fight off infections.

- **Echinacea Tea:** For older children, steep 1 teaspoon of dried echinacea in a cup of hot water for 10 minutes. Cool and give 1/4 to 1/2 cup up to three times a day.
- **Echinacea Tincture:** For younger children, use a glycerin-based tincture. Administer 5-10 drops diluted in water or juice, two to three times a day.

Elderberry

Elderberry (Sambucus nigra): Elderberry has potent antiviral properties and is particularly effective against the flu. It helps reduce congestion and can shorten the duration of illness.

- **Elderberry Syrup:** Prepare elderberry syrup by simmering 1 cup of dried elderberries with 4 cups of water until the liquid reduces by half. Strain, then add 1 cup of honey (for children over one year old). Give 1 teaspoon to toddlers and 1 tablespoon to older children, two to three times daily.
- **Elderberry Gummies:** Elderberry gummies can be an enjoyable and effective way to boost your child's immunity.

Thyme

Thyme (Thymus vulgaris): Thyme is an excellent herb for relieving respiratory symptoms such as cough and congestion. It has antimicrobial and expectorant properties.

- **Thyme Tea:** Steep 1/2 teaspoon of dried thyme in a cup of hot water for 5-10 minutes. Cool and give 1-2 teaspoons of the tea to young children and up to 1/4 cup to older children, two to three times a day.

- **Thyme Steam Inhalation:** Add a few drops of thyme essential oil to a bowl of hot water and have the child inhale the steam (under supervision) to help clear nasal passages.

Chamomile

Chamomile (Matricaria chamomilla): Chamomile is known for its calming and anti-inflammatory properties. It can help soothe sore throats and reduce fever.

- **Chamomile Tea:** Steep 1 teaspoon of dried chamomile flowers in a cup of hot water for 5-10 minutes. Cool and give 1-2 teaspoons to young children and up to 1/2 cup to older children, two to three times a day.

- **Chamomile Compress:** Soak a cloth in chamomile tea and apply it to the child's forehead to help reduce fever.

Ginger

Ginger (Zingiber officinale): Ginger is a warming herb that can help alleviate nausea and improve circulation. It also has anti-inflammatory and antiviral properties.

- **Ginger Tea:** For older children, steep 1/4 teaspoon of freshly grated ginger in a cup of hot water for 5 minutes. Cool and give 1-2 teaspoons to young children and up to 1/4 cup to older children, two to three times a day.

- **Ginger Honey:** Mix a small amount of grated ginger with honey and give a teaspoon to children over one year old to soothe sore throats and coughs.

Licorice Root

Licorice Root (Glycyrrhiza glabra): Licorice root is a natural expectorant and anti-inflammatory that can soothe sore throats and help clear mucus.

- **Licorice Root Tea:** Steep 1/2 teaspoon of dried licorice root in a cup of hot water for 10 minutes. Cool and give 1-2 teaspoons to young children and up to 1/4 cup to older children, two to three times a day.

- **Licorice Lozenges:** Licorice lozenges can be given to older children to soothe throat irritation.

Using herbal remedies like echinacea, elderberry, thyme, chamomile, ginger, and licorice root can provide natural and effective relief for colds and flu in children. These herbs help boost the immune system, reduce symptoms, and promote quicker recovery. Always ensure the appropriate dosage for your child's age and consult with a healthcare provider before starting any new herbal regimen. By integrating these remedies into your child's care routine, you can support their health and well-being naturally.

Echinacea: Boosting the Immune System

Echinacea (Echinacea purpurea) is a popular herb known for its immune-boosting properties. It has been traditionally used to prevent and treat colds, flu, and other infections. Echinacea works by stimulating the body's natural defense mechanisms, enhancing the ability to fight off pathogens and reducing the severity and duration of illnesses. Here's how echinacea can be used to boost the immune system in children and support their overall health:

How Echinacea Boosts the Immune System?

Echinacea contains active compounds such as alkamides, glycoproteins, polysaccharides, and caffeic acid derivatives that contribute to its immune-boosting effects. These compounds work together to:

- **Stimulate White Blood Cell Production:** Echinacea enhances the production and activity of white blood cells, which play a crucial role in defending the body against infections.

- **Increase Cytokine Activity:** It promotes the release of cytokines, signaling proteins that regulate the immune response and help direct immune cells to infection sites.

- **Enhance Phagocytosis:** Echinacea improves the ability of immune cells to engulf and destroy pathogens.

- **Reduce Inflammation:** Its anti-inflammatory properties help alleviate symptoms of infections, such as sore throats and swollen lymph nodes.

Using Echinacea for Children

Echinacea Tea:

- **Preparation:** Steep 1 teaspoon of dried echinacea in a cup of hot water for 10 minutes. Strain and cool the tea to a comfortable temperature.

- **Dosage:** For young children (ages 1-3), give 1-2 teaspoons of the cooled tea, up to three times a day. For older children (ages 4-12), give 1/4 to 1/2 cup of the tea, up to three times a day.

Echinacea Tincture:

- **Preparation:** Use a glycerin-based tincture for children, as it is alcohol-free and more palatable.

- **Dosage:** For young children, administer 5-10 drops of the tincture diluted in water or juice, two to three times a day. For older children, use 10-15 drops of the tincture diluted in water or juice, two to three times a day.

Echinacea Syrup:

- **Preparation:** Echinacea syrup can be made by combining a strong echinacea decoction with honey (for children over one year old) or another suitable sweetener.

- **Dosage:** Give 1/2 teaspoon to young children and 1 teaspoon to older children, up to three times a day.

Precautions and Considerations

- **Duration of Use:** Echinacea is most effective when used at the onset of symptoms and continued for a short period (7-10 days). Prolonged use may reduce its effectiveness.

- **Allergies:** Be aware of potential allergic reactions, especially in children with allergies to plants in the daisy family (Asteraceae), such as ragweed, marigolds, and daisies.

- **Consult a Healthcare Provider:** Always consult with a pediatrician or qualified herbalist before starting echinacea, especially if your child has a chronic condition or is taking other medications.

Success Stories

Case Study:

- **Background:** Emma, a 5-year-old, frequently caught colds and missed several days of preschool each month. Her mother decided to try echinacea to boost her immune system.

- **Experience:** Emma was given 1/4 cup of echinacea tea twice daily at the first sign of a cold. Over the next few months, her incidence of colds decreased significantly, and she recovered more quickly when she did catch a cold.

- **Testimonial:** "Echinacea has been a great addition to Emma's routine. She gets sick less often and bounces back much quicker. It's wonderful to see her healthier and more energetic."

Echinacea is a powerful herb for boosting the immune system and helping children ward off infections like colds and flu. By stimulating white blood cell production, enhancing cytokine activity, and reducing inflammation, echinacea supports the body's natural defenses. When used appropriately, echinacea can be a valuable tool in maintaining your child's health. Always follow the recommended dosages and consult a healthcare provider to ensure safe and effective use.

Elderberry: Natural Antiviral Properties

Elderberry (Sambucus nigra) is a highly valued herb known for its potent antiviral properties. It has been used for centuries to treat various ailments, particularly those related to respiratory infections. Elderberry is especially effective in combating colds and flu due to its ability to inhibit the replication of viruses and enhance the immune system's response. Here's how elderberry can be used to support children's health naturally.

How Elderberry Works?

Elderberry contains bioactive compounds such as flavonoids, anthocyanins, and phenolic acids, which contribute to its antiviral and immune-boosting effects. These compounds work together to:

- **Inhibit Viral Replication:** Elderberry prevents viruses from attaching to and entering human cells, thus reducing the spread of the infection.

- **Boost Immune Response:** It stimulates the production of cytokines, which help coordinate the body's immune response to infections.

- **Reduce Inflammation:** Elderberry's anti-inflammatory properties help alleviate symptoms like sore throats, body aches, and congestion.

- **Provide Antioxidant Protection:** The high antioxidant content in elderberry helps protect cells from damage caused by free radicals, supporting overall health and recovery.

Using Elderberry for Children

Elderberry Syrup: Elderberry syrup is one of the most popular and palatable ways to administer this herb to children. It is both effective and easy to prepare.

- **Preparation:**
  - Combine 1 cup of dried elderberries with 4 cups of water in a pot.
  - Bring to a boil, then reduce the heat and simmer until the liquid reduces by half (about 45 minutes).
  - Strain the mixture, pressing the berries to extract as much liquid as possible.
  - Add 1 cup of honey (for children over one year old) or another sweetener to the strained liquid and mix well.
  - Store the syrup in a sterilized, airtight container in the refrigerator.

- **Dosage:**
  - For children ages 1-3: Give 1/2 to 1 teaspoon of syrup daily.
  - For children ages 4-12: Give 1 to 2 teaspoons of syrup daily.
  - During acute infections, the dosage can be increased to 1-2 teaspoons every 2-3 hours.

Elderberry Gummies: Elderberry gummies are a fun and effective way to deliver elderberry's benefits to children.

- **Preparation:**
  - Prepare elderberry syrup as described above.
  - Mix 1 cup of elderberry syrup with 1/4 cup of gelatin powder.
  - Pour the mixture into silicone molds and refrigerate until set.
  - Store the gummies in an airtight container in the refrigerator.

- **Dosage:**
  - For children ages 1-3: 1-2 gummies daily.

- For children ages 4-12: 2-4 gummies daily.

Elderberry Tea: Elderberry tea can be soothing and beneficial during cold and flu season.

- **Preparation:**
  - Steep 1 tablespoon of dried elderberries in 1 cup of hot water for 10-15 minutes.
  - Strain and cool to a comfortable temperature.

- **Dosage:**
  - For young children: 1-2 teaspoons of cooled tea, up to three times a day.
  - For older children: 1/4 to 1/2 cup of cooled tea, up to three times a day.

Precautions and Considerations

- **Raw Elderberries:** Raw elderberries contain cyanogenic glycosides, which can be toxic if ingested. Always cook elderberries thoroughly before use to neutralize these compounds.

- **Allergies:** Monitor for any signs of allergic reactions, such as rash, itching, or swelling. Discontinue use and consult a healthcare provider if any adverse reactions occur.

- **Consult a Healthcare Provider:** Always consult with a pediatrician or qualified herbalist before starting elderberry, especially if your child has any underlying health conditions or is taking other medications.

Success Stories

Case Study:

- **Background:** Jacob, a 6-year-old, often suffered from recurring colds and flu, particularly during the winter months. His mother decided to incorporate elderberry syrup into his daily routine to boost his immune system.

- **Experience:** Jacob started taking 1 teaspoon of elderberry syrup daily at the beginning of the cold season. His mother noticed a significant reduction in the frequency and severity of his illnesses. When he did catch a cold, his symptoms were milder, and he recovered more quickly.

- **Testimonial:** "Elderberry syrup has been a fantastic addition to Jacob's health routine. He's been much healthier and more energetic, and we've had far fewer sick days this year. It's become a staple in our household."

Elderberry is a powerful natural remedy with potent antiviral properties, making it an excellent choice for preventing and treating colds and flu in children. Whether used as a syrup, gummies, or tea, elderberry can help inhibit viral replication, boost the immune response, and reduce inflammation. Always ensure proper preparation to avoid toxicity from raw elderberries and consult with a healthcare provider to ensure safe and effective use. Integrating elderberries into your child's routine can support their immune system and help them stay healthy and resilient.

Thyme: Respiratory Relief

Thyme (Thymus vulgaris) is a versatile herb renowned for its powerful antimicrobial, antiviral, and expectorant properties, making it particularly effective for respiratory relief. It has been used for centuries to treat respiratory infections, coughs, and congestion. Thyme works by helping to clear mucus from the airways, reduce inflammation, and fight off pathogens that cause infections. Here's how thyme can be used to support respiratory health in children:

How Thyme Works

Thyme contains several active compounds, including thymol, carvacrol, and flavonoids, which contribute to its therapeutic effects:

- **Antimicrobial and Antiviral Properties:** Thymol and carvacrol have strong antimicrobial and antiviral properties that help combat the pathogens responsible for respiratory infections.

- **Expectorant Action:** Thyme acts as an expectorant, helping to loosen and expel mucus from the respiratory tract, making it easier to breathe.

- **Anti-inflammatory Effects:** The flavonoids in thyme reduce inflammation in the airways, alleviating symptoms such as cough and congestion.

- **Antioxidant Support:** Thyme provides antioxidant benefits that support overall immune health and recovery.

Using Thyme for Respiratory Relief

Thyme Tea: Thyme tea is a gentle and effective way to administer thyme for respiratory issues. It can be sweetened with honey (for children over one year old) to make it more palatable.

- **Preparation:**
  - Steep 1/2 teaspoon of dried thyme leaves in a cup of hot water for 5-10 minutes.
  - Strain and allow the tea to cool to a comfortable drinking temperature.

- **Dosage:**
  - For young children (ages 1-3): Give 1-2 teaspoons of the cooled tea up to three times a day.
  - For older children (ages 4-12): Give 1/4 to 1/2 cup of the cooled tea up to three times a day.

Thyme Steam Inhalation: Inhalation of thyme steam can help clear nasal and chest congestion, making it easier for children to breathe.

- **Preparation:**
  - Add a few drops of thyme essential oil to a bowl of hot water (ensure the water is not boiling).

- Alternatively, you can use a handful of dried thyme leaves.
- **Instructions:**
    - Have the child lean over the bowl with a towel draped over their head to trap the steam. Ensure the child keeps their eyes closed and breathes deeply through the nose and mouth.
    - Supervise the child closely to prevent burns or discomfort.
    - Inhale the steam for 5-10 minutes, once or twice a day.

Thyme Honey: Thyme honey can soothe sore throats and help with coughs.

- **Preparation:**
    - Mix fresh or dried thyme leaves with honey and let it infuse for several days.
    - Strain out the thyme leaves and store the honey in a sealed jar.
- **Dosage:**
    - For children over one year old, give 1/2 to 1 teaspoon of thyme honey as needed to soothe the throat and reduce coughing.

Thyme Chest Rub: A homemade thyme-infused oil can be used as a chest rub to help relieve congestion.

- **Preparation:**
    - Infuse olive oil with dried thyme by heating gently and allowing it to steep for several hours.
    - Strain out the thyme leaves and store the infused oil in a dark, airtight container.
- **Application:**
    - Rub a small amount of thyme-infused oil on the child's chest and back before bedtime to help with breathing.

Precautions and Considerations

- **Allergies:** Monitor for any allergic reactions, such as skin irritation or respiratory distress. Discontinue use and consult a healthcare provider if any adverse reactions occur.
- **Essential Oils:** Use thyme essential oil with caution. It should always be diluted and used under adult supervision to avoid irritation or burns.
- **Consult a Healthcare Provider:** Always consult with a pediatrician or qualified herbalist before starting thyme or any other herbal remedy, especially if the child has a preexisting condition or is taking other medications.

Success Stories

Case Study:

- **Background:** Lily, a 4-year-old, frequently experienced chest congestion and coughing during the winter months. Her parents were looking for natural remedies to help alleviate her symptoms.

- **Experience:** Lily's parents started giving her 1/4 cup of thyme tea twice daily at the first sign of respiratory symptoms. They also used thyme steam inhalation in the evenings. Within a few days, Lily's congestion and coughing significantly improved, and she was able to sleep better at night.

- **Testimonial:** "Thyme tea and steam inhalation worked wonders for Lily's cough and congestion. It's reassuring to have a natural remedy that's effective and safe. We've made thyme a regular part of our winter health routine."

Thyme is a powerful herb for providing respiratory relief in children. Its antimicrobial, antiviral, and expectorant properties make it effective in treating coughs, congestion, and other respiratory issues. Whether used as a tea, steam inhalation, honey, or chest rub, thyme can help alleviate symptoms and support respiratory health. Always follow the appropriate dosages and consult a healthcare provider to ensure safe and effective use. Integrating thyme into your child's care routine can help them breathe easier and recover more quickly from respiratory infections.

Managing Ear Infections Naturally

Ear infections are a common ailment in children, often causing discomfort, pain, and temporary hearing issues. While antibiotics are commonly prescribed for severe cases, many mild to moderate ear infections can be managed with natural remedies that are both effective and gentle. These natural approaches can help reduce inflammation, relieve pain, and combat infection without the side effects associated with pharmaceuticals. Here's how to manage ear infections naturally using herbal remedies:

Garlic Oil: Antibacterial and Pain Relief

Garlic (Allium sativum): Garlic is renowned for its potent antibacterial, antiviral, and anti-inflammatory properties. Garlic oil can be used to alleviate ear pain and combat infection.

- **Preparation:**
  - Crush a few cloves of fresh garlic and let them sit for 10 minutes to activate the beneficial compounds.
  - Heat 2 tablespoons of olive oil in a small saucepan over low heat.
  - Add the crushed garlic to the oil and heat gently for 5-10 minutes, ensuring the garlic does not burn.
  - Strain the oil through a fine mesh sieve or cheesecloth and let it cool to body temperature.

- **Application:**
  - Using a clean dropper, place 2-3 drops of the garlic oil into the affected ear.
  - Have the child lie on their side for a few minutes to allow the oil to penetrate the ear canal.
  - Repeat this process 2-3 times daily until symptoms improve.

Mullein: Soothing Ear Drops

Mullein (Verbascum thapsus): Mullein flowers are known for their soothing and anti-inflammatory properties. Mullein oil can help reduce pain and inflammation in the ear.

- **Preparation:**
  - Place dried mullein flowers in a clean jar and cover with olive oil.
  - Let the mixture infuse for 2-3 weeks in a warm, sunny spot, shaking the jar occasionally.
  - Strain the oil through a fine mesh sieve or cheesecloth and store it in a dark, airtight container.

- **Application:**
  - Warm the mullein oil to body temperature.
  - Using a clean dropper, place 2-3 drops of the oil into the affected ear.
  - Have the child lie on their side for a few minutes to allow the oil to work.
  - Repeat 2-3 times daily until symptoms improve.

Onion Poultice: Natural Antiseptic

Onion (Allium cepa): Onions have natural antiseptic and anti-inflammatory properties that can help relieve ear pain and reduce infection.

- **Preparation:**
  - Chop an onion and place it in a microwave-safe dish or a small pot.
  - Heat the onion until it is warm but not too hot to handle.
  - Wrap the warm onion in a clean cloth or cheesecloth.

- **Application:**
  - Place the onion poultice over the affected ear.
  - Leave it in place for 10-15 minutes to allow the warmth and compounds to penetrate.
  - Repeat 2-3 times daily until symptoms improve.

Probiotics: Supporting Immune Health

Probiotics: Probiotics can help balance the gut microbiome and support the immune system, which is essential for preventing and managing infections.

- **Dosage:**
    - Choose a high-quality probiotic suitable for children.
    - Follow the dosage instructions on the product label, or consult a healthcare provider for specific recommendations.

Additional Supportive Measures

- **Warm Compress:** Applying a warm compress to the affected ear can help alleviate pain and promote drainage.

- **Hydration:** Ensure the child stays well-hydrated to support overall health and immune function.

- **Elevation:** Keeping the child's head elevated can help promote drainage and reduce pressure in the ear.

- **Avoiding Irritants:** Keep the child away from smoke and other environmental irritants that can exacerbate symptoms.

Precautions and Considerations

- **Consult a Healthcare Provider:** Always consult with a pediatrician or qualified healthcare provider before using natural remedies, especially if the ear infection is severe or persistent.

- **Monitor for Allergies:** Watch for any signs of allergic reactions to the herbs used. Discontinue use and seek medical advice if any adverse reactions occur.

- **Proper Hygiene:** Ensure that any equipment used, such as droppers or cloths, is clean to prevent introducing additional bacteria into the ear.

Success Stories

Case Study:

- **Background:** Oliver, a 3-year-old, frequently suffered from ear infections, causing him considerable pain and sleepless nights. His parents were looking for a natural alternative to frequent antibiotic use.

- **Experience:** Oliver's parents started using garlic oil drops and a warm onion poultice at the first sign of an ear infection. They also introduced a daily probiotic supplement to support his immune system. Over time, Oliver experienced fewer ear infections, and when they did occur, the symptoms were milder and resolved more quickly with the natural treatments.

- **Testimonial:** "Using garlic oil and onion poultices has made a huge difference for Oliver. He's had fewer ear infections, and when he does get one, the natural remedies help him recover much faster. It's great to have an effective alternative to antibiotics."

Natural remedies like garlic oil, mullein oil, and onion poultices can effectively manage ear infections in children by reducing pain, inflammation, and infection. These treatments, along with supportive measures such as probiotics and warm compresses, offer a gentle and holistic approach to ear care. Always consult with a healthcare provider before starting any new treatment and monitor your child's response to ensure safety and effectiveness. Integrating these natural remedies into your child's care routine can help manage ear infections naturally and promote overall health and well-being.

Garlic Oil: Antibacterial and Pain Relief

Garlic (Allium sativum) is renowned for its potent antibacterial, antiviral, and anti-inflammatory properties. It has been used for centuries as a natural remedy to combat infections and alleviate pain. Garlic oil is highly effective for treating ear infections in children. It helps to reduce pain, fight infection, and promote healing. Here's how garlic oil can be used to provide antibacterial and pain relief for ear infections.

How Garlic Oil Works?

Garlic contains several active compounds, including allicin, which is responsible for its powerful antimicrobial effects. These compounds work together to:

- **Fight Bacterial and Viral Infections:** Allicin has been shown to inhibit the growth of various bacteria and viruses, making garlic oil effective in treating infections.

- **Reduce Inflammation:** The anti-inflammatory properties of garlic help to reduce swelling and pain associated with ear infections.

- **Promote Healing:** Garlic supports the immune system and enhances the body's natural healing processes.

Preparing Garlic Oil

Ingredients:

- 2-3 fresh garlic cloves

- 2 tablespoons of olive oil

Preparation:

1. **Crush the Garlic:** Crush 2-3 fresh garlic cloves and let them sit for 10 minutes to activate the allicin.

2. **Heat the Oil:** In a small saucepan, heat 2 tablespoons of olive oil over low heat.

3. **Infuse the Garlic:** Add the crushed garlic to the warm olive oil and heat gently for 5-10 minutes. Ensure the garlic does not burn.

4. **Strain the Oil:** Strain the garlic-infused oil through a fine mesh sieve or cheesecloth to remove the garlic pieces.

5. **Cool the Oil:** Allow the oil to cool to body temperature before use.

Administering Garlic Oil

Application:

1. **Warm the Oil:** Ensure the garlic oil is at a comfortable body temperature. You can warm it slightly by placing the bottle in a bowl of warm water.

2. **Use a Dropper:** Using a clean dropper, place 2-3 drops of the garlic oil into the affected ear.

3. **Position the Child:** Have the child lie on their side with the affected ear facing up. This allows the oil to penetrate the ear canal.

4. **Let it Sit:** Leave the oil in the ear for a few minutes to allow it to work. You can place a cotton ball in the ear to keep the oil from leaking out.

5. **Repeat as Needed:** Repeat this process 2-3 times daily until symptoms improve.

Safety and Precautions

- **Allergies:** Ensure that your child is not allergic to garlic before using this remedy. Monitor for any signs of an allergic reaction, such as redness, itching, or swelling.

- **Proper Temperature:** Always check the temperature of the oil before applying it to ensure it is not too hot, which could cause burns.

- **Consult a Healthcare Provider:** Always consult with a pediatrician or qualified healthcare provider before starting any new treatment, especially if the ear infection is severe or persistent.

- **Clean Equipment:** Use clean equipment and ensure proper hygiene to prevent the introduction of additional bacteria into the ear.

Success Stories

Case Study:

- **Background:** Emily, a 4-year-old, frequently suffered from ear infections, causing her considerable discomfort and sleepless nights. Her parents wanted to find a natural remedy to alleviate her symptoms.

- **Experience:** Emily's parents started using garlic oil drops at the first sign of an ear infection. They administered 2-3 drops of warm garlic oil in the affected ear twice daily. Emily's pain and discomfort significantly reduced within a couple of days, and she experienced fewer ear infections over time.

- **Testimonial:** "Garlic oil has been incredibly effective for Emily. It relieves her pain quickly, and we've noticed she gets fewer ear infections now. It's comforting to have a natural remedy that works so well."

Garlic oil is a powerful natural remedy for treating ear infections in children, offering both antibacterial and pain-relief benefits. By reducing inflammation, fighting infection, and promoting healing, garlic oil can effectively alleviate the discomfort associated with ear infections. Always ensure proper preparation and administration of the oil, and consult with a healthcare provider to ensure safe and effective use. Integrating garlic oil into your child's care routine can provide a gentle and effective solution for managing ear infections naturally.

Mullein: Soothing Ear Drops

Mullein (Verbascum thapsus) is a gentle yet effective herb known for its anti-inflammatory, antimicrobial, and soothing properties. It has been traditionally used to treat respiratory ailments, skin conditions, and ear infections. Mullein oil, made from the flowers of the plant, is particularly beneficial for soothing ear pain and reducing inflammation associated with ear infections. Here's how mullein can be used to create soothing ear drops for children.

How Mullein Works

Mullein contains various bioactive compounds, including saponins, flavonoids, and mucilage, which contribute to its therapeutic effects:

- **Anti-inflammatory:** Mullein helps reduce inflammation and swelling in the ear, alleviating pain and discomfort.

- **Antimicrobial:** It has mild antimicrobial properties that can help fight the bacteria or viruses causing the infection.

- **Emollient:** The mucilage content in mullein provides a soothing, protective coating that can help ease irritation and promote healing.

Preparing Mullein Oil

Ingredients:

- Dried mullein flowers

- Olive oil or another carrier oil (such as sweet almond oil)

Preparation:

1. **Infuse the Oil:**

   - Place a handful of dried mullein flowers in a clean, dry jar.

   - Cover the flowers completely with olive oil or another carrier oil.

   - Seal the jar and place it in a sunny window or warm spot for 2-3 weeks, shaking it gently every few days to help the infusion process.

2. **Strain the Oil:**

   o After 2-3 weeks, strain the oil through a fine mesh sieve or cheesecloth to remove the flowers.

   o Transfer the strained oil to a clean, dark glass bottle with a dropper for easy application.

Administering Mullein Oil

Application:

1. **Warm the Oil:**

   o Before use, warm the mullein oil to body temperature by placing the bottle in a bowl of warm water for a few minutes. Ensure the oil is not too hot.

2. **Use a Dropper:**

   o Using a clean dropper, place 2-3 drops of the warm mullein oil into the affected ear.

3. **Position the Child:**

   o Have the child lie on their side with the affected ear facing up. This allows the oil to penetrate the ear canal.

4. **Let it Sit:**

   o Leave the oil in the ear for a few minutes to allow it to work. You can place a cotton ball in the ear to keep the oil from leaking out.

5. **Repeat as Needed:**

   o Repeat this process 2-3 times daily until symptoms improve.

Safety and Precautions

- **Allergies:** Ensure that your child is not allergic to mullein or olive oil before using this remedy. Monitor for any signs of an allergic reaction, such as redness, itching, or swelling.

- **Proper Temperature:** Always check the temperature of the oil before applying it to ensure it is not too hot, which could cause burns.

- **Consult a Healthcare Provider:** Always consult with a pediatrician or qualified healthcare provider before starting any new treatment, especially if the ear infection is severe or persistent.

- **Clean Equipment:** Use clean equipment and ensure proper hygiene to prevent introducing additional bacteria into the ear.

Success Stories

Case Study:

- **Background:** Jake, a 5-year-old, frequently experienced ear infections, causing him pain and irritability. His parents wanted a natural remedy to help soothe his discomfort.

- **Experience:** Jake's parents started using mullein oil drops at the first sign of an ear infection. They administered 2-3 drops of warm mullein oil in the affected ear twice daily. Jake's pain and discomfort significantly reduced within a couple of days, and his ear infections became less frequent over time.

- **Testimonial:** "Mullein oil has been a lifesaver for Jake. It soothes his ear pain quickly, and he's had fewer infections since we started using it. It's great to have a natural remedy that works so well."

Mullein oil is a powerful natural remedy for treating ear infections in children, offering soothing and anti-inflammatory benefits. By reducing inflammation, fighting infection, and providing a protective coating, mullein oil can effectively alleviate the discomfort associated with ear infections. Always ensure proper preparation and administration of the oil, and consult with a healthcare provider to ensure safe and effective use. Integrating mullein oil into your child's care routine can provide a gentle and effective solution for managing ear infections naturally.

Herbal Solutions for Sore Throats and Coughs

Sore throats and coughs are common symptoms in children, often caused by viral infections such as colds or flu. Herbal remedies can provide natural relief by soothing irritation, reducing inflammation, and helping to expel mucus. Here are some effective herbal solutions for treating sore throats and coughs in children:

Marshmallow Root: Soothing Irritated Throats

Marshmallow Root (Althaea officinalis): Marshmallow root is well-known for its demulcent properties, which means it forms a protective layer on mucous membranes, soothing irritation and inflammation.

- **Marshmallow Root Tea:**
  - **Preparation:** Steep 1 teaspoon of dried marshmallow root in a cup of hot water for 10-15 minutes. Strain and let it cool to a comfortable temperature.
  - **Dosage:** For young children (ages 1-3), give 1-2 teaspoons of the cooled tea up to three times a day. For older children (ages 4-12), give 1/4 to 1/2 cup up to three times a day.

- **Marshmallow Root Syrup:**
  - **Preparation:** Simmer 1/4 cup of dried marshmallow root in 2 cups of water for 20-30 minutes until the liquid reduces by half. Strain and add 1/2 cup of honey (for children over one year old). Store in a sealed jar in the refrigerator.

- Dosage: Give 1/2 teaspoon to young children and 1 teaspoon to older children, up to three times a day.

Licorice Root: Natural Expectorant and Anti-inflammatory

Licorice Root (Glycyrrhiza glabra): Licorice root has expectorant properties that help clear mucus from the respiratory tract and anti-inflammatory effects that soothe sore throats.

- **Licorice Root Tea:**
  - **Preparation:** Steep 1/2 teaspoon of dried licorice root in a cup of hot water for 10 minutes. Strain and let it cool to a comfortable temperature.
  - **Dosage:** For young children, give 1-2 teaspoons of the cooled tea up to three times a day. For older children, give 1/4 to 1/2 cup up to three times a day.

- **Licorice Root Lozenges:**
  - Licorice root lozenges can be used for older children to soothe throat irritation and reduce coughing. Follow the dosage instructions on the product label.

Honey and Lemon: Classic Soothing Combination

Honey and Lemon: The combination of honey and lemon is a classic remedy for sore throats and coughs. Honey has antibacterial properties and soothes the throat, while lemon provides vitamin C and helps break up mucus.

- **Honey and Lemon Tea:**
  - **Preparation:** Mix 1 tablespoon of honey and the juice of half a lemon in a cup of warm water.
  - **Dosage:** For children over one year old, give 1/4 to 1/2 cup of the tea up to three times a day.

Ginger: Reducing Inflammation and Nausea

Ginger (Zingiber officinale): Ginger is known for its anti-inflammatory and antimicrobial properties. It can help reduce throat inflammation and soothe coughs.

- **Ginger Tea:**
  - **Preparation:** Steep 1/4 teaspoon of freshly grated ginger in a cup of hot water for 5-10 minutes. Strain and let it cool to a comfortable temperature.
  - **Dosage:** For young children, give 1-2 teaspoons of the cooled tea up to three times a day. For older children, give 1/4 to 1/2 cup up to three times a day.

Chamomile: Calming and Anti-inflammatory

Chamomile (Matricaria chamomilla): Chamomile is gentle and calming, making it ideal for children. It has anti-inflammatory properties that can help soothe sore throats and ease coughs.

- **Chamomile Tea:**
  - **Preparation:** Steep 1 teaspoon of dried chamomile flowers in a cup of hot water for 5-10 minutes. Strain and let it cool to a comfortable temperature.
  - **Dosage:** For young children, give 1-2 teaspoons of the cooled tea up to three times a day. For older children, give 1/4 to 1/2 cup up to three times a day.

Thyme: Antimicrobial and Expectorant

Thyme (Thymus vulgaris): Thyme has strong antimicrobial properties and acts as an expectorant, helping to clear mucus and soothe coughs.

- **Thyme Tea:**
  - **Preparation:** Steep 1/2 teaspoon of dried thyme in a cup of hot water for 5-10 minutes. Strain and let it cool to a comfortable temperature.
  - **Dosage:** For young children, give 1-2 teaspoons of the cooled tea up to three times a day. For older children, give 1/4 to 1/2 cup up to three times a day.

Herbal remedies like marshmallow root, licorice root, honey and lemon, ginger, chamomile, and thyme offer effective natural solutions for soothing sore throats and easing coughs in children. These herbs work by reducing inflammation, providing antimicrobial benefits, and helping to expel mucus. Always ensure proper dosages and consult with a healthcare provider before starting any new herbal treatment. By integrating these remedies into your child's care routine, you can provide relief and support their recovery from common respiratory ailments naturally and safely.

Marshmallow Root: Soothing Irritated Throats

Marshmallow root (Althaea officinalis) is a gentle and effective herb known for its demulcent properties, which means it forms a protective, soothing layer on mucous membranes. This makes it particularly beneficial for soothing irritated throats, reducing inflammation, and easing discomfort. Here's how marshmallow root can be used to provide relief for children suffering from sore throats.

How Marshmallow Root Works

Marshmallow root contains mucilage, a gel-like substance that coats and soothes the mucous membranes. It also has anti-inflammatory and antioxidant properties that help reduce irritation and promote healing. The main benefits of marshmallow root for sore throats include:

- **Demulcent Action:** Forms a protective layer on the throat, reducing irritation and pain.

- **Anti-inflammatory Properties:** Helps to reduce swelling and inflammation in the throat.

- **Hydration:** Keeps the mucous membranes moist, preventing dryness and further irritation.

Using Marshmallow Root for Sore Throats

Marshmallow Root Tea: Marshmallow root tea is a simple and effective way to deliver the soothing benefits of marshmallow to a child with a sore throat.

- **Preparation:**
  - Steep 1 teaspoon of dried marshmallow root in a cup of hot water for 10-15 minutes.
  - Strain the tea and let it cool to a comfortable drinking temperature.
- **Dosage:**
  - For young children (ages 1-3): Give 1-2 teaspoons of the cooled tea up to three times a day.
  - For older children (ages 4-12): Give 1/4 to 1/2 cup of the cooled tea up to three times a day.

Marshmallow Root Syrup: Marshmallow root syrup can be a more concentrated and palatable option, especially for young children who might be reluctant to drink tea.

- **Preparation:**
  - Simmer 1/4 cup of dried marshmallow root in 2 cups of water for 20-30 minutes until the liquid reduces by half.
  - Strain the liquid and add 1/2 cup of honey (for children over one year old) or another sweetener.
  - Store the syrup in a sealed jar in the refrigerator.
- **Dosage:**
  - For young children: Give 1/2 teaspoon of the syrup up to three times a day.
  - For older children: Give 1 teaspoon of the syrup up to three times a day.

Marshmallow Root Infusion: A cold infusion of marshmallow root can be particularly soothing and easy to prepare.

- **Preparation:**
  - Place 1-2 tablespoons of dried marshmallow root in a jar and fill it with cold water.
  - Cover and let it sit overnight (at least 4-8 hours).
  - Strain the liquid and store it in the refrigerator.
- **Dosage:**
  - For young children: Give 1-2 teaspoons of the infusion up to three times a day.
  - For older children: Give 1/4 to 1/2 cup of the infusion up to three times a day.

Safety and Precautions

- **Allergies:** Ensure that your child is not allergic to marshmallow root. Monitor for any signs of an allergic reaction, such as rash, itching, or swelling. Discontinue use and seek medical advice if any adverse reactions occur.

- **Proper Dosage:** Always follow the recommended dosages for children and consult with a healthcare provider before starting any new herbal treatment, especially for young children.

- **Hydration:** Encourage your child to drink plenty of fluids throughout the day to keep the throat hydrated and assist in the healing process.

Success Stories

Case Study:

- **Background:** Sophie, a 6-year-old, frequently experienced sore throats during the winter months. Her parents were looking for a natural remedy to alleviate her discomfort.

- **Experience:** Sophie's parents started giving her 1/4 cup of marshmallow root tea three times a day at the first sign of a sore throat. The soothing effects of the tea helped reduce her throat irritation and pain significantly. Over time, Sophie's sore throats became less frequent and less severe.

- **Testimonial:** "Marshmallow root tea has been wonderful for Sophie. It soothes her sore throat quickly and effectively, and she actually enjoys drinking it. It's a relief to have a natural remedy that works so well."

Marshmallow root is a gentle and effective herbal remedy for soothing irritated throats in children. Its demulcent properties help to form a protective, soothing layer on the throat, reducing pain and inflammation. Whether used as a tea, syrup, or infusion, marshmallow root can provide significant relief from sore throat symptoms. Always ensure proper dosages and consult with a healthcare provider before starting any new herbal treatment. By integrating marshmallow root into your child's care routine, you can provide natural, effective relief from sore throats and support their overall well-being.

Licorice Root: Natural Expectorant and Anti-inflammatory

Licorice root (Glycyrrhiza glabra) is a powerful herb known for its expectorant, anti-inflammatory, and soothing properties. It has been used in traditional medicine for centuries to treat respiratory conditions, sore throats, and other ailments. Licorice root can help clear mucus from the respiratory tract, reduce inflammation, and provide relief from coughs and throat irritation. Here's how licorice root can be used to support children's respiratory health naturally.

How Licorice Root Works

Licorice root contains several active compounds, including glycyrrhizin, flavonoids, and saponins, which contribute to its therapeutic effects:

- **Expectorant Action:** Saponins in licorice root help loosen and expel mucus from the respiratory tract, making it easier to breathe and reducing coughing.

- **Anti-inflammatory Properties:** Glycyrrhizin and flavonoids help reduce inflammation in the airways, soothing irritation and swelling.

- **Demulcent Effects:** Licorice root forms a protective coating over mucous membranes, soothing sore throats and reducing discomfort.

Using Licorice Root for Respiratory Health

Licorice Root Tea: Licorice root tea is an effective way to deliver the benefits of this herb to children suffering from coughs and sore throats.

- **Preparation:**
  - Steep 1/2 teaspoon of dried licorice root in a cup of hot water for 10 minutes.
  - Strain the tea and let it cool to a comfortable drinking temperature.

- **Dosage:**
  - For young children (ages 1-3): Give 1-2 teaspoons of the cooled tea up to three times a day.
  - For older children (ages 4-12): Give 1/4 to 1/2 cup of the cooled tea up to three times a day.

Licorice Root Syrup: Licorice root syrup can be a more concentrated and palatable option, especially for young children who might be reluctant to drink tea.

- **Preparation:**
  - Simmer 1/4 cup of dried licorice root in 2 cups of water for 20-30 minutes until the liquid reduces by half.
  - Strain the liquid and add 1/2 cup of honey (for children over one year old) or another sweetener.
  - Store the syrup in a sealed jar in the refrigerator.

- **Dosage:**
  - For young children: Give 1/2 teaspoon of the syrup up to three times a day.
  - For older children: Give 1 teaspoon of the syrup up to three times a day.

Licorice Root Lozenges: Licorice root lozenges can be used to soothe throat irritation and reduce coughing in older children.

- **Preparation:**

- o Licorice root lozenges are often available in health food stores or can be made at home by combining licorice root extract with a binding agent such as honey or glycerin.

- o Follow the dosage instructions on the product label or consult a healthcare provider for specific recommendations.

Licorice Root Steam Inhalation: Steam inhalation with licorice root can help clear congestion and soothe inflamed airways.

- **Preparation:**

  - o Add a few drops of licorice root extract or a small amount of dried licorice root to a bowl of hot water.

  - o Allow the child to inhale the steam (under supervision) for 5-10 minutes. Ensure the water is not too hot to avoid burns.

Safety and Precautions

- **Allergies:** Ensure that your child is not allergic to licorice root. Monitor for any signs of an allergic reaction, such as rash, itching, or swelling. Discontinue use and seek medical advice if any adverse reactions occur.

- **Proper Dosage:** Always follow the recommended dosages for children and consult with a healthcare provider before starting any new herbal treatment, especially for young children.

- **Duration of Use:** Licorice root should not be used continuously for extended periods, as excessive use can lead to side effects such as increased blood pressure or potassium depletion. Limit use to a few weeks and consult a healthcare provider for guidance.

Success Stories

Case Study:

- **Background:** Noah, a 7-year-old, frequently experienced persistent coughs and sore throats during the winter months. His parents wanted to find a natural remedy to alleviate his symptoms.

- **Experience:** Noah's parents started giving him 1/4 cup of licorice root tea three times a day at the first sign of a cough. The soothing and expectorant effects of the tea helped reduce his coughing and throat irritation significantly. Over time, Noah's respiratory symptoms became less frequent and less severe.

- **Testimonial:** "Licorice root tea has been a fantastic remedy for Noah. It soothes his cough quickly and effectively, and he enjoys drinking it. It's reassuring to have a natural remedy that works so well."

Licorice root is a powerful natural remedy for treating respiratory conditions in children, offering both expectorant and anti-inflammatory benefits. By loosening and expelling mucus, reducing inflammation, and soothing irritated throats, licorice root can effectively alleviate the discomfort associated with coughs and sore throats. Always ensure proper preparation and dosages, and consult with a healthcare provider before starting any new herbal treatment. Integrating licorice root into your child's care routine can provide natural, effective relief from respiratory symptoms and support their overall health and well-being.

BOOK 16:

Herbs for Cognitive Development Support: You absolutely must know them

Cognitive development in children is a crucial aspect of their overall growth and well-being. It encompasses the progression of learning, memory, problem-solving, and decision-making abilities. As children grow, their brains undergo rapid changes and development, requiring adequate nutrition and support to ensure optimal functioning. While a balanced diet and healthy lifestyle are fundamental, certain herbs can provide additional benefits to support cognitive development. These herbs have been traditionally used to enhance memory, improve concentration, and promote overall brain health. This chapter explores the various herbs known for their cognitive benefits and how they can be safely incorporated into a child's routine to support and enhance their cognitive development naturally.

Enhancing Memory and Concentration

Memory and concentration are vital components of cognitive development, playing a crucial role in a child's ability to learn, retain information, and perform well academically and in daily activities. Certain herbs have been found to enhance these cognitive functions by supporting brain health, improving blood flow to the brain, and providing essential nutrients. Here are some herbs that can be beneficial for enhancing memory and concentration in children:

Ginkgo Biloba: Improving Blood Flow to the Brain

Ginkgo Biloba: Ginkgo biloba is one of the oldest living tree species and has been used for centuries in traditional medicine. It is well-known for its ability to improve blood flow, particularly to the brain, which can enhance cognitive function.

- **Benefits:**
  - Enhances memory and cognitive processing
  - Improves concentration and attention span
  - Provides antioxidant protection to brain cells
- **Usage:**

- Ginkgo Biloba Tea: Steep 1 teaspoon of dried ginkgo leaves in a cup of hot water for 5-10 minutes. Let it cool and give 1/4 cup to older children (ages 6 and up) up to twice daily.
- Ginkgo Biloba Capsules: Follow the dosage instructions on the product label, typically starting with a low dose to ensure tolerance.

Bacopa Monnieri: Supporting Cognitive Function

Bacopa Monnieri: Bacopa monnieri, also known as Brahmi, is an herb traditionally used in Ayurvedic medicine to enhance cognitive function and memory. It is particularly effective in supporting brain health and improving learning capabilities.

- **Benefits:**
  - Boosts memory retention and recall
  - Enhances cognitive performance and learning ability
  - Reduces anxiety and stress, which can improve concentration
- **Usage:**
  - **Bacopa Tea:** Steep 1/2 teaspoon of dried bacopa leaves in a cup of hot water for 5-10 minutes. Let it cool and give 1-2 teaspoons to young children and 1/4 cup to older children (ages 6 and up) up to twice daily.
  - **Bacopa Capsules:** Follow the dosage instructions on the product label, ensuring it is suitable for children.

Gotu Kola: Enhancing Brain Function

Gotu Kola (Centella Asiatica): Gotu kola is another Ayurvedic herb known for its ability to enhance brain function, improve memory, and support mental clarity. It helps increase circulation and oxygen supply to the brain.

- **Benefits:**
  - Improves memory and cognitive function
  - Enhances mental clarity and focus
  - Supports overall brain health
- **Usage:**
  - **Gotu Kola Tea:** Steep 1/2 teaspoon of dried gotu kola leaves in a cup of hot water for 5-10 minutes. Let it cool and give 1-2 teaspoons to young children and 1/4 cup to older children (ages 6 and up) up to twice daily.
  - **Gotu Kola Capsules:** Follow the dosage instructions on the product label, ensuring it is appropriate for children.

Lemon Balm: Calming and Focusing

Lemon Balm (Melissa officinalis): Lemon balm is a gentle herb known for its calming effects. It helps reduce anxiety and improve mood, which can enhance concentration and cognitive performance.

- **Benefits:**
    - Reduces anxiety and stress
    - Improves mood and promotes relaxation
    - Enhances concentration and mental clarity

- **Usage:**
    - **Lemon Balm Tea:** Steep 1 teaspoon of dried lemon balm leaves in a cup of hot water for 5-10 minutes. Let it cool and give 1-2 teaspoons to young children and 1/4 cup to older children up to twice daily.

Rosemary: Stimulating Memory and Mental Clarity

Rosemary (Rosmarinus officinalis): Rosemary is an aromatic herb that has been associated with improved memory and mental clarity. It stimulates brain function and enhances cognitive performance.

- **Benefits:**
    - Boosts memory and cognitive performance
    - Enhances mental clarity and focus
    - Provides antioxidant support to brain cells

- **Usage:**
    - **Rosemary Tea:** Steep 1/2 teaspoon of dried rosemary leaves in a cup of hot water for 5-10 minutes. Let it cool and give 1-2 teaspoons to young children and 1/4 cup to older children up to twice daily.
    - **Aromatherapy:** Diffuse rosemary essential oil in a well-ventilated room to create a stimulating environment for study and focus.

Herbs such as Ginkgo Biloba, Bacopa Monnieri, Gotu Kola, Lemon Balm, and Rosemary can effectively enhance memory and concentration in children. These herbs support brain health, improve blood flow to the brain, reduce anxiety, and provide essential nutrients that boost cognitive function. Always ensure proper dosages and consult with a healthcare provider before incorporating new herbs into your child's routine. By integrating these herbal remedies, you can support your child's cognitive development naturally and help them achieve their full potential in learning and daily activities.

Ginkgo Biloba: Improving Blood Flow to the Brain

Ginkgo biloba is one of the oldest living tree species and has been used for thousands of years in traditional medicine to enhance cognitive function and memory. This herb is particularly valued for its ability to improve blood flow to the brain, which is essential for maintaining healthy cognitive functions such as memory, focus, and mental clarity. Here's how ginkgo biloba can be used to support cognitive development in children.

How Ginkgo Biloba Works?

Ginkgo biloba contains several active compounds, including flavonoids and terpenoids, which contribute to its therapeutic effects:

- **Improving Blood Flow:** Ginkgo biloba helps dilate blood vessels and reduce blood viscosity, thereby improving blood circulation, particularly to the brain.

- **Antioxidant Properties:** The flavonoids in ginkgo biloba provide powerful antioxidant protection, helping to combat oxidative stress and protect brain cells from damage.

- **Neuroprotective Effects:** Ginkgo biloba supports overall brain health by protecting neurons and enhancing neurotransmitter function, which is crucial for learning and memory.

Using Ginkgo Biloba for Cognitive Support

Ginkgo Biloba Tea: Ginkgo biloba tea is a simple and effective way to deliver the cognitive benefits of this herb to children.

- **Preparation:**

  - Steep 1 teaspoon of dried ginkgo biloba leaves in a cup of hot water for 5-10 minutes.

  - Strain the tea and let it cool to a comfortable drinking temperature.

- **Dosage:**

  - For older children (ages 6 and up): Give 1/4 cup of the cooled tea up to twice daily.

Ginkgo Biloba Capsules: Ginkgo biloba capsules can be a convenient alternative, especially for older children who can swallow capsules.

- **Dosage:**

  - Follow the dosage instructions on the product label. It is typically recommended to start with a low dose to ensure tolerance and then adjust as needed.

Ginkgo Biloba Tincture: Ginkgo biloba tincture can be another effective form of administration.

- **Preparation:**

  - Use a glycerin-based tincture for children, as it is alcohol-free and more palatable.

- **Dosage:**

- For older children: Use 5-10 drops of the tincture diluted in water or juice up to twice daily.

Safety and Precautions

- **Allergies:** Ensure that your child is not allergic to ginkgo biloba. Monitor for any signs of an allergic reaction, such as rash, itching, or swelling. Discontinue use and seek medical advice if any adverse reactions occur.

- **Proper Dosage:** Always follow the recommended dosages for children and consult with a healthcare provider before starting any new herbal treatment, especially for young children.

- **Potential Side Effects:** While ginkgo biloba is generally safe, some children may experience mild side effects such as stomach upset, headache, or dizziness. If any of these occur, reduce the dosage or discontinue use.

- **Interactions:** Ginkgo biloba may interact with certain medications, such as blood thinners. Consult a healthcare provider if your child is taking any medications.

Success Stories

Case Study:

- **Background:** Emma, a 10-year-old, had difficulty focusing in school and often struggled with memory retention. Her parents sought a natural remedy to help improve her cognitive function.

- **Experience:** Emma's parents started giving her 1/4 cup of ginkgo biloba tea twice daily. Over the next few weeks, they noticed significant improvements in her concentration and memory. Emma reported feeling more alert and able to focus better in class.

- **Testimonial:** "Ginkgo biloba tea has made a noticeable difference for Emma. She's more focused and her memory has improved. It's great to see her doing better in school with the help of a natural remedy."

Ginkgo biloba is a powerful herb that can significantly enhance cognitive function in children by improving blood flow to the brain, providing antioxidant protection, and supporting overall brain health. Whether used as a tea, capsule, or tincture, ginkgo biloba can help boost memory, concentration, and mental clarity. Always ensure proper dosages and consult with a healthcare provider before incorporating ginkgo biloba into your child's routine. By integrating this herb, you can support your child's cognitive development and help them achieve their full potential in learning and daily activities.

Bacopa Monnieri: Supporting Cognitive Function

Bacopa monnieri, commonly known as Brahmi, is a revered herb in Ayurvedic medicine, traditionally used to enhance cognitive function, memory, and learning. It has gained recognition for its ability to support brain health and improve cognitive performance, making it an excellent choice for children who need a natural boost in their mental abilities. Here's how Bacopa monnieri can be used to support cognitive function in children.

How Bacopa Monnieri Works

Bacopa monnieri contains several bioactive compounds, including bacosides, which are primarily responsible for its cognitive-enhancing effects:

- **Neuroprotective Properties:** Bacosides help protect brain cells from damage and support the repair of damaged neurons, enhancing overall brain function.

- **Memory Enhancement:** Bacopa monnieri improves memory retention and recall by enhancing synaptic communication and promoting the growth of dendrites, which are involved in learning and memory.

- **Anti-Anxiety Effects:** Bacopa monnieri helps reduce anxiety and stress, which can improve concentration and cognitive performance.

- **Antioxidant Activity:** The herb provides strong antioxidant protection, reducing oxidative stress and supporting long-term brain health.

Using Bacopa Monnieri for Cognitive Support

Bacopa Monnieri Tea: Bacopa monnieri tea is a simple and effective way to deliver the cognitive benefits of this herb to children.

- **Preparation:**
  - Steep 1/2 teaspoon of dried bacopa monnieri leaves in a cup of hot water for 5-10 minutes.
  - Strain the tea and let it cool to a comfortable drinking temperature.

- **Dosage:**
  - For young children (ages 4-6): Give 1-2 teaspoons of the cooled tea up to twice daily.
  - For older children (ages 7 and up): Give 1/4 cup of the cooled tea up to twice daily.

Bacopa Monnieri Syrup: Bacopa monnieri syrup can be a more concentrated and palatable option, especially for younger children who might be reluctant to drink tea.

- **Preparation:**
  - Simmer 1/4 cup of dried bacopa monnieri leaves in 2 cups of water for 20-30 minutes until the liquid reduces by half.
  - Strain the liquid and add 1/2 cup of honey (for children over one year old) or another sweetener.
  - Store the syrup in a sealed jar in the refrigerator.

- **Dosage:**
  - For young children: Give 1/2 teaspoon of the syrup up to twice daily.
  - For older children: Give 1 teaspoon of the syrup up to twice daily.

Bacopa Monnieri Capsules: Bacopa monnieri capsules can be a convenient alternative, especially for older children who can swallow capsules.

- **Dosage:**
  - Follow the dosage instructions on the product label, typically starting with a low dose to ensure tolerance and then adjusting as needed.

Safety and Precautions

- **Allergies:** Ensure that your child is not allergic to bacopa monnieri. Monitor for any signs of an allergic reaction, such as rash, itching, or swelling. Discontinue use and seek medical advice if any adverse reactions occur.

- **Proper Dosage:** Always follow the recommended dosages for children and consult with a healthcare provider before starting any new herbal treatment, especially for young children.

- **Potential Side Effects:** While bacopa monnieri is generally safe, some children may experience mild side effects such as stomach upset or dry mouth. If any of these occur, reduce the dosage or discontinue use.

- **Interactions:** Bacopa monnieri may interact with certain medications, such as those for thyroid conditions. Consult a healthcare provider if your child is taking any medications.

Success Stories

Case Study:

- **Background:** James, an 8-year-old, struggled with attention and memory in school, affecting his academic performance. His parents were looking for a natural way to support his cognitive function.

- **Experience:** James's parents started giving him 1/4 cup of bacopa monnieri tea twice daily. Over the next few weeks, they noticed significant improvements in his attention span and memory recall. James reported feeling more focused and capable in his studies.

- **Testimonial:** "Bacopa monnieri tea has been a game-changer for James. He's more focused and his memory has improved. It's wonderful to see him more confident and performing better in school."

Bacopa monnieri is a powerful herb that can significantly enhance cognitive function in children by supporting brain health, improving memory retention, and reducing anxiety. Whether used as a tea, syrup, or capsule, bacopa monnieri can help boost cognitive performance and support overall mental well-being. Always ensure proper dosages and consult with a healthcare provider before incorporating bacopa monnieri into your child's routine. By integrating this herb, you can support your child's cognitive development and help them achieve their full potential in learning and daily activities.

Supporting Emotional Well-being

Emotional well-being is crucial for the overall health and development of children. It encompasses a child's ability to understand, manage, and express emotions, as well as their capacity to form healthy relationships and cope with stress. Herbal remedies can provide gentle and natural support for emotional well-being, helping to reduce anxiety, improve mood, and promote relaxation.

Chamomile: Calming and Relaxing

Chamomile (Matricaria chamomilla) is a well-known herb that has been used for centuries to promote relaxation and reduce anxiety. Its calming effects are especially beneficial for children who may experience nervousness, restlessness, or difficulty sleeping. Chamomile contains apigenin, a compound that binds to certain receptors in the brain, promoting a sense of calm and reducing anxiety. A warm cup of chamomile tea before bed can help soothe a child's nerves and prepare them for restful sleep. Additionally, chamomile's gentle nature makes it suitable for young children, providing a safe and effective way to support their emotional well-being.

Lemon Balm: Uplifting and Soothing

Lemon balm (Melissa officinalis) is another excellent herb for supporting emotional well-being in children. Known for its uplifting and soothing properties, lemon balm helps to alleviate anxiety, improve mood, and enhance cognitive function. Its mild sedative effects can help calm an anxious mind and promote a sense of relaxation. Lemon balm is particularly useful for children who experience mood swings or who need help winding down after a busy day. A tea made from lemon balm leaves can be a delightful and effective way to help children feel more balanced and at ease.

Lavender: Reducing Stress and Anxiety

Lavender (Lavandula angustifolia) is renowned for its stress-relieving and anxiety-reducing properties. The soothing aroma of lavender can help calm the mind and body, making it an ideal herb for promoting emotional well-being in children. Lavender can be used in various forms, such as essential oils, teas, or even dried flowers placed under a pillow. For children, a few drops of lavender essential oil in a diffuser can create a calming atmosphere in their room, helping them to relax and sleep better. Lavender tea can also be a gentle way to reduce stress and promote a sense of tranquility.

Passionflower: Easing Anxiety and Promoting Relaxation

Passionflower (Passiflora incarnata) is known for its ability to ease anxiety and promote relaxation without causing drowsiness. It works by increasing the levels of gamma-aminobutyric acid (GABA) in the brain, a neurotransmitter that helps regulate mood and reduce anxiety.

Passionflower can be particularly helpful for children who struggle with feelings of anxiety or who have difficulty unwinding before bedtime. A mild tea made from passionflower can be an effective way to help children feel more relaxed and emotionally balanced.

Holy Basil: Enhancing Emotional Balance

Holy basil (Ocimum sanctum), also known as Tulsi, is revered in Ayurvedic medicine for its adaptogenic properties, which help the body adapt to stress and promote emotional balance. Holy basil can help reduce anxiety, improve mood, and enhance overall mental clarity. It is particularly beneficial for children who may feel overwhelmed by stress or who need support in managing their emotions. A tea made from holy basil leaves can provide a comforting and balancing effect, helping children to feel more centered and resilient.

Supporting the emotional well-being of children is essential for their overall development and quality of life. Herbs such as chamomile, lemon balm, lavender, passionflower, and holy basil offer gentle and effective ways to promote relaxation, reduce anxiety, and enhance mood. Incorporating these herbs into a child's daily routine, whether through teas, aromatherapy, or other preparations, can provide natural support for their emotional health. Always ensure proper dosages and consult with a healthcare provider before starting any new herbal regimen. By integrating these herbs, you can help foster a nurturing environment that supports your child's emotional well-being and overall happiness.

Lemon Balm: Calming Anxiety

Lemon balm (Melissa officinalis) is a versatile herb known for its calming and soothing properties, making it an excellent natural remedy for alleviating anxiety and promoting emotional well-being in children. Its mild sedative effects and pleasant lemony scent can help reduce stress, improve mood, and enhance cognitive function. Here's how lemon balm can be used to calm anxiety and support emotional health in children.

How Lemon Balm Works

Lemon balm contains several active compounds, including rosmarinic acid, flavonoids, and essential oils, which contribute to its therapeutic effects:

- **Calming and Sedative Effects:** Lemon balm has mild sedative properties that help to relax the nervous system, making it effective in reducing anxiety and stress.

- **Antioxidant Properties:** The antioxidants in lemon balm help protect the brain from oxidative stress, which can negatively impact emotional health.

- **Mood Enhancement:** Lemon balm can improve mood and cognitive function, helping children feel more balanced and focused.

Using Lemon Balm to Calm Anxiety

Lemon Balm Tea: Lemon balm tea is a simple and effective way to deliver the calming benefits of this herb to children.

- **Preparation:**

- Steep 1 teaspoon of dried lemon balm leaves in a cup of hot water for 5-10 minutes.
- Strain the tea and let it cool to a comfortable drinking temperature.

- **Dosage:**
  - For young children (ages 4-6): Give 1-2 teaspoons of the cooled tea up to twice daily.
  - For older children (ages 7 and up): Give 1/4 cup of the cooled tea up to twice daily.

Lemon Balm Syrup: Lemon balm syrup can be a more concentrated and palatable option, especially for younger children who might be reluctant to drink tea.

- **Preparation:**
  - Simmer 1/4 cup of dried lemon balm leaves in 2 cups of water for 20-30 minutes until the liquid reduces by half.
  - Strain the liquid and add 1/2 cup of honey (for children over one year old) or another sweetener.
  - Store the syrup in a sealed jar in the refrigerator.

- **Dosage:**
  - For young children: Give 1/2 teaspoon of the syrup up to twice daily.
  - For older children: Give 1 teaspoon of the syrup up to twice daily.

Lemon Balm Essential Oil: Lemon balm essential oil can be used in aromatherapy to create a calming environment for children.

- **Preparation:**
  - Add a few drops of lemon balm essential oil to a diffuser in the child's room.
  - Alternatively, dilute a few drops of the essential oil in a carrier oil (such as almond or coconut oil) and use it for a gentle massage or apply to pulse points.

- **Usage:**
  - Use the diffuser or apply the diluted oil before bedtime or during times of anxiety to help calm and relax the child.

Lemon Balm Infused Bath: A lemon balm-infused bath can provide a soothing and calming experience for children.

- **Preparation:**

- Add a handful of dried lemon balm leaves to a muslin bag or cheesecloth and tie it securely.
- Place the bag in a warm bath and let it steep for a few minutes.
- Allow the child to soak in the bath for 15-20 minutes.

Safety and Precautions

- **Allergies:** Ensure that your child is not allergic to lemon balm. Monitor for any signs of an allergic reaction, such as rash, itching, or swelling. Discontinue use and seek medical advice if any adverse reactions occur.

- **Proper Dosage:** Always follow the recommended dosages for children and consult with a healthcare provider before starting any new herbal treatment, especially for young children.

- **Potential Side Effects:** Lemon balm is generally safe, but some children may experience mild side effects such as stomach upset or drowsiness. If any of these occur, reduce the dosage or discontinue use.

Success Stories

Case Study:

- **Background:** Sarah, a 7-year-old, often experienced anxiety and had trouble winding down before bedtime. Her parents were looking for a natural remedy to help calm her nerves.

- **Experience:** Sarah's parents started giving her 1/4 cup of lemon balm tea twice daily, particularly before bedtime. They also used lemon balm essential oil in a diffuser in her room. Over the next few weeks, they noticed a significant reduction in Sarah's anxiety levels, and she was able to relax and sleep better.

- **Testimonial:** "Lemon balm has been wonderful for Sarah. It helps her feel more relaxed and she sleeps so much better. We love that it's a natural remedy that's safe and effective."

Lemon balm is a powerful yet gentle herb that can effectively calm anxiety and promote emotional well-being in children. Whether used as a tea, syrup, essential oil, or infused bath, lemon balm provides soothing and calming effects that help reduce stress and improve mood. Always ensure proper dosages and consult with a healthcare provider before incorporating lemon balm into your child's routine. By integrating this herb, you can support your child's emotional health and help them navigate stress and anxiety more comfortably.

Chamomile: Promoting Relaxation and Reducing Hyperactivity

Chamomile (Matricaria chamomilla) is one of the most well-known and widely used herbs for promoting relaxation and reducing hyperactivity, especially in children. Its gentle, calming effects make it an ideal remedy for children who experience anxiety, restlessness, or difficulty winding down. Chamomile is also highly regarded for its ability to soothe digestive issues and promote restful sleep, making it a versatile herb for overall well-being.

Promoting Relaxation

Chamomile contains several active compounds, including apigenin, a flavonoid that binds to specific receptors in the brain, producing a calming effect. This helps to reduce anxiety and stress, promoting a sense of relaxation. For children who struggle with anxiety or find it difficult to relax after a busy day, a warm cup of chamomile tea can be a simple yet effective remedy. The gentle sedative properties of chamomile help ease the mind and body, making it easier for children to transition into a more relaxed state. Chamomile's pleasant taste and mild nature make it a favorite among parents looking for a natural way to calm their children.

Reducing Hyperactivity

Hyperactivity in children can be challenging to manage and can interfere with their ability to focus and perform daily tasks. Chamomile can help reduce hyperactivity by calming the nervous system and promoting a balanced state of mind. The soothing effects of chamomile can help children who are overly energetic or easily overstimulated to feel more grounded and centered. Regular use of chamomile, whether in the form of tea, tincture, or bath, can help maintain a sense of calm and reduce instances of hyperactivity, leading to improved behavior and focus.

Chamomile Tea

Chamomile tea is one of the most common and effective ways to use this herb. It's easy to prepare and can be given to children as part of their bedtime routine to help them unwind.

- **Preparation:**
    - Steep 1 teaspoon of dried chamomile flowers in a cup of hot water for 5-10 minutes.
    - Strain the tea and let it cool to a comfortable drinking temperature.
- **Dosage:**
    - For young children (ages 2-4): Give 1-2 teaspoons of the cooled tea up to twice daily.
    - For older children (ages 5-12): Give 1/4 to 1/2 cup of the cooled tea up to twice daily.

Chamomile Bath

A chamomile-infused bath can be a soothing way to help children relax before bedtime. The warm water combined with the calming properties of chamomile can create a perfect environment for winding down.

- **Preparation:**

- Add a handful of dried chamomile flowers to a muslin bag or cheesecloth and tie it securely.
- Place the bag in a warm bath and let it steep for a few minutes.
- Allow the child to soak in the bath for 15-20 minutes.

Chamomile Tincture

Chamomile tincture can be a more concentrated form of this herb, suitable for older children who may need stronger support.

- **Preparation:**
    - Use a glycerin-based tincture for children, as it is alcohol-free and more palatable.
- **Dosage:**
    - For older children: Use 5-10 drops of the tincture diluted in water or juice up to twice daily.

Safety and Precautions

- **Allergies:** Ensure that your child is not allergic to chamomile, especially if they have allergies to other plants in the Asteraceae family, such as ragweed. Monitor for any signs of an allergic reaction, such as rash, itching, or swelling. Discontinue use and seek medical advice if any adverse reactions occur.

- **Proper Dosage:** Always follow the recommended dosages for children and consult with a healthcare provider before starting any new herbal treatment, especially for young children.

- **Potential Side Effects:** Chamomile is generally safe, but some children may experience mild side effects such as stomach upset or drowsiness. If any of these occur, reduce the dosage or discontinue use.

Success Stories

Case Study:

- **Background:** Jack, a 6-year-old, often struggled with hyperactivity and had difficulty relaxing before bedtime. His parents were looking for a natural remedy to help him calm down.

- **Experience:** Jack's parents started giving him 1/4 cup of chamomile tea each evening before bed. They also prepared a chamomile-infused bath for him twice a week. Over the next few weeks, they noticed a significant improvement in Jack's ability to relax and his hyperactivity levels decreased.

- **Testimonial:** "Chamomile tea and baths have made a huge difference for Jack. He's able to calm down much more easily, and bedtime has become a lot less stressful. We're so happy to have found a natural solution that works."

Chamomile is a gentle yet powerful herb that can effectively promote relaxation and reduce hyperactivity in children. Its calming effects help ease anxiety and stress, making it easier for children to unwind and prepare for restful sleep. Whether used as a tea, tincture, or in a soothing bath, chamomile provides a natural and safe way to support your child's emotional well-being and overall health. Always ensure proper dosages and consult with a healthcare provider before incorporating chamomile into your child's routine. By integrating this herb, you can help create a peaceful and balanced environment that supports your child's relaxation and emotional stability.

Herbal Teas and Tinctures for Study Time

Herbal teas and tinctures can provide a natural and effective way to support children's focus, memory, and cognitive function during study time. Certain herbs are known for their ability to enhance mental clarity, reduce stress, and promote a calm yet alert state of mind, making them ideal for supporting academic performance. Here are some beneficial herbal teas and tinctures that can be incorporated into a child's study routine to help them concentrate and perform better academically.

Ginkgo Biloba Tea: Enhancing Memory and Focus

Ginkgo Biloba (Ginkgo biloba): Ginkgo biloba is renowned for its ability to improve blood flow to the brain, which enhances memory and cognitive function. It is particularly useful for improving focus and mental clarity, making it an excellent choice for study time.

- **Preparation:**
    - Steep 1 teaspoon of dried ginkgo biloba leaves in a cup of hot water for 5-10 minutes.
    - Strain the tea and let it cool to a comfortable drinking temperature.

- **Dosage:**
    - For older children (ages 6 and up): Give 1/4 cup of the cooled tea up to twice daily.

Lemon Balm Tea: Reducing Anxiety and Enhancing Concentration

Lemon Balm (Melissa officinalis): Lemon balm is known for its calming and soothing properties, which can help reduce anxiety and improve mood. It also enhances cognitive function and concentration, making it a great herb for study time.

- **Preparation:**
    - Steep 1 teaspoon of dried lemon balm leaves in a cup of hot water for 5-10 minutes.
    - Strain the tea and let it cool to a comfortable drinking temperature.

- **Dosage:**

- For young children (ages 4-6): Give 1-2 teaspoons of the cooled tea up to twice daily.

- For older children (ages 7 and up): Give 1/4 cup of the cooled tea up to twice daily.

Peppermint Tea: Boosting Alertness and Mental Clarity

Peppermint (Mentha piperita): Peppermint is known for its refreshing and invigorating properties. It can help boost alertness, enhance mental clarity, and improve overall cognitive function, making it a perfect choice for study sessions.

- **Preparation:**
  - Steep 1 teaspoon of dried peppermint leaves in a cup of hot water for 5-10 minutes.
  - Strain the tea and let it cool to a comfortable drinking temperature.

- **Dosage:**
  - For young children (ages 4-6): Give 1-2 teaspoons of the cooled tea up to twice daily.
  - For older children (ages 7 and up): Give 1/4 cup of the cooled tea up to twice daily.

Rosemary Tea: Stimulating Memory and Cognitive Performance

Rosemary (Rosmarinus officinalis): Rosemary is an aromatic herb that has been associated with improved memory and cognitive performance. Its stimulating properties can help enhance mental clarity and focus during study time.

- **Preparation:**
  - Steep 1/2 teaspoon of dried rosemary leaves in a cup of hot water for 5-10 minutes.
  - Strain the tea and let it cool to a comfortable drinking temperature.

- **Dosage:**
  - For young children (ages 4-6): Give 1-2 teaspoons of the cooled tea up to twice daily.
  - For older children (ages 7 and up): Give 1/4 cup of cooled tea up to twice daily.

Bacopa Monnieri Tincture: Supporting Cognitive Function

Bacopa Monnieri (Bacopa monnieri): Bacopa monnieri, also known as Brahmi, is a traditional Ayurvedic herb known for its ability to enhance cognitive function and memory. It can be particularly beneficial for improving learning and focus.

- **Preparation:**
  - Use a glycerin-based tincture for children, as it is alcohol-free and more palatable.
- **Dosage:**
  - For young children (ages 4-6): Use 5 drops of tincture diluted in water or juice up to twice daily.
  - For older children (ages 7 and up): Use 10 drops of the tincture diluted in water or juice up to twice daily.

Holy Basil Tincture: Promoting Mental Clarity and Emotional Balance

Holy Basil (Ocimum sanctum): Holy basil, also known as Tulsi, is revered in Ayurvedic medicine for its adaptogenic properties. It helps the body adapt to stress and promotes mental clarity and emotional balance, making it ideal for supporting cognitive function during study time.

- **Preparation:**
  - Use a glycerin-based tincture for children, as it is alcohol-free and more palatable.
- **Dosage:**
  - For young children (ages 4-6): Use 5 drops of the tincture diluted in water or juice up to twice daily.
  - For older children (ages 7 and up): Use 10 drops of the tincture diluted in water or juice up to twice daily.

Incorporating herbal teas and tinctures into a child's study routine can provide significant benefits for their cognitive function, memory, and concentration. Herbs such as ginkgo biloba, lemon balm, peppermint, rosemary, bacopa monnieri, and holy basil offer natural support to enhance mental clarity, reduce anxiety, and promote overall cognitive health. Always ensure proper dosages and consult with a healthcare provider before starting any new herbal regimen. By integrating these herbal remedies, you can help create an optimal environment for learning and academic success.

Creating Blends for Focus and Calm

Creating herbal blends that promote focus and calm can be an effective way to support children's cognitive and emotional well-being. Combining herbs that enhance mental clarity, reduce anxiety, and promote relaxation can provide a balanced approach to help children concentrate during study time and stay calm in stressful situations. Here are some well-balanced herbal blends that can be prepared as teas or tinctures to support focus and calm.

Focus and Calm Tea Blend

This tea blend combines the calming properties of chamomile and lemon balm with the cognitive-enhancing benefits of ginkgo biloba and peppermint. It is designed to help children stay focused and calm during study sessions or other activities that require concentration.

Ingredients:

- 1 part chamomile (Matricaria chamomilla)
- 1 part lemon balm (Melissa officinalis)
- 1/2 part ginkgo biloba (Ginkgo biloba)
- 1/2 part peppermint (Mentha piperita)

Preparation:

1. **Mix the Herbs:** Combine the dried chamomile, lemon balm, ginkgo biloba, and peppermint in a jar or airtight container. Shake well to mix the herbs thoroughly.
2. **Steep the Tea:** Use 1 teaspoon of the herb blend per cup of hot water. Steep for 5-10 minutes.
3. **Strain and Cool:** Strain the tea and let it cool to a comfortable drinking temperature.

Dosage:

- For young children (ages 4-6): Give 1-2 teaspoons of the cooled tea up to twice daily.
- For older children (ages 7 and up): Give 1/4 to 1/2 cup of the cooled tea up to twice daily.

Concentration and Relaxation Tea Blend

This tea blend combines the stress-relieving properties of holy basil and lemon balm with the memory-enhancing effects of rosemary and the calming nature of chamomile. It is ideal for helping children stay calm and focused during study time.

Ingredients:

- 1 part holy basil (Ocimum sanctum)
- 1 part lemon balm (Melissa officinalis)
- 1/2 part rosemary (Rosmarinus officinalis)
- 1 part chamomile (Matricaria chamomilla)

Preparation:

1. **Mix the Herbs:** Combine the dried holy basil, lemon balm, rosemary, and chamomile in a jar or airtight container. Shake well to mix the herbs thoroughly.
2. **Steep the Tea:** Use 1 teaspoon of the herb blend per cup of hot water. Steep for 5-10 minutes.

3. **Strain and Cool:** Strain the tea and let it cool to a comfortable drinking temperature.

Dosage:

- For young children (ages 4-6): Give 1-2 teaspoons of the cooled tea up to twice daily.

- For older children (ages 7 and up): Give 1/4 to 1/2 cup of the cooled tea up to twice daily.

Focus and Calm Tincture Blend

This tincture blend combines the cognitive benefits of bacopa monnieri and ginkgo biloba with the calming effects of chamomile and lemon balm. It is a convenient and potent way to support focus and calm in children.

Ingredients:

- 1 part bacopa monnieri (Bacopa monnieri)

- 1 part ginkgo biloba (Ginkgo biloba)

- 1 part chamomile (Matricaria chamomilla)

- 1 part lemon balm (Melissa officinalis)

Preparation:

1. **Mix the Herbs:** Combine the glycerin-based tinctures of bacopa monnieri, ginkgo biloba, chamomile, and lemon balm in a dark glass bottle with a dropper. Shake well to mix the tinctures thoroughly.

Dosage:

- For young children (ages 4-6): Use 5 drops of the tincture blend diluted in water or juice up to twice daily.

- For older children (ages 7 and up): Use 10 drops of the tincture blend diluted in water or juice up to twice daily.

Tips for Success

1. **Quality Ingredients:** Use high-quality, organic herbs to ensure the best therapeutic effects.

2. **Consistency:** For optimal results, use the herbal blends consistently. It may take some time for the full benefits to be realized.

3. **Hydration:** Encourage children to stay well-hydrated, as proper hydration is crucial for cognitive function.

4. **Monitoring:** Monitor the child's response to the herbal blends and adjust dosages if necessary. Consult with a healthcare provider if you have any concerns.

Creating herbal blends for focus and calm can provide children with natural support for their cognitive and emotional well-being. Blends that combine herbs such as chamomile, lemon balm, ginkgo biloba, peppermint, rosemary, holy basil, and bacopa monnieri can enhance mental clarity, reduce anxiety, and promote relaxation. Always ensure proper dosages and consult with a healthcare provider before starting any new herbal regimen. By integrating these herbal blends into your child's routine, you can help them achieve better focus and emotional balance, supporting their overall health and academic success.

Herbal Remedies for Childhood Allergies

Childhood allergies can cause significant discomfort and impact a child's overall well-being, affecting their daily activities, sleep, and school performance. Common symptoms include sneezing, runny nose, itchy eyes, and skin rashes. While conventional medications are available to manage these symptoms, many parents seek natural alternatives to avoid potential side effects. Herbal remedies offer a gentle and effective approach to alleviate allergy symptoms and support the immune system. This chapter explores various herbs known for their anti-inflammatory, antihistamine, and immune-boosting properties, providing natural solutions to help manage and reduce the impact of childhood allergies.

Managing Seasonal Allergies Naturally

Seasonal allergies, also known as hay fever or allergic rhinitis, are common in children and can cause symptoms such as sneezing, runny nose, itchy eyes, and congestion. These symptoms can significantly affect a child's quality of life, disrupting their sleep, concentration, and overall comfort. Natural remedies can provide relief from these symptoms and help manage seasonal allergies without the side effects associated with conventional medications. Here are some effective herbal and natural remedies for managing seasonal allergies in children.

Stinging Nettle: Natural Antihistamine

Stinging Nettle (Urtica dioica): Stinging nettle is a powerful natural antihistamine that can help reduce allergy symptoms such as sneezing and itching. It works by inhibiting the production of histamine, the compound responsible for allergic reactions.

- **Preparation:**
    - Steep 1 teaspoon of dried stinging nettle leaves in a cup of hot water for 5-10 minutes.
    - Strain the tea and let it cool to a comfortable drinking temperature.
- **Dosage:**
    - For young children (ages 4-6): Give 1-2 teaspoons of the cooled tea up to twice daily.
    - For older children (ages 7 and up): Give 1/4 cup of the cooled tea up to twice daily.

Butterbur: Reducing Inflammation

Butterbur (Petasites hybridus): Butterbur is known for its anti-inflammatory properties, which can help reduce nasal congestion and other allergy symptoms. It is particularly effective in managing hay fever symptoms.

- **Preparation:**
  - Use a standardized butterbur supplement or extract, ensuring it is free from pyrrolizidine alkaloids (PAs), which can be toxic.

- **Dosage:**
  - Follow the dosage instructions on the product label, and consult with a healthcare provider to ensure it is appropriate for children.

Quercetin: Natural Antioxidant and Antihistamine

Quercetin: Quercetin is a natural flavonoid found in many fruits and vegetables. It has strong antioxidant and anti-inflammatory properties and acts as a natural antihistamine, helping to reduce allergy symptoms.

- **Sources:**
  - Quercetin can be found in apples, onions, berries, and leafy greens. It is also available in supplement form.

- **Dosage:**
  - Consult with a healthcare provider for appropriate quercetin dosages for children if using supplements.

Local Honey: Building Immunity to Pollen

Local Honey: Consuming local honey can help build immunity to local pollen, potentially reducing the severity of seasonal allergies. The theory is that small amounts of pollen in the honey can help desensitize the immune system over time.

- **Usage:**
  - Give 1/2 to 1 teaspoon of local honey daily for children over one year old. Do not give honey to infants under one year due to the risk of botulism.

Eyebright: Alleviating Eye Symptoms

Eyebright (Euphrasia officinalis): Eyebright is traditionally used to alleviate symptoms affecting the eyes, such as redness, itching, and watering, which are common in seasonal allergies.

- **Preparation:**
  - Steep 1/2 teaspoon of dried eyebright in a cup of hot water for 5-10 minutes.

- Strain the tea and let it cool. Use the cooled tea as an eye wash or compress.

- **Dosage:**

  - For eye washes, use the tea to gently rinse the eyes. For compresses, soak a clean cloth in the tea and apply it to closed eyelids for 10-15 minutes.

Rooibos Tea: Anti-inflammatory and Antioxidant

Rooibos (Aspalathus linearis): Rooibos tea is caffeine-free and rich in antioxidants. It has anti-inflammatory properties that can help reduce allergy symptoms.

- **Preparation:**

  - Steep 1 teaspoon of rooibos tea leaves in a cup of hot water for 5-10 minutes.

  - Strain the tea and let it cool to a comfortable drinking temperature.

- **Dosage:**

  - For young children (ages 4-6): Give 1-2 teaspoons of the cooled tea up to twice daily.

  - For older children (ages 7 and up): Give 1/4 cup of the cooled tea up to twice daily.

Safety and Precautions

- **Allergies:** Ensure that your child is not allergic to any of the herbs used. Monitor for any signs of an allergic reaction, such as rash, itching, or swelling. Discontinue use and seek medical advice if any adverse reactions occur.

- **Proper Dosage:** Always follow the recommended dosages for children and consult with a healthcare provider before starting any new herbal treatment, especially for young children.

- **Consult a Healthcare Provider:** Always consult with a healthcare provider before using any new herbs or supplements to ensure they are appropriate for your child's specific health needs and conditions.

Natural remedies such as stinging nettle, butterbur, quercetin, local honey, eyebright, and rooibos tea can provide effective relief from seasonal allergy symptoms in children. These herbs and natural substances help reduce inflammation, act as natural antihistamines, and support overall immune health. Always ensure proper dosages and consult with a healthcare provider before incorporating new herbal remedies into your child's routine. By using these natural approaches, you can help manage your child's seasonal allergies and improve their overall comfort and well-being.

Nettle: Reducing Histamine Reactions

Stinging nettle (Urtica dioica) is a potent herb known for its antihistamine and anti-inflammatory properties, making it an excellent natural remedy for managing allergies. Histamine is a compound released by the immune system during allergic reactions, causing symptoms such as itching, sneezing, and swelling. Nettle works by inhibiting the production of histamine and reducing inflammation, providing relief from these uncomfortable symptoms. Here's how nettle can be used to reduce histamine reactions in children suffering from allergies.

How Nettle Works

Nettle contains several bioactive compounds that contribute to its therapeutic effects:

- **Antihistamine Properties:** Nettle inhibits the release of histamine from mast cells, which helps reduce the severity of allergic reactions.

- **Anti-inflammatory Effects:** The herb contains anti-inflammatory compounds such as flavonoids, which help reduce swelling and inflammation associated with allergies.

- **Rich in Nutrients:** Nettle is rich in vitamins and minerals, including vitamin C, iron, and potassium, which support overall immune health.

Using Nettle for Allergy Relief

Nettle Tea: Nettle tea is a simple and effective way to administer nettle to children. The tea helps reduce histamine levels and alleviate allergy symptoms.

- **Preparation:**
    - Steep 1 teaspoon of dried nettle leaves in a cup of hot water for 5-10 minutes.
    - Strain the tea and let it cool to a comfortable drinking temperature.

- **Dosage:**
    - For young children (ages 4-6): Give 1-2 teaspoons of the cooled tea up to twice daily.
    - For older children (ages 7 and up): Give 1/4 cup of the cooled tea up to twice daily.

Nettle Tincture: A nettle tincture can be a more concentrated and convenient form, especially for children who may not like the taste of nettle tea.

- **Preparation:**
    - Use a glycerin-based tincture for children, as it is alcohol-free and more palatable.

- **Dosage:**
    - For young children (ages 4-6): Use 5 drops of the tincture diluted in water or juice up to twice daily.
    - For older children (ages 7 and up): Use 10 drops of the tincture diluted in water or juice up to twice daily.

Nettle Infused Honey: Combining the benefits of nettle with the soothing properties of honey can create a tasty and effective remedy for allergies.

- **Preparation:**
  - Fill a jar halfway with dried nettle leaves.
  - Pour honey over the nettle leaves until the jar is full.
  - Seal the jar and let it sit for 2-3 weeks, occasionally turning it to ensure the honey infuses with the nettle.
  - Strain the honey to remove the nettle leaves.

- **Dosage:**
  - For children over one year old, give 1/2 to 1 teaspoon of nettle-infused honey daily.

Safety and Precautions

- **Allergies:** Ensure that your child is not allergic to nettle. Monitor for any signs of an allergic reaction, such as rash, itching, or swelling. Discontinue use and seek medical advice if any adverse reactions occur.

- **Proper Dosage:** Always follow the recommended dosages for children and consult with a healthcare provider before starting any new herbal treatment, especially for young children.

- **Consult a Healthcare Provider:** Always consult with a healthcare provider before using a nettle to ensure it is appropriate for your child's specific health needs and conditions.

Success Stories

Case Study:

- **Background:** Lily, a 9-year-old, frequently experienced severe seasonal allergies, causing her significant discomfort and disrupting her daily activities. Her parents sought a natural remedy to help manage her symptoms.

- **Experience:** Lily's parents started giving her 1/4 cup of nettle tea twice daily during allergy season. They also used a glycerin-based nettle tincture for convenience when on the go. Over the next few weeks, they noticed a significant reduction in Lily's allergy symptoms, including less sneezing and itching.

- **Testimonial:** "Nettle tea and tincture have been incredibly effective for Lily's allergies. She's much more comfortable and can enjoy outdoor activities again. It's wonderful to have a natural remedy that works so well."

Stinging nettle is a powerful herb that can effectively reduce histamine reactions and alleviate allergy symptoms in children. Its antihistamine and anti-inflammatory properties make it a natural and safe alternative to conventional allergy medications. Whether used as a tea, tincture, or infused honey, nettle provides significant relief from seasonal allergies. Always ensure proper dosages and consult with a healthcare provider before incorporating nettle into your child's routine. By integrating nettle, you can help manage your child's allergies naturally and improve their overall well-being.

Butterbur: Alleviating Allergy Symptoms

Butterbur (Petasites hybridus) is a traditional herbal remedy known for its potent anti-inflammatory and antihistamine properties, making it highly effective in alleviating allergy symptoms. It has been used for centuries to treat various ailments, including headaches, asthma, and allergies. Butterbur works by inhibiting the production of histamines and leukotrienes, compounds involved in allergic reactions, thus reducing symptoms such as sneezing, nasal congestion, and itchy eyes. Here's how butterbur can be used to manage allergy symptoms in children.

How Butterbur Works

Butterbur contains several active compounds, including petasin and isopetasin, which contribute to its therapeutic effects:

- **Antihistamine Properties:** Butterbur inhibits the release of histamines, reducing allergic reactions such as sneezing, itching, and runny nose.

- **Anti-inflammatory Effects:** The herb reduces inflammation in the nasal passages, alleviating symptoms of nasal congestion and sinus pressure.

- **Bronchodilator Effects:** Butterbur can help open up the airways, making it beneficial for children with asthma or respiratory issues related to allergies.

Using Butterbur for Allergy Relief

Butterbur Extract: Butterbur is most commonly used in the form of standardized extracts, which are processed to remove pyrrolizidine alkaloids (PAs), compounds that can be toxic to the liver. Always choose butterbur supplements labeled "PA-free" to ensure safety.

- **Dosage:**
  - **For Young Children (Ages 6-9):** Use 25-50 mg of standardized butterbur extract twice daily. Consult with a healthcare provider to determine the appropriate dosage based on the child's weight and health condition.

  - **For Older Children (Ages 10 and Up):** Use 50-75 mg of standardized butterbur extract twice daily.

Safety and Precautions

- **Allergies:** Ensure that your child is not allergic to butterbur. Monitor for any signs of an allergic reaction, such as rash, itching, or swelling. Discontinue use and seek medical advice if any adverse reactions occur.

- **Proper Dosage:** Always follow the recommended dosages for children and consult with a healthcare provider before starting any new herbal treatment, especially for young children.

- **PA-Free Products:** Only use butterbur products that are labeled "PA-free" to avoid potential liver toxicity from pyrrolizidine alkaloids.

- **Consult a Healthcare Provider:** Always consult with a healthcare provider before using butterbur to ensure it is appropriate for your child's specific health needs and conditions.

Success Stories

Case Study:

- **Background:** Ethan, an 11-year-old, suffered from severe seasonal allergies that caused frequent sneezing, nasal congestion, and itchy eyes. His parents were looking for a natural remedy to help manage his symptoms.

- **Experience:** Ethan's parents started giving him 50 mg of standardized PA-free butterbur extract twice daily at the onset of allergy season. Over the next few weeks, they noticed a significant reduction in his allergy symptoms. Ethan was able to participate in outdoor activities without being hindered by his allergies.

- **Testimonial:** "Butterbur has been a game-changer for Ethan's allergies. His symptoms have significantly decreased, and he's much more comfortable during allergy season. We're thrilled to have found a natural remedy that works so well."

Butterbur is a highly effective herbal remedy for alleviating allergy symptoms in children, thanks to its potent antihistamine and anti-inflammatory properties. By inhibiting the release of histamines and reducing inflammation, butterbur can significantly reduce symptoms such as sneezing, nasal congestion, and itchy eyes. Always ensure proper dosages, choose PA-free products, and consult with a healthcare provider before incorporating butterbur into your child's routine. By using butterbur, you can help manage your child's allergies naturally and improve their overall comfort and well-being.

Treating Skin Allergies and Eczema

Skin allergies and eczema are common conditions in children that can cause significant discomfort and distress. Symptoms such as itching, redness, dryness, and inflammation can disrupt sleep, affect mood, and impact a child's overall quality of life. While conventional treatments are available, many parents seek natural remedies to avoid potential side effects and provide gentle, effective relief. Herbal remedies offer promising solutions for treating skin allergies and eczema by soothing inflammation, hydrating the skin, and promoting healing. Here are some effective herbs and natural treatments for managing these conditions in children.

Chamomile: Soothing and Anti-inflammatory

Chamomile (Matricaria chamomilla) is renowned for its calming and anti-inflammatory properties, making it an excellent choice for treating skin allergies and eczema. The herb contains compounds like bisabolol and chamazulene, which help reduce inflammation and promote healing. Chamomile can be used topically as a compress or added to bathwater to soothe irritated skin.

- **Chamomile Compress:** Steep 1-2 teaspoons of dried chamomile flowers in a cup of hot water for 10 minutes. Strain the liquid and allow it to cool. Soak a clean cloth in the chamomile tea and apply it to the affected areas for 15-20 minutes.
- **Chamomile Bath:** Add a handful of dried chamomile flowers to a muslin bag or cheesecloth and secure it. Place the bag in warm bathwater and let it steep for a few minutes. Allow the child to soak in the chamomile-infused bath for 15-20 minutes to soothe and hydrate the skin.

Calendula: Healing and Moisturizing

Calendula (Calendula officinalis) is a gentle herb known for its powerful healing and moisturizing properties. It is particularly effective for treating eczema and other skin conditions due to its ability to promote tissue repair and reduce inflammation. Calendula can be used as an infused oil, cream, or salve to provide relief from itching and dryness.

- **Calendula Infused Oil:** Fill a jar with dried calendula flowers and cover them with a carrier oil such as olive or coconut oil. Seal the jar and place it in a sunny spot for 2-3 weeks, shaking it occasionally. Strain the oil and apply it to the affected areas several times a day to moisturize and heal the skin.
- **Calendula Cream or Salve:** Look for calendula-based creams or salves at health food stores or make your own by combining calendula-infused oil with beeswax and shea butter. Apply the cream or salve to the affected areas to soothe and protect the skin.

Oatmeal: Anti-inflammatory and Hydrating

Oatmeal is a well-known remedy for soothing irritated and inflamed skin. It contains avenanthramides, compounds that reduce inflammation and itching. Oatmeal baths are particularly effective for providing relief from eczema and skin allergies.

- **Oatmeal Bath:** Grind 1 cup of plain oatmeal into a fine powder using a blender or food processor. Add the oatmeal powder to warm bathwater and stir well to disperse it evenly. Allow the child to soak in the oatmeal bath for 15-20 minutes. Rinse with lukewarm water and gently pat the skin dry.

Aloe Vera: Cooling and Healing

Aloe vera (Aloe barbadensis) is known for its cooling and healing properties. It helps to soothe irritated skin, reduce inflammation, and promote healing. Aloe vera gel can be applied directly to the affected areas to provide immediate relief from itching and redness.

- **Aloe Vera Gel:** Cut a fresh aloe vera leaf and scoop out the gel. Apply the gel directly to the affected areas several times a day. For convenience, you can also use store-bought aloe vera gel, ensuring it is pure and free from additives.

Evening Primrose Oil: Moisturizing and Anti-inflammatory

Evening primrose oil (Oenothera biennis) is rich in gamma-linolenic acid (GLA), an essential fatty acid that has anti-inflammatory properties and helps maintain healthy skin. It can be applied topically or taken internally to support skin health and reduce eczema symptoms.

- **Topical Application:** Apply evening primrose oil directly to the affected areas to moisturize and reduce inflammation.

- **Internal Use:** Consult a healthcare provider for the appropriate dosage of evening primrose oil supplements for children to support overall skin health.

Treating skin allergies and eczema in children with natural remedies can provide effective relief while avoiding the side effects of conventional treatments. Herbs such as chamomile, calendula, oatmeal, aloe vera, and evening primrose oil offer soothing, anti-inflammatory, and healing properties that help manage symptoms and promote healthy skin. Always ensure proper dosages and consult with a healthcare provider before starting any new herbal regimen. By incorporating these natural treatments, you can help alleviate your child's discomfort and improve their overall skin health.

Calendula: Healing and Soothing the Skin

Calendula (Calendula officinalis), also known as marigold, is a gentle and effective herb renowned for its healing and soothing properties. Traditionally used in herbal medicine, calendula is particularly beneficial for treating skin conditions such as eczema, dermatitis, and minor wounds. Its anti-inflammatory, antimicrobial, and antioxidant qualities make it an excellent choice for promoting skin health and alleviating discomfort associated with skin ailments.

Promoting Tissue Repair

One of the key benefits of calendula is its ability to promote tissue repair and accelerate the healing process. Calendula contains high levels of flavonoids and triterpenoids, which contribute to its potent anti-inflammatory and regenerative properties. These compounds help reduce inflammation and stimulate the production of collagen, essential for wound healing and tissue repair. Applying calendula to minor cuts, scrapes, and burns can speed up the healing process and minimize scarring. Its gentle nature makes it suitable for use on sensitive skin, including the delicate skin of children.

Moisturizing and Hydrating

Calendula is also known for its moisturizing and hydrating effects, making it a valuable remedy for dry and irritating skin conditions such as eczema. The herb helps to soothe dryness and provide much-needed hydration, creating a protective barrier on the skin that locks in moisture. This barrier helps to prevent further irritation and promotes a healthy skin environment. Using calendula-infused oils, creams, or salves can provide continuous moisture and relief from the itching and discomfort associated with dry skin conditions. Regular application can help restore the skin's natural balance and improve overall skin health.

Anti-inflammatory and Antimicrobial Properties

Calendula's anti-inflammatory properties are beneficial for reducing redness, swelling, and irritation. These properties make it an effective remedy for inflammatory skin conditions like dermatitis and allergic reactions. Additionally, calendula has antimicrobial qualities that help prevent infection in minor wounds and cuts. The herb's ability to combat bacteria and fungi makes it an excellent choice for maintaining skin hygiene and preventing complications from skin injuries. This dual action of reducing inflammation and preventing infection makes calendula a comprehensive treatment for various skin issues.

Calendula Infused Oil

Calendula-infused oil is a versatile and easy-to-make remedy that can be used to treat a wide range of skin conditions. To prepare calendula-infused oil, fill a jar with dried calendula flowers and cover them with a carrier oil such as olive or coconut oil. Seal the jar and place it in a sunny spot for 2-3 weeks, shaking it occasionally to ensure thorough infusion. After the infusion period, strain the oil and store it in a dark, airtight container. This infused oil can be applied directly to the skin to soothe and heal dry, irritated, or inflamed areas.

Calendula Creams and Salves

For more targeted application, calendula can be incorporated into creams and salves. These products combine the healing properties of calendula with other beneficial ingredients like beeswax and shea butter to create a protective and nourishing treatment for the skin. Calendula creams and salves are particularly useful for treating eczema, dermatitis, and other chronic skin conditions. They provide a concentrated dose of calendula's healing properties and create a barrier that protects the skin from environmental irritants while locking in moisture.

Calendula is a powerful yet gentle herb that offers significant benefits for skin health. Its healing, soothing, and moisturizing properties make it an effective treatment for a variety of skin conditions, including eczema, dermatitis, and minor wounds. Whether used as an infused oil, cream, or salve, calendula provides comprehensive care for irritated and damaged skin. By incorporating calendula into your skincare routine, you can promote faster healing, reduce inflammation, and maintain healthy, hydrated skin. Always consult with a healthcare provider before starting any new herbal treatment to ensure it is appropriate for your specific needs.

Chickweed: Reducing Itchiness and Inflammation

Chickweed (Stellaria media) is a small, flowering plant often considered a common weed, but it holds remarkable healing properties, particularly for skin conditions. This unassuming herb is celebrated in herbal medicine for its ability to reduce itchiness and inflammation, making it an excellent remedy for eczema, rashes, and other irritating skin issues. Chickweed's soothing and anti-inflammatory qualities provide natural relief, promoting comfort and skin health without the side effects often associated with conventional treatments.

Soothing Itchiness

Chickweed is particularly effective at alleviating itchiness, a common and distressing symptom of many skin conditions. The herb contains saponins, which have gentle cleansing properties that help soothe the skin. These compounds, along with other phytochemicals present in chickweed, can calm irritated nerve endings, reducing the sensation of itchiness. Applying chickweed as a topical treatment can bring immediate relief to itchy skin, whether from eczema, insect bites, or allergic reactions. Its mild nature makes it suitable for sensitive skin, including that of children, providing a natural solution for itch relief.

Anti-inflammatory Properties

The anti-inflammatory properties of chickweed make it a powerful herb for reducing swelling and redness associated with skin inflammation. Chickweed contains high levels of vitamins and minerals, including vitamin C and flavonoids, which contribute to its anti-inflammatory effects. These nutrients help to reduce the production of inflammatory cytokines, thereby calming inflamed skin and promoting healing. Regular use of chickweed in the form of salves, ointments, or poultices can help manage chronic inflammatory skin conditions, providing ongoing relief and improving overall skin health.

Chickweed Poultice

A chickweed poultice is a simple and effective way to harness the herb's soothing properties. To make a poultice, crush fresh chickweed leaves to release their juices, then apply the crushed leaves directly to the affected area. Cover the poultice with a clean cloth or bandage and leave it in place for 15-20 minutes. This application can be repeated several times a day to relieve itchiness and reduce inflammation. The fresh juice of chickweed is particularly potent and can be used on various skin irritations, providing immediate cooling and soothing effects.

Chickweed Infused Oil and Salve

Chickweed-infused oil and salve are versatile preparations that can be used for long-term management of skin conditions. To make chickweed-infused oil, fill a jar with fresh chickweed and cover it with a carrier oil such as olive or sunflower oil. Let the mixture steep in a sunny window for 2-3 weeks, shaking it occasionally to ensure thorough infusion. Strain the oil and store it in a dark, airtight container. This oil can be applied directly to the skin or used as a base for making a salve by mixing it with melted beeswax. Chickweed salve provides a protective barrier on the skin, locking in moisture and delivering the herb's healing properties.

Enhancing Skin Healing

Beyond reducing itchiness and inflammation, chickweed also promotes overall skin healing. Its emollient properties help to soften and moisturize the skin, aiding in the repair of damaged tissues. This makes chickweed an excellent choice for treating minor wounds, cuts, and abrasions, as well as chronic conditions like psoriasis and eczema. The herb's ability to support skin regeneration and maintain hydration ensures that the skin remains healthy and resilient, reducing the frequency and severity of flare-ups.

Chickweed is a powerful yet gentle herb that offers significant benefits for reducing itchiness and inflammation in various skin conditions. Its soothing, anti-inflammatory, and healing properties make it an effective natural remedy for managing eczema, rashes, and other irritating skin issues. Whether used as a poultice, infused oil, or salve, chickweed provides immediate and lasting relief, promoting healthy and comfortable skin. By incorporating chickweed into your skincare routine, you can harness its natural benefits to maintain skin health and alleviate discomfort naturally. Always consult with a healthcare provider before starting any new herbal treatment to ensure it is appropriate for your specific needs.

Respiratory Support for Allergies

Respiratory allergies, often triggered by pollen, dust, mold, or pet dander, can cause symptoms such as congestion, sneezing, coughing, and shortness of breath. These symptoms can significantly impact a child's quality of life, affecting sleep, school performance, and overall comfort. While conventional medications are available, many parents seek natural alternatives to manage these symptoms without the side effects. Herbal remedies can provide effective respiratory support for allergies by reducing inflammation, clearing mucus, and enhancing overall respiratory health.

Mullein: Clearing Mucus and Reducing Inflammation

Mullein (Verbascum thapsus) is an herb traditionally used for respiratory conditions. Its leaves and flowers contain saponins, which help to expel mucus, and mucilage, which soothes the respiratory tract. Mullein's anti-inflammatory properties reduce swelling in the airways, making breathing easier. For children experiencing congestion and coughing due to allergies, mullein tea or tincture can provide significant relief.

- **Mullein Tea:** Steep 1 teaspoon of dried mullein leaves in a cup of hot water for 10 minutes. Strain and let it cool to a comfortable temperature. For young children, give 1-2 teaspoons up to three times a day. For older children, give 1/4 to 1/2 cup up to three times a day.

Nettle: Natural Antihistamine

Nettle (Urtica dioica) is well-known for its antihistamine properties, making it a powerful herb for managing respiratory allergies. Nettle inhibits the release of histamines, which are responsible for allergic reactions. Regular use of nettle can reduce symptoms such as sneezing, runny nose, and congestion.

- **Nettle Tea:** Steep 1 teaspoon of dried nettle leaves in a cup of hot water for 5-10 minutes. Strain and let it cool to a comfortable drinking temperature. For young children, give 1-2 teaspoons up to twice daily. For older children, give 1/4 cup up to twice daily.

Licorice Root: Anti-inflammatory and Immune Support

Licorice root (Glycyrrhiza glabra) has anti-inflammatory and immune-boosting properties that are beneficial for managing respiratory allergies. It helps to reduce inflammation in the airways, soothe irritation, and support the body's immune response. Licorice root also has expectorant properties, helping to clear mucus from the respiratory tract.

- **Licorice Root Tea:** Steep 1/2 teaspoon of dried licorice root in a cup of hot water for 10 minutes. Strain and let it cool. For young children, give 1-2 teaspoons up to twice daily. For older children, give 1/4 cup up to twice daily. Note: Licorice root should be used in moderation and not for extended periods due to potential side effects like increased blood pressure.

Thyme: Antimicrobial and Expectorant

Thyme (Thymus vulgaris) is an herb with strong antimicrobial and expectorant properties, making it effective for treating respiratory conditions associated with allergies. It helps to clear mucus, reduce coughing, and fight off respiratory infections. Thyme can be used in teas or inhalations to support respiratory health.

- **Thyme Tea:** Steep 1/2 teaspoon of dried thyme leaves in a cup of hot water for 5-10 minutes. Strain and let it cool. For young children, give 1-2 teaspoons up to twice daily. For older children, give 1/4 cup up to twice daily.

- **Thyme Inhalation:** Add a few drops of thyme essential oil to a bowl of hot water. Have the child inhale the steam (under supervision) to help clear congestion and soothe the airways.

Eucalyptus: Clearing Airways and Reducing Congestion

Eucalyptus (Eucalyptus globulus) is widely used for its ability to clear airways and reduce congestion. Its active component, eucalyptol, has decongestant and anti-inflammatory properties. Eucalyptus can be used in steam inhalations or diffused as an essential oil to provide respiratory relief.

- **Eucalyptus Inhalation:** Add a few drops of eucalyptus essential oil to a bowl of hot water. Have the child inhale the steam (under supervision) to help clear nasal and chest congestion.

- **Diffusing Eucalyptus:** Use a diffuser to release eucalyptus essential oil into the air, creating a decongesting environment that can help alleviate respiratory symptoms.

Herbal remedies such as mullein, nettle, licorice root, thyme, and eucalyptus provide effective respiratory support for managing allergies in children. These herbs help reduce inflammation, clear mucus, and support overall respiratory health, providing natural relief from symptoms like congestion, sneezing, and coughing. Always ensure proper dosages and consult with a healthcare provider before starting any new herbal regimen. By incorporating these herbs into your child's care routine, you can help manage respiratory allergies naturally and improve their overall well-being.

Mullein: Clearing Respiratory Passages

Mullein (Verbascum thapsus) is a versatile herb traditionally used to support respiratory health. Its leaves and flowers contain compounds that make it particularly effective at clearing respiratory passages, soothing irritated tissues, and promoting overall lung health. Mullein's expectorant and anti-inflammatory properties make it an excellent choice for managing respiratory conditions, including those triggered by allergies.

Expectorant Properties

Mullein is well-known for its expectorant properties, which help to expel mucus and clear the respiratory passages. The herb contains saponins, natural detergents that thin mucus and make it easier to cough up. This is especially beneficial for children suffering from congestion and productive coughs, as it helps to clear the airways and facilitate easier breathing. Regular use of mullein can help reduce the buildup of mucus in the lungs and bronchi, promoting a healthier respiratory system.

Soothing Inflammation

In addition to its expectorant effects, mullein is also highly effective at soothing inflammation in the respiratory tract. The herb contains mucilage, a gelatinous substance that coats and protects the mucous membranes, reducing irritation and inflammation. This is particularly beneficial for children who experience chronic respiratory conditions like asthma or bronchitis, where inflammation can exacerbate symptoms and cause discomfort. Mullein's anti-inflammatory properties help to calm the respiratory passages, making it easier for children to breathe comfortably.

Antimicrobial Benefits

Mullein also possesses antimicrobial properties that help combat infections in the respiratory system. The herb's antibacterial and antiviral effects can help reduce the duration and severity of respiratory infections, making it a valuable ally during cold and flu season. By supporting the body's ability to fight off pathogens, mullein helps maintain a healthier respiratory environment, preventing secondary infections that can complicate allergic reactions or chronic conditions.

Mullein Tea

One of the most effective ways to utilize mullein for respiratory health is by preparing mullein tea. This gentle yet potent remedy can be easily administered to children to help clear their respiratory passages and soothe irritation.

- **Preparation:**
  - Steep 1 teaspoon of dried mullein leaves in a cup of hot water for 10 minutes.
  - Strain the tea through a fine mesh sieve or cheesecloth to remove any fine hairs from the mullein leaves, which can be irritating if ingested.
  - Let the tea cool to a comfortable drinking temperature.
- **Dosage:**
  - For young children (ages 4-6): Give 1-2 teaspoons of the cooled tea up to three times a day.
  - For older children (ages 7 and up): Give 1/4 to 1/2 cup of the cooled tea up to three times a day.

Mullein Steam Inhalation

For more immediate relief of congestion and respiratory discomfort, mullein steam inhalation can be highly effective. This method helps to open up the airways and reduce mucus buildup.

- **Preparation:**
    - Add a handful of dried mullein leaves to a pot of boiling water.
    - Remove the pot from heat and allow it to cool slightly.
    - Have the child lean over the pot with a towel draped over their head to trap the steam. Ensure the child keeps their eyes closed and breathes deeply.

- **Instructions:**
    - Supervise the child closely to prevent burns or discomfort.
    - Inhale the steam for 5-10 minutes, once or twice a day.

Mullein Infused Oil

Mullein-infused oil can be used as a chest rub to provide relief from respiratory discomfort and congestion. The oil helps to soothe the airways and promote easier breathing.

- **Preparation:**
    - Fill a jar with dried mullein flowers and cover them with olive oil.
    - Seal the jar and place it in a warm, sunny spot for 2-3 weeks, shaking it occasionally.
    - Strain the oil through a fine mesh sieve or cheesecloth and store it in a dark, airtight container.

- **Application:**
    - Rub a small amount of mullein-infused oil on the child's chest and back before bedtime to help with breathing and reduce congestion.

Mullein is a powerful herb that offers significant benefits for clearing respiratory passages and supporting overall lung health. Its expectorant, anti-inflammatory, and antimicrobial properties make it an ideal natural remedy for managing respiratory conditions in children. Whether used as a tea, steam inhalation, or infused oil, mullein provides effective relief from congestion and irritation, promoting easier breathing and enhanced respiratory comfort. Always ensure proper dosages and consult with a healthcare provider before incorporating mullein into your child's care routine. By using mullein, you can help maintain healthy respiratory passages and improve your child's overall well-being.

Licorice Root: Easing Breathing and Reducing Inflammation

Licorice root (Glycyrrhiza glabra) is a well-established herb in traditional medicine, known for its ability to ease breathing and reduce inflammation, making it an excellent remedy for respiratory conditions. Its unique combination of active compounds, such as glycyrrhizin, flavonoids, and saponins, provides significant therapeutic benefits for children suffering from allergies, asthma, bronchitis, and other respiratory ailments. Here's how licorice root can support respiratory health by easing breathing and reducing inflammation.

Easing Breathing

Licorice root helps to ease breathing by acting as a natural expectorant, which means it helps to loosen and expel mucus from the respiratory tract. This is particularly beneficial for children dealing with congestion and a productive cough. The saponins in licorice root help to break down and thin mucus, making it easier to cough up and clear from the airways. This clearing of mucus can alleviate the feeling of chest tightness and shortness of breath, providing much-needed relief for children with respiratory issues.

Reducing Inflammation

Inflammation of the airways is a common issue in many respiratory conditions, including asthma and bronchitis. Licorice root has powerful anti-inflammatory properties that can help to reduce this inflammation and soothe the respiratory tract. The active compound glycyrrhizin has been shown to inhibit inflammatory enzymes and cytokines, which play a key role in the inflammatory response. By reducing inflammation, licorice root can help to open up the airways, making breathing easier and more comfortable for children.

Supporting Immune Function

Licorice root also supports the immune system, helping the body to fight off infections that can exacerbate respiratory conditions. Its antiviral and antibacterial properties help to protect the respiratory tract from infections, while its immune-boosting effects enhance the body's ability to recover from illness. This dual action of supporting the immune system and reducing inflammation makes licorice root a comprehensive remedy for respiratory health.

Licorice Root Tea

One of the most effective ways to use licorice root for respiratory health is by preparing licorice root tea. This warm, soothing beverage can provide immediate relief from respiratory discomfort and help to reduce inflammation in the airways.

- **Preparation:**
    - Steep 1/2 teaspoon of dried licorice root in a cup of hot water for 10 minutes.
    - Strain the tea and let it cool to a comfortable drinking temperature.
- **Dosage:**
    - For young children (ages 4-6): Give 1-2 teaspoons of the cooled tea up to twice daily.
    - For older children (ages 7 and up): Give 1/4 cup of the cooled tea up to twice daily.

Licorice Root Tincture

A licorice root tincture is another effective form of this herb, providing a concentrated dose of its beneficial compounds. Tinctures are convenient and can be easily added to water or juice.

- **Preparation:**
  - Use a glycerin-based tincture for children, as it is alcohol-free and more palatable.

- **Dosage:**
  - For young children (ages 4-6): Use 5 drops of the tincture diluted in water or juice up to twice daily.
  - For older children (ages 7 and up): Use 10 drops of the tincture diluted in water or juice up to twice daily.

Safety and Precautions

- **Allergies:** Ensure that your child is not allergic to licorice root. Monitor for any signs of an allergic reaction, such as rash, itching, or swelling. Discontinue use and seek medical advice if any adverse reactions occur.

- **Proper Dosage:** Always follow the recommended dosages for children and consult with a healthcare provider before starting any new herbal treatment, especially for young children.

- **Potential Side Effects:** Licorice root should be used in moderation and not for extended periods due to potential side effects such as increased blood pressure and potassium depletion. Consult with a healthcare provider for appropriate usage and duration.

- **Consult a Healthcare Provider:** Always consult with a healthcare provider before using licorice root to ensure it is appropriate for your child's specific health needs and conditions.

Success Stories

Case Study:

- **Background:** Jamie, a 10-year-old with chronic bronchitis, often struggled with persistent coughing and shortness of breath. His parents sought a natural remedy to help ease his breathing and reduce inflammation.

- **Experience:** Jamie's parents started giving him 1/4 cup of licorice root tea twice daily. They also used a glycerin-based licorice root tincture for convenience. Over the next few weeks, they noticed significant improvements in Jamie's symptoms. His coughing reduced, and he could breathe more comfortably.

- **Testimonial:** "Licorice root tea and tincture have been incredibly effective for Jamie's bronchitis. His symptoms have improved noticeably, and he's much more comfortable. We're thrilled to have found a natural remedy that works so well."

Licorice root is a powerful herb that offers significant benefits for easing breathing and reducing inflammation in children with respiratory conditions. Its expectorant, anti-inflammatory, and immune-supporting properties make it an excellent natural remedy for managing symptoms of allergies, asthma, bronchitis, and other respiratory ailments. Whether used as a tea or tincture, licorice root provides effective relief and promotes overall respiratory health. Always ensure proper dosages and consult with a healthcare provider before incorporating licorice root into your child's care routine. By using licorice root, you can help support your child's respiratory health naturally and improve their overall well-being.

Natural Treatments for Colic and Digestive Issues

Colic and digestive issues are common concerns for parents, particularly during the early months of a child's life. These conditions can cause significant discomfort for infants and stress for their caregivers. Colic, characterized by prolonged periods of crying and fussiness, is often linked to digestive discomfort and gas. Similarly, digestive issues such as bloating, constipation, and indigestion can affect children of all ages, impacting their well-being and overall health. While conventional treatments are available, many parents seek natural remedies to alleviate these symptoms gently and effectively. This chapter explores various natural treatments for colic and digestive issues, highlighting safe and soothing herbal remedies that can provide relief and support healthy digestion in children.

Herbal Solutions for Colic Relief

Colic can be a distressing condition for both infants and their parents, characterized by prolonged periods of crying and discomfort, often due to digestive issues and gas. While the exact cause of colic is not well understood, natural herbal remedies can provide gentle and effective relief. These herbs work by soothing the digestive tract, reducing gas, and promoting overall digestive health. Here are some effective herbal solutions for colic relief.

Fennel: Soothing Digestive Discomfort

Fennel (Foeniculum vulgare) is a well-known remedy for relieving gas and bloating, making it an excellent choice for colic relief. The herb contains anethole, a compound that has antispasmodic properties, helping to relax the muscles of the gastrointestinal tract and reduce discomfort.

- **Fennel Tea:**
  - **Preparation:** Steep 1/2 teaspoon of crushed fennel seeds in a cup of hot water for 5-10 minutes. Strain and let it cool to room temperature.
  - **Dosage:** For infants, give 1-2 teaspoons of fennel tea up to three times a day. For older children, give 1/4 to 1/2 cup up to twice daily.

Chamomile: Calming and Anti-inflammatory

Chamomile (Matricaria chamomilla) is widely used for its calming and anti-inflammatory properties. It can help soothe the digestive system, reduce gas, and alleviate discomfort associated with colic.

- **Chamomile Tea:**
  - **Preparation:** Steep 1 teaspoon of dried chamomile flowers in a cup of hot water for 5-10 minutes. Strain and let it cool to room temperature.
  - **Dosage:** For infants, give 1-2 teaspoons of chamomile tea up to three times a day. For older children, give 1/4 to 1/2 cup up to twice daily.

Ginger: Reducing Gas and Spasms

Ginger (Zingiber officinale) has been traditionally used to treat various digestive issues, including colic. It helps reduce gas and intestinal spasms, providing relief from colic symptoms.

- **Ginger Tea:**
  - **Preparation:** Steep a few slices of fresh ginger in a cup of hot water for 5-10 minutes. Strain and let it cool to room temperature.
  - **Dosage:** For infants, give 1-2 teaspoons of ginger tea up to three times a day. For older children, give 1/4 cup up to twice daily.

Dill: Reducing Gas and Improving Digestion

Dill (Anethum graveolens) is another herb known for its digestive benefits, particularly in reducing gas and soothing the digestive tract.

- **Dill Water:**
  - **Preparation:** Boil 1 teaspoon of dill seeds in a cup of water for 10 minutes. Strain and let it cool to room temperature.
  - **Dosage:** For infants, give 1-2 teaspoons of dill water up to three times a day. For older children, give 1/4 cup up to twice daily.

Peppermint: Alleviating Gas and Cramping

Peppermint (Mentha piperita) is effective in alleviating gas and cramping, making it a helpful herb for colic relief. Its antispasmodic properties help to relax the muscles of the digestive tract.

- **Peppermint Tea:**
  - **Preparation:** Steep 1/2 teaspoon of dried peppermint leaves in a cup of hot water for 5-10 minutes. Strain and let it cool to room temperature.
  - **Dosage:** For infants, give 1-2 teaspoons of peppermint tea up to three times a day. For older children, give 1/4 to 1/2 cup up to twice daily.

Safety and Precautions

- **Allergies:** Ensure that your child is not allergic to any of the herbs used. Monitor for any signs of an allergic reaction, such as rash, itching, or swelling. Discontinue use and seek medical advice if any adverse reactions occur.

- **Proper Dosage:** Always follow the recommended dosages for infants and children, and consult with a healthcare provider before starting any new herbal treatment.

- **Consult a Healthcare Provider:** Always consult with a healthcare provider before using herbal remedies, especially for infants, to ensure safety and appropriateness for your child's specific health needs.

Herbal remedies such as fennel, chamomile, ginger, dill, and peppermint offer gentle and effective solutions for relieving colic symptoms in infants and children. These herbs work by soothing the digestive tract, reducing gas, and promoting overall digestive health. Always ensure proper dosages and consult with a healthcare provider before incorporating these remedies into your child's care routine. By using these herbal solutions, you can provide natural relief from colic and improve your child's comfort and well-being.

Fennel: Easing Gas and Bloating

Fennel (Foeniculum vulgare) has been used for centuries as a natural remedy for various digestive issues, particularly gas and bloating. This aromatic herb is rich in essential oils, such as anethole, which contribute to its carminative (gas-relieving) and antispasmodic properties. Fennel is a safe and effective herb for easing digestive discomfort in both infants and children, making it a popular choice for treating colic and other gastrointestinal disturbances.

Carminative Properties

Fennel's carminative properties help to prevent and reduce the formation of gas in the gastrointestinal tract. The essential oils in fennel, particularly anethole, work by relaxing the smooth muscles of the digestive system. This relaxation helps to release trapped gas, alleviating discomfort and reducing bloating. For children who suffer from colic or frequent episodes of gas, fennel can provide quick and gentle relief. By easing the tension in the digestive tract, fennel helps to create a more comfortable environment in the stomach and intestines, allowing gas to pass more easily and reducing the overall sensation of bloating.

Antispasmodic Effects

In addition to its carminative properties, fennel also has significant antispasmodic effects. This means it can help to relieve muscle spasms and cramps in the digestive tract, which are often associated with gas and bloating. The soothing action of fennel on the digestive muscles helps to prevent the painful contractions that can cause discomfort and distress in children. This makes fennel an ideal remedy not only for colic but also for other digestive disorders that involve spasms and cramping, such as irritable bowel syndrome (IBS).

Safe and Gentle for Infants

One of the most notable benefits of fennel is its safety and gentleness, making it suitable for use in infants. Fennel has been traditionally used to treat colic in babies, offering a natural alternative to pharmaceutical treatments. Fennel tea can be easily prepared and administered to infants to help alleviate their digestive discomfort. The mild flavor of fennel makes it well-tolerated by young children, ensuring that they can receive its benefits without resistance.

- **Fennel Tea Preparation:**
  - Steep 1/2 teaspoon of crushed fennel seeds in a cup of hot water for 5-10 minutes.
  - Strain the tea and let it cool to room temperature.
  - For infants, give 1-2 teaspoons of fennel tea up to three times a day.
  - For older children, give 1/4 to 1/2 cup up to twice daily.

Additional Health Benefits

Beyond its digestive benefits, fennel is also rich in nutrients such as vitamin C, fiber, and potassium. These nutrients contribute to overall health and well-being, supporting the immune system and promoting healthy digestion. The antioxidant properties of fennel help to protect the cells in the digestive tract from oxidative stress and inflammation, further enhancing its beneficial effects.

Practical Applications

Fennel can be incorporated into the diet in various forms, including as a tea, in soups, or as a spice in cooking. For parents looking for a more convenient option, fennel extracts and supplements are also available. When using fennel for digestive relief, it is important to start with small doses and observe how the child responds, gradually increasing the amount if needed.

Fennel is a highly effective and natural remedy for easing gas and bloating in infants and children. Its carminative and antispasmodic properties make it ideal for relieving digestive discomfort, reducing gas formation, and soothing muscle spasms in the gastrointestinal tract. Safe and gentle for use even in infants, fennel provides a reliable solution for parents seeking natural treatments for their children's digestive issues. By incorporating fennel into the daily routine, parents can help promote healthy digestion and alleviate discomfort, ensuring their children's overall well-being. Always consult with a healthcare provider before starting any new herbal treatment to ensure it is appropriate for your child's specific health needs.

Catnip: Soothing Digestive Discomfort

Catnip (Nepeta cataria) is an herb well-known for its effects on cats, but it also offers significant therapeutic benefits for humans, particularly for soothing digestive discomfort. Historically used in traditional medicine, catnip is valued for its calming, antispasmodic, and carminative properties, making it an effective remedy for digestive issues such as colic, gas, and indigestion. Its gentle nature makes it suitable for use in children, providing a natural and safe way to alleviate digestive discomfort.

Calming and Relaxing Properties

Catnip contains nepetalactone, a compound that provides calming and sedative effects, which are beneficial for soothing the digestive system. This calming effect helps to relax the muscles of the gastrointestinal tract, reducing spasms and cramping that can cause discomfort and pain. For children experiencing colic or other forms of digestive distress, catnip can provide gentle relief by easing tension and promoting relaxation.

Antispasmodic Effects

One of the key benefits of catnip is its antispasmodic properties, which help to reduce muscle spasms in the digestive tract. These spasms can lead to sharp, painful cramps and contribute to conditions like colic and irritable bowel syndrome (IBS). By relieving these spasms, catnip helps to soothe the digestive tract and reduce the frequency and intensity of cramps. This makes it an excellent choice for managing chronic digestive issues that involve muscle spasms and discomfort.

Carminative Properties

Catnip also has carminative properties, which means it helps to expel gas from the digestive system and prevent the formation of new gas bubbles. This can be particularly beneficial for children who suffer from bloating and gas-related discomfort. By aiding in the expulsion of gas, catnip helps to reduce the pressure and pain associated with bloating, leading to a more comfortable and settled stomach.

Catnip Tea for Digestive Relief

Catnip tea is a simple and effective way to utilize the herb's benefits for digestive health. The tea can be easily prepared and administered to children to help soothe their digestive discomfort.

- **Catnip Tea Preparation:**
    - Steep 1 teaspoon of dried catnip leaves in a cup of hot water for 5-10 minutes.
    - Strain the tea and let it cool to room temperature.
    - For infants, give 1-2 teaspoons of catnip tea up to three times a day.
    - For older children, give 1/4 to 1/2 cup up to twice daily.

The mild flavor of catnip tea makes it well-tolerated by children, and its gentle nature ensures that it provides relief without causing additional discomfort.

Additional Health Benefits

In addition to its digestive benefits, catnip also offers other health advantages. It can help reduce anxiety and promote better sleep, which are important for overall well-being. The calming effects of catnip can be particularly useful for children who are prone to stress or have trouble sleeping, further supporting their digestive health by promoting a more relaxed state.

Practical Applications

Catnip can be used in various forms, including as a tea, in tinctures, or even as a dried herb added to foods. When using catnip for digestive relief, it is important to start with small doses and observe how the child responds, gradually increasing the amount if needed. This ensures that the herb is effective without causing any adverse reactions.

Catnip is a highly effective and natural remedy for soothing digestive discomfort in children. Its calming, antispasmodic, and carminative properties make it ideal for relieving conditions such as colic, gas, and indigestion. Safe and gentle, catnip provides a reliable solution for parents seeking natural treatments for their children's digestive issues. By incorporating catnip into the daily routine, parents can help promote healthy digestion and alleviate discomfort, ensuring their children's overall well-being. Always consult with a healthcare provider before starting any new herbal treatment to ensure it is appropriate for your child's specific health needs.

Supporting Healthy Digestion

Healthy digestion is crucial for overall well-being, especially in children. A well-functioning digestive system ensures that nutrients are effectively absorbed, waste is efficiently eliminated, and discomforts such as bloating, gas, and constipation are minimized. Supporting healthy digestion involves a combination of proper diet, lifestyle habits, and the use of natural remedies that promote digestive health. Here are some key strategies and herbal solutions to support healthy digestion in children.

Balanced Diet

A balanced diet rich in fiber, fruits, vegetables, whole grains, and lean proteins is fundamental for healthy digestion. Fiber helps to keep the digestive tract moving, preventing constipation and promoting regular bowel movements. Foods rich in fiber include apples, pears, berries, carrots, broccoli, oats, and whole grains. Additionally, ensuring children stay hydrated by drinking plenty of water helps to soften stool and support overall digestive function.

Probiotics

Probiotics are beneficial bacteria that support gut health by maintaining a healthy balance of gut flora. These can be found in fermented foods such as yogurt, kefir, sauerkraut, and kimchi, or taken as supplements. Probiotics help to improve digestion, enhance nutrient absorption, and strengthen the immune system. Including probiotics in a child's diet can help prevent digestive issues such as diarrhea and constipation, promoting a healthy digestive environment.

Regular Physical Activity

Regular physical activity helps to stimulate the digestive system and promote regular bowel movements. Encouraging children to engage in daily activities such as walking, playing sports, or simply playing outside can significantly improve their digestive health. Physical activity helps to move food through the digestive tract more efficiently, reducing the risk of constipation and promoting overall digestive function.

Herbal Remedies for Healthy Digestion

Several herbs can support healthy digestion by soothing the digestive tract, reducing inflammation, and promoting the efficient breakdown of food. Here are some effective herbal remedies for supporting healthy digestion in children:

Ginger: Promoting Digestion and Reducing Nausea

Ginger (Zingiber officinale) is widely used for its digestive benefits. It helps to stimulate digestive enzymes, improve the breakdown of food, and reduce nausea. Ginger's anti-inflammatory properties also help to soothe the digestive tract, making it an excellent remedy for indigestion and upset stomach.

- **Ginger Tea:**

  - Steep a few slices of fresh ginger in a cup of hot water for 5-10 minutes. Strain and let it cool to a comfortable drinking temperature.

  - For young children, give 1-2 teaspoons of ginger tea up to twice daily. For older children, give 1/4 cup up to twice daily.

Peppermint: Easing Digestive Discomfort

Peppermint (Mentha piperita) is known for its ability to ease digestive discomfort and reduce symptoms of bloating, gas, and indigestion. Its antispasmodic properties help to relax the muscles of the digestive tract, making it an effective remedy for relieving stomach cramps and promoting healthy digestion.

- **Peppermint Tea:**

  - Steep 1 teaspoon of dried peppermint leaves in a cup of hot water for 5-10 minutes. Strain and let it cool to a comfortable drinking temperature.

  - For young children, give 1-2 teaspoons of peppermint tea up to twice daily. For older children, give 1/4 cup up to twice daily.

Chamomile: Soothing the Digestive Tract

Chamomile (Matricaria chamomilla) is a gentle herb that helps to soothe the digestive tract, reduce inflammation, and alleviate symptoms of indigestion and gas. Its calming effects also help to reduce stress and anxiety, which can negatively impact digestion.

- **Chamomile Tea:**

  - Steep 1 teaspoon of dried chamomile flowers in a cup of hot water for 5-10 minutes. Strain and let it cool to a comfortable drinking temperature.

  - For young children, give 1-2 teaspoons of chamomile tea up to twice daily. For older children, give 1/4 cup up to twice daily.

Fennel: Reducing Gas and Bloating

Fennel (Foeniculum vulgare) is particularly effective at reducing gas and bloating. Its carminative properties help to expel gas from the digestive tract and soothe intestinal discomfort.

- **Fennel Tea:**
  - Steep 1/2 teaspoon of crushed fennel seeds in a cup of hot water for 5-10 minutes. Strain and let it cool to a comfortable drinking temperature.
  - For young children, give 1-2 teaspoons of fennel tea up to three times a day. For older children, give 1/4 cup up to twice daily.

Conclusion

Supporting healthy digestion in children involves a holistic approach that includes a balanced diet, regular physical activity, probiotics, and the use of gentle herbal remedies. Herbs like ginger, peppermint, chamomile, and fennel can provide effective relief from digestive discomfort and promote overall digestive health. By incorporating these strategies and remedies into your child's daily routine, you can help ensure their digestive system functions optimally, leading to better health and well-being. Always consult with a healthcare provider before starting any new herbal treatment to ensure it is appropriate for your child's specific health needs.

Ginger: Reducing Nausea and Promoting Digestion

Ginger (Zingiber officinale) is a widely revered herb with a long history of use in traditional medicine for its powerful digestive benefits. Known for its distinctive spicy flavor and aromatic qualities, ginger is particularly effective in reducing nausea and promoting healthy digestion. Its versatility and efficacy make it a popular choice for alleviating digestive discomfort in both children and adults.

Reducing Nausea

One of the most well-known benefits of ginger is its ability to reduce nausea. Ginger contains bioactive compounds such as gingerol and shogaol, which have strong antiemetic (anti-nausea) properties. These compounds work by enhancing the digestive process and regulating stomach function, thereby reducing the occurrence of nausea and vomiting. For children who experience nausea due to motion sickness, indigestion, or illness, ginger can provide quick and natural relief. A small amount of ginger tea or ginger-infused water can help soothe the stomach and prevent nausea from escalating.

Promoting Digestion

Ginger not only alleviates nausea but also significantly promotes digestion. It stimulates the production of digestive enzymes and increases gastric motility, which helps to move food more efficiently through the digestive tract. This enhanced digestive process prevents the buildup of gas and bloating, common causes of discomfort in children. By improving overall digestive function, ginger helps to ensure that nutrients are properly absorbed, and waste is efficiently eliminated, promoting a healthier digestive system.

Anti-inflammatory Properties

The anti-inflammatory properties of ginger further support its role in digestive health. Inflammation in the digestive tract can lead to a variety of issues, including indigestion, bloating, and discomfort. The gingerols and shogaols in ginger help to reduce inflammation in the gut, providing relief from these symptoms. This makes ginger particularly useful for children with conditions such as irritable bowel syndrome (IBS) or other inflammatory digestive disorders.

Ginger Tea for Digestive Health

Ginger tea is one of the most effective and easily prepared forms of ginger for promoting digestive health. The warm tea can provide immediate soothing effects on the stomach and is gentle enough for children to consume.

- **Preparation:**

    - Steep a few slices of fresh ginger or 1/2 teaspoon of grated ginger in a cup of hot water for 5-10 minutes.

    - Strain the tea and let it cool to a comfortable drinking temperature.

    - For young children, give 1-2 teaspoons of ginger tea up to twice daily. For older children, give 1/4 cup up to twice daily.

Incorporating Ginger into the Diet

In addition to ginger tea, there are various ways to incorporate ginger into a child's diet to support digestion. Fresh ginger can be added to soups, stir-fries, and smoothies, providing both flavor and digestive benefits. Ginger-infused water, made by adding slices of fresh ginger to a water bottle, is another convenient way to ensure children receive its benefits throughout the day. Ginger candies or chews can also be a tasty and effective option for reducing nausea and promoting digestion.

Practical Considerations

While ginger is generally safe for most children, it is important to start with small amounts and observe any reactions. Some children may be sensitive to the spiciness of ginger, so adjusting the quantity based on the child's tolerance is key. Always consult with a healthcare provider before introducing ginger or any new herbal remedy to ensure it is appropriate for your child's specific health needs.

Ginger is a powerful and versatile herb that offers significant benefits for reducing nausea and promoting digestion in children. Its antiemetic, digestive stimulant, and anti-inflammatory properties make it an ideal natural remedy for various digestive issues. Whether used in the form of tea, incorporated into meals, or consumed as a snack, ginger provides gentle and effective relief from digestive discomfort. By integrating ginger into your child's diet, you can help support their digestive health and overall well-being. Always consult with a healthcare provider to ensure the appropriate use of ginger for your child's specific health needs.

Peppermint: Calming the Stomach

Peppermint (Mentha piperita) is a popular herb known for its refreshing aroma and soothing properties, especially when it comes to digestive health. With a long history of use in traditional medicine, peppermint is highly effective in calming the stomach and alleviating a range of digestive issues, from indigestion to irritable bowel syndrome (IBS). Its ability to relax the gastrointestinal tract and reduce symptoms of discomfort makes peppermint an essential herb for promoting digestive health in both children and adults.

Antispasmodic Properties

One of the key benefits of peppermint is its strong antispasmodic properties. The menthol in peppermint oil helps to relax the smooth muscles of the gastrointestinal tract, which can alleviate spasms and cramping. This makes peppermint particularly effective for conditions like IBS, where muscle spasms in the intestines can cause significant pain and discomfort. By relaxing these muscles, peppermint helps to ease the digestive process, reducing the frequency and severity of cramps.

Relieving Indigestion and Gas

Peppermint is also well-known for its ability to relieve indigestion and gas. The herb stimulates bile flow, which is crucial for the digestion of fats, and helps to expedite the digestive process. This can prevent the build-up of gas and reduce feelings of bloating and fullness. For children who experience frequent episodes of indigestion or gas, peppermint can provide quick and effective relief. Drinking peppermint tea or using peppermint oil can help to soothe the stomach and promote more comfortable digestion.

Cooling and Soothing Effects

The cooling and soothing effects of peppermint make it ideal for calming the stomach and reducing nausea. Peppermint's menthol content provides a cooling sensation that can alleviate nausea and vomiting, making it a valuable remedy for children suffering from motion sickness or upset stomachs. Peppermint tea is a gentle and pleasant way to deliver these benefits, offering both hydration and digestive relief.

Peppermint Tea for Digestive Health

Peppermint tea is one of the most popular and effective ways to use peppermint for digestive health. The tea is easy to prepare and provides a soothing, aromatic experience that can help calm the stomach and alleviate digestive discomfort.

- **Preparation:**
    - Steep 1 teaspoon of dried peppermint leaves in a cup of hot water for 5-10 minutes.
    - Strain the tea and let it cool to a comfortable drinking temperature.
    - For young children, give 1-2 teaspoons of peppermint tea up to twice daily. For older children, give 1/4 cup up to twice daily.

Peppermint Oil Applications

Peppermint oil can be used in various ways to support digestive health. While it should not be ingested directly in its pure form, diluted peppermint oil can be used in aromatherapy or applied topically to the abdomen.

- **Aromatherapy:**
  - Add a few drops of peppermint oil to a diffuser to fill the room with its soothing scent. This can help alleviate nausea and promote relaxation.

- **Topical Application:**
  - Dilute a few drops of peppermint oil in a carrier oil (such as almond or coconut oil) and gently massage it onto the child's abdomen. This can help relieve stomach cramps and discomfort.

Practical Considerations

While peppermint is generally safe, it is important to use it appropriately, especially in children. Start with small amounts and monitor for any adverse reactions. Peppermint oil should always be diluted before topical use to avoid skin irritation. Additionally, individuals with gastroesophageal reflux disease (GERD) or severe acid reflux should use peppermint with caution, as it can sometimes exacerbate these conditions.

Peppermint is a highly effective herb for calming the stomach and alleviating various digestive issues. Its antispasmodic, carminative, and soothing properties make it an excellent natural remedy for conditions like indigestion, gas, and IBS. Whether used as a tea, in aromatherapy, or as a diluted topical oil, peppermint provides significant relief from digestive discomfort. By incorporating peppermint into your child's digestive health routine, you can help promote more comfortable and efficient digestion. Always consult with a healthcare provider before starting any new herbal treatment to ensure it is appropriate for your child's specific health needs.

Remedies for Constipation and Diarrhea

Digestive issues such as constipation and diarrhea are common problems that can cause significant discomfort in children. While these conditions are often temporary, they can impact a child's overall well-being and quality of life. Fortunately, several natural remedies can help alleviate these issues by promoting healthy bowel movements and supporting digestive health. Here are some effective herbal and dietary solutions for managing constipation and diarrhea in children.

Remedies for Constipation

Constipation is characterized by infrequent or difficult bowel movements and can be accompanied by abdominal pain and bloating. Here are some natural remedies to relieve constipation:

1. Prune Juice: Natural Laxative

Prune juice is a well-known natural laxative that helps to relieve constipation. Prunes are high in fiber and sorbitol, a sugar alcohol that softens stools and promotes bowel movements.

- **Dosage:** For young children, start with a small amount (1-2 ounces) of prune juice, and increase gradually if needed. For older children, give 4-6 ounces as required.

2. Flaxseed: Promoting Regularity

Flaxseed is rich in fiber and omega-3 fatty acids, which help to promote regular bowel movements. Ground flaxseed can be easily added to a child's diet.

- **Usage:** Add 1 teaspoon of ground flaxseed to a smoothie, yogurt, or oatmeal. Ensure the child drinks plenty of water to help the fiber work effectively.

3. Aloe Vera Juice: Soothing and Laxative

Aloe vera juice has natural laxative properties and helps soothe the digestive tract, making it effective for relieving constipation.

- **Dosage:** Give 1-2 teaspoons of aloe vera juice mixed with water or juice once daily. Use with caution, as excessive use can lead to diarrhea.

4. Chamomile Tea: Gentle Relief

Chamomile tea is known for its calming and soothing effects on the digestive system. It can help relieve constipation by relaxing the muscles in the intestines.

- **Preparation:** Steep 1 teaspoon of dried chamomile flowers in a cup of hot water for 5-10 minutes. Strain and let it cool to a comfortable drinking temperature.
- **Dosage:** For young children, give 1-2 teaspoons of chamomile tea up to twice daily. For older children, give 1/4 cup up to twice daily.

Remedies for Diarrhea

Diarrhea involves frequent, loose, or watery bowel movements and can lead to dehydration if not managed properly. Here are some natural remedies to help manage diarrhea:

1. BRAT Diet: Binding and Bland Foods

The BRAT diet (Bananas, Rice, Applesauce, Toast) consists of bland, binding foods that help to firm up stools and reduce the frequency of bowel movements.

- **Usage:** Offer small amounts of these foods to the child throughout the day. Ensure they stay hydrated by drinking clear fluids.

2. Ginger Tea: Reducing Inflammation

Ginger tea can help reduce inflammation in the intestines and alleviate the symptoms of diarrhea. It also aids in digestion and soothes the stomach.

- **Preparation:** Steep a few slices of fresh ginger in a cup of hot water for 5-10 minutes. Strain and let it cool to a comfortable drinking temperature.
- **Dosage:** For young children, give 1-2 teaspoons of ginger tea up to twice daily. For older children, give 1/4 cup up to twice daily.

3. Peppermint Tea: Calming the Stomach

Peppermint tea has antispasmodic properties that can help calm the stomach and intestines, reducing the frequency of bowel movements.

- **Preparation:** Steep 1 teaspoon of dried peppermint leaves in a cup of hot water for 5-10 minutes. Strain and let it cool to a comfortable drinking temperature.

- **Dosage:** For young children, give 1-2 teaspoons of peppermint tea up to twice daily. For older children, give 1/4 cup up to twice daily.

4. Probiotics: Restoring Gut Flora

Probiotics help to restore the balance of good bacteria in the gut, which can be disrupted during episodes of diarrhea. Probiotic-rich foods include yogurt, kefir, and fermented foods, or they can be taken as supplements.

- **Dosage:** Follow the dosage instructions on the probiotic supplement or include probiotic-rich foods in the child's diet daily.

Hydration and Electrolyte Balance

Maintaining proper hydration and electrolyte balance is crucial for both constipation and diarrhea. Encourage children to drink plenty of water and consider oral rehydration solutions (ORS) if diarrhea leads to significant fluid loss. ORS can be purchased commercially or made at home by mixing 1 liter of water with 6 teaspoons of sugar and 1/2 teaspoon of salt.

Managing constipation and diarrhea in children can be effectively achieved with a combination of dietary adjustments, hydration, and natural remedies. Prune juice, flaxseed, aloe vera, and chamomile can provide relief from constipation, while the BRAT diet, ginger, peppermint, and probiotics can help manage diarrhea. Always ensure proper dosages and consult with a healthcare provider before starting any new herbal treatment to ensure it is appropriate for your child's specific health needs. By using these natural remedies, you can help support your child's digestive health and overall well-being.

Slippery Elm: Gentle Relief for Constipation

Slippery elm (Ulmus rubra), also known as red elm or Indian elm, is a tree native to North America, and its inner bark has been used for centuries in traditional medicine to treat various ailments, particularly digestive issues. This herb is highly regarded for its soothing and mucilaginous properties, making it an excellent natural remedy for constipation, especially in children. Slippery elm provides gentle relief by coating and soothing the digestive tract, promoting regular bowel movements without causing harsh side effects.

Mucilaginous Properties

The inner bark of slippery elm contains mucilage, a gel-like substance that becomes slippery when mixed with water. This mucilage is what makes slippery elm particularly effective for easing constipation. When ingested, the mucilage coats the lining of the intestines, creating a soothing and protective layer. This action helps to reduce irritation and inflammation, making the passage of stool more comfortable. The slippery texture also helps to soften the stool, making it easier to pass and reducing the strain associated with constipation.

Promoting Regular Bowel Movements

Slippery elm not only soothes the digestive tract but also promotes regular bowel movements. The mucilage in slippery elm acts as a gentle bulk-forming laxative. It absorbs water and expands in the intestines, adding bulk to the stool and stimulating peristalsis, the wave-like muscle contractions that move food through the digestive tract. This natural mechanism helps to encourage regular bowel movements without the harsh effects of stimulant laxatives, making it safe and effective for children who need gentle relief from constipation.

Soothing and Healing

In addition to its laxative effects, slippery elm has soothing and healing properties that benefit the entire digestive system. The mucilage can help to heal irritated or inflamed tissues in the gastrointestinal tract, making it useful for conditions like irritable bowel syndrome (IBS) and inflammatory bowel disease (IBD). For children who experience frequent digestive discomfort, slippery elm can provide ongoing relief and support digestive health.

Slippery Elm Preparation and Dosage

Slippery elm is typically prepared as a powder, which can be easily mixed into water or other liquids to create a soothing drink.

- **Slippery Elm Drink:**
  - **Preparation:** Mix 1 teaspoon of slippery elm powder into a cup of warm water, stirring well to dissolve. Let it sit for a few minutes until it thickens slightly.
  - **Dosage:** For young children, give 1-2 teaspoons of the slippery elm mixture up to twice daily. For older children, give 1/4 to 1/2 cup up to twice daily.

The mild, slightly sweet flavor of slippery elm makes it palatable for children, and it can also be mixed with a small amount of honey or fruit juice to enhance the taste.

Practical Considerations

While slippery elm is generally safe for most children, it is important to start with small amounts and observe how the child responds. As with any herbal remedy, it is essential to consult with a healthcare provider before introducing slippery elm to ensure it is appropriate for the child's specific health needs. Additionally, slippery elm should be taken separately from other medications, as its mucilaginous properties can potentially interfere with the absorption of other drugs.

Slippery elm offers gentle and effective relief for constipation, making it an ideal natural remedy for children. Its mucilaginous properties soothe and protect the digestive tract, while its bulk-forming action promotes regular bowel movements. By incorporating slippery elm into the child's routine, parents can provide a safe and soothing solution for constipation and support overall digestive health. Always consult with a healthcare provider before starting any new herbal treatment to ensure it is appropriate for the child's specific health needs. Slippery elm can be a valuable addition to a natural health regimen, offering comfort and relief for children experiencing digestive discomfort.

Blackberry Leaf: Managing Diarrhea Naturally

Blackberry leaf (Rubus fruticosus) is a time-honored herbal remedy known for its ability to manage diarrhea naturally. Rich in tannins, blackberry leaves have astringent properties that help to tighten and tone the tissues of the digestive tract, reducing inflammation and excessive fluid secretion. This makes blackberry leaf an effective and gentle option for treating diarrhea, particularly in children.

Astringent Properties

The astringent properties of blackberry leaf are primarily due to its high tannin content. Tannins are plant compounds that bind to proteins and other organic compounds, which helps to contract and tighten bodily tissues. In the digestive tract, this action helps to reduce the secretion of fluids into the intestines, thereby firming up stools and reducing the frequency of bowel movements. For children suffering from diarrhea, this astringent effect can provide quick and effective relief by restoring normal stool consistency.

Anti-inflammatory Effects

In addition to its astringent properties, blackberry leaf also has anti-inflammatory effects that help to soothe the digestive tract. The tannins and flavonoids in blackberry leaves reduce inflammation and irritation in the intestines, which can be particularly beneficial for children experiencing discomfort from diarrhea. By calming the inflammation, blackberry leaf helps to alleviate pain and cramping associated with diarrhea, promoting a more comfortable recovery.

Antimicrobial Benefits

Blackberry leaf contains antimicrobial compounds that can help fight off the pathogens that often cause diarrhea. These compounds can inhibit the growth of bacteria and viruses in the digestive tract, contributing to faster resolution of diarrheal episodes. This makes blackberry leaf not only a remedy for symptom relief but also a supportive treatment to address the underlying cause of diarrhea.

Blackberry Leaf Tea for Diarrhea

One of the most effective ways to use blackberry leaf for managing diarrhea is by preparing blackberry leaf tea. The tea is easy to prepare and gentle enough for children to consume.

- **Blackberry Leaf Tea:**
    - **Preparation:** Steep 1 teaspoon of dried blackberry leaves in a cup of hot water for 10 minutes. Strain and let it cool to a comfortable drinking temperature.
    - **Dosage:** For young children, give 1-2 teaspoons of the cooled tea up to three times a day. For older children, give 1/4 to 1/2 cup up to three times a day.

Blackberry Leaf Tincture

For a more concentrated form, blackberry leaf tincture can be used. Tinctures are convenient and can be easily administered in small, precise doses.

- **Blackberry Leaf Tincture:**
  - **Dosage:** For young children, use 5 drops of the tincture diluted in water or juice up to three times a day. For older children, use 10 drops up to three times a day.

Safety and Precautions

While blackberry leaf is generally safe for children, it is important to start with small doses and monitor for any adverse reactions. As with any herbal remedy, consulting with a healthcare provider before use is essential, especially if the child is taking other medications or has underlying health conditions.

Hydration and Electrolyte Balance

When managing diarrhea, it is crucial to ensure that the child remains hydrated and maintains proper electrolyte balance. Diarrhea can lead to significant fluid and electrolyte loss, so providing oral rehydration solutions (ORS) alongside blackberry leaf tea can help. ORS can be purchased commercially or made at home by mixing 1 liter of water with 6 teaspoons of sugar and 1/2 teaspoon of salt.

Blackberry leaf is an effective and natural remedy for managing diarrhea in children. Its astringent, anti-inflammatory, and antimicrobial properties help to reduce excessive fluid secretion, soothe the digestive tract, and combat pathogens. Whether used as a tea or tincture, blackberry leaf provides gentle relief from diarrhea and supports the overall recovery of digestive health. Always consult with a healthcare provider before starting any new herbal treatment to ensure it is appropriate for your child's specific health needs. By incorporating blackberry leaf into your child's care routine, you can provide a natural and effective solution for diarrhea, promoting comfort and well-being.

BOOK 17:

DIY Herbal Preparations: Complete Guide to Tinctures, Oils, and Salves

Tinctures, Infusions, and Decoctions

The art of herbal medicine encompasses various methods of extracting the beneficial properties of plants, each tailored to specific needs and uses. Tinctures, infusions, and decoctions are three fundamental techniques that allow us to harness the healing power of herbs in different ways. Tinctures involve using alcohol or glycerin to extract and preserve the active compounds of herbs, resulting in a potent and long-lasting remedy. Infusions, on the other hand, use hot water to draw out the delicate constituents of flowers, leaves, and other soft plant parts, creating soothing teas that are ideal for daily use. Decoctions employ prolonged boiling to extract the more robust compounds from roots, barks, and seeds, making them perfect for treating chronic conditions. Understanding these methods is crucial for anyone interested in creating their own herbal remedies, as each technique offers unique benefits and applications. This chapter will introduce you to the basics of tinctures, infusions, and decoctions, guiding you through their preparation and use to enhance your herbal medicine practice.

Understanding and Making Tinctures

Tinctures are concentrated herbal extracts made by soaking herbs in alcohol or glycerin. This method of extraction is highly effective at preserving the active constituents of herbs, resulting in a potent remedy that has a long shelf life. Tinctures are an excellent way to utilize the medicinal properties of herbs, providing a convenient and efficient form of herbal medicine. They can be easily administered in small, precise doses, making them ideal for both acute and chronic conditions.

The Basics of Tinctures

The process of making tinctures involves steeping herbs in a solvent, typically alcohol, for a period of time to extract the active compounds. Alcohol is the most common solvent used because it effectively draws out both water-soluble and alcohol-soluble components from the herbs. However, for those who prefer an alcohol-free option, glycerin can be used as an alternative, though it may not be as effective in extracting certain compounds.

Benefits of Tinctures

Tinctures offer several advantages over other forms of herbal medicine. They are highly concentrated, meaning that a small amount can deliver a significant therapeutic effect. This makes tinctures particularly useful for individuals who need to take herbs regularly or in larger doses. Additionally, tinctures have a long shelf life, often lasting several years if stored properly, which makes them a cost-effective and practical choice for maintaining a home apothecary. Their liquid form allows for easy absorption and rapid onset of effects, providing quick relief in acute situations.

Making Your Own Tinctures

Creating your own tinctures at home is a straightforward process that allows you to customize your remedies to suit your specific needs. Here is a step-by-step guide to making a basic tincture:

1. Selecting and Preparing Herbs: Choose fresh or dried herbs that are free from contaminants. Fresh herbs should be chopped finely to increase the surface area for extraction, while dried herbs can be used as they are.

2. Choosing a Solvent: Decide whether you will use alcohol or glycerin as your solvent. For alcohol-based tinctures, high-proof vodka or brandy (at least 40% alcohol by volume) is typically used. For glycerin-based tinctures, ensure you use food-grade glycerin.

3. Combining Herbs and Solvent: Place the prepared herbs in a clean glass jar. Pour the chosen solvent over the herbs, ensuring they are completely submerged. The general ratio is one part herb to five parts solvent for dried herbs, or one part herb to two parts solvent for fresh herbs.

4. Steeping Process: Seal the jar tightly and store it in a cool, dark place. Shake the jar daily to ensure the herbs are thoroughly mixed with the solvent. Allow the mixture to steep for 4-6 weeks to ensure maximum extraction of the herbal compounds.

5. Straining and Bottling: After the steeping period, strain the mixture through a fine mesh strainer or cheesecloth to remove the plant material. Pour the liquid tincture into dark glass bottles with dropper tops for easy dispensing. Label the bottles with the name of the herb and the date of preparation.

6. Dosage and Usage: Tinctures are usually taken in small doses, typically 1-2 dropperfuls (about 20-40 drops) diluted in water or juice, 2-3 times a day. Always follow dosage recommendations specific to the herb and individual needs.

Safety and Precautions

While tinctures are generally safe and effective, it is important to use them responsibly. Always research the specific herbs you are using to understand their potential effects and interactions. Consult with a healthcare provider, especially if you are pregnant, nursing, or taking other medications. Properly label and store tinctures out of reach of children.

Tinctures are a powerful and versatile form of herbal medicine that can easily be made at home. By understanding the basics of tincture preparation and the benefits they offer, you can create customized herbal remedies that are both potent and convenient. With a little time and effort, tinctures can become a valuable addition to your natural health regimen, providing you with an effective means of harnessing the healing power of herbs.

Herbal Infusions: Benefits and Preparation

Herbal infusions are a simple yet potent way to extract the medicinal properties of herbs. This method involves steeping plant material, typically flowers, leaves, or other soft parts, in hot water to draw out the active constituents. Herbal infusions are commonly enjoyed as teas and offer a gentle, effective means of delivering the therapeutic benefits of herbs. They are easy to prepare and can be a soothing and enjoyable part of a daily health regimen.

Benefits of Herbal Infusions

1. Nutrient-Rich: Herbal infusions are rich in vitamins, minerals, and other phytonutrients that are easily absorbed by the body. Herbs such as nettle, alfalfa, and red clover provide essential nutrients like iron, calcium, and magnesium, supporting overall health and wellness.

2. Hydrating and Detoxifying: Infusions contribute to daily fluid intake, promoting hydration. Herbs like dandelion and burdock root have gentle diuretic properties, supporting the body's natural detoxification processes by aiding kidney and liver function.

3. Calming and Relaxing: Certain herbs, such as chamomile, lemon balm, and lavender, have calming effects on the nervous system. Infusions made from these herbs can help reduce stress, promote relaxation, and improve sleep quality.

4. Digestive Support: Herbs like peppermint, ginger, and fennel can be infused to create teas that soothe the digestive tract, alleviate indigestion, and reduce gas and bloating. These herbs are particularly beneficial for children and adults with sensitive stomachs.

5. Immune Boosting: Infusions made from herbs like echinacea, elderberry, and astragalus can support the immune system, helping to prevent and alleviate symptoms of colds and flu. These immune-boosting herbs are rich in antioxidants and have antiviral properties.

Preparation of Herbal Infusions

Making an herbal infusion is a straightforward process that requires minimal equipment. Here's how to prepare a basic herbal infusion:

1. Selecting Herbs: Choose high-quality dried or fresh herbs. For optimal medicinal benefits, ensure the herbs are organic and free from contaminants. Common herbs used for infusions include chamomile, nettle, peppermint, and lemon balm.

2. Measuring Herbs: For a standard infusion, use 1-2 tablespoons of dried herbs per cup of water. If using fresh herbs, increase the amount to 2-4 tablespoons per cup of water, as fresh herbs contain more water and require a higher quantity to achieve the same potency.

3. Boiling Water: Bring fresh, filtered water to a boil. The quality of water is important, as it affects the taste and therapeutic properties of the infusion.

4. Steeping: Place the herbs in a teapot, heatproof jar, or infuser. Pour the boiling water over the herbs, cover the container to retain the volatile oils, and let it steep for 10-15 minutes for most herbs. For a stronger infusion, you can steep the herbs for up to 4 hours.

5. Straining: After steeping, strain the infusion using a fine mesh strainer, cheesecloth, or a specialized tea strainer to remove the plant material. This ensures a smooth, pleasant tea without any debris.

6. Serving: Pour the strained infusion into a cup and enjoy. You can sweeten your infusion with honey, maple syrup, or another natural sweetener if desired. Infusions can be enjoyed hot or cold, depending on personal preference.

7. Storing: If you make a larger batch, store the remaining infusion in a sealed container in the refrigerator. It will stay fresh for up to 48 hours. Reheat gently before drinking, if desired.

Popular Herbal Infusion Combinations

1. Relaxing Blend:

- Chamomile
- Lemon Balm
- Lavender

2. Digestive Support:

- Peppermint
- Fennel
- Ginger

3. Immune Boosting:

- Echinacea
- Elderberry
- Astragalus

4. Nutrient-Rich Blend:

- Nettle
- Red Clover
- Alfalfa

Herbal infusions are a versatile and beneficial way to incorporate the healing properties of herbs into your daily routine. They provide essential nutrients, support hydration, promote relaxation, aid digestion, and boost the immune system. The simple preparation process makes herbal infusions an accessible and enjoyable form of natural medicine. By incorporating a variety of herbs, you can tailor infusions to meet your specific health needs and enjoy the wide-ranging benefits they offer. Always consult with a healthcare provider before introducing new herbs into your routine to ensure they are appropriate for your specific health needs.

Herbal Decoctions: Benefits and Preparation

Herbal decoctions are a traditional method of extracting the medicinal properties of tougher plant materials such as roots, barks, seeds, and some berries. Unlike infusions, which involve steeping herbs in hot water for a short period, decoctions require simmering these denser parts of the plant for a longer time to fully extract their beneficial compounds. Decoctions are particularly valued for their ability to draw out a wide range of active ingredients, making them highly effective for various therapeutic purposes.

Benefits of Herbal Decoctions

1. Enhanced Extraction: Decoctions are especially effective for extracting minerals, starches, and other robust compounds that are not easily released through simple steeping. This makes them ideal for utilizing the full therapeutic potential of herbs like dandelion root, licorice root, and cinnamon bark.

2. Potent Medicinal Properties: Due to the extended simmering process, decoctions tend to be more concentrated than infusions. This concentration allows for a more potent remedy, which can be beneficial for addressing chronic health issues such as digestive disorders, respiratory problems, and immune system support.

3. Versatile Applications: Herbal decoctions can be used in various ways, including as a base for other herbal preparations like syrups and tinctures. They can also be incorporated into soups and broths, adding both medicinal benefits and rich flavors to everyday meals.

4. Improved Bioavailability: The prolonged cooking process in decoctions helps to break down plant cell walls, enhancing the bioavailability of the herbs' active constituents. This means that the body can more readily absorb and utilize these compounds, leading to more effective healing outcomes.

Preparation of Herbal Decoctions

Creating an herbal decoction requires a bit more time and effort compared to making an infusion, but the results are well worth it. Here's a step-by-step guide to preparing a basic herbal decoction:

1. Selecting Herbs: Choose high-quality, dried or fresh roots, barks, seeds, or berries. Common herbs used for decoctions include ginger root, dandelion root, burdock root, and cinnamon bark.

2. Measuring Herbs: For a standard decoction, use about 1-2 tablespoons of dried herbs per cup of water. If using fresh herbs, increase the amount to 3-4 tablespoons per cup of water, as fresh herbs contain more water and may require a higher quantity to achieve the same potency.

3. Boiling Water: Place the measured herbs in a saucepan and add the appropriate amount of cold water. Bring the mixture to a gentle boil.

4. Simmering: Once the water reaches a boil, reduce the heat to a low simmer. Cover the saucepan with a lid to prevent evaporation and maintain the integrity of the volatile compounds. Simmer the mixture for 20-45 minutes, depending on the herb. Some herbs may require longer simmering times to fully extract their beneficial properties.

5. Straining: After simmering, remove the saucepan from heat and let the decoction cool slightly. Strain the liquid through a fine mesh strainer, cheesecloth, or a specialized tea strainer to remove the plant material. This ensures a smooth, clear decoction without any debris.

6. Serving: Pour the strained decoction into a cup and enjoy. Decoctions can be consumed hot or cold, depending on personal preference. You can sweeten your decoction with honey, maple syrup, or another natural sweetener if desired.

7. Storing: If you make a larger batch, store the remaining decoction in a sealed container in the refrigerator. It will stay fresh for up to 72 hours. Reheat gently before drinking, if desired.

Popular Herbal Decoction Combinations

1. Digestive Health:

- Ginger Root
- Dandelion Root
- Licorice Root

2. Immune Support:

- Astragalus Root
- Echinacea Root
- Elderberry

3. Respiratory Relief:

- Marshmallow Root
- Elecampane Root
- Cinnamon Bark

4. Detoxification:

- Burdock Root
- Dandelion Root
- Yellow Dock Root

Herbal decoctions are a powerful and effective way to extract the medicinal properties of tougher plant materials, offering enhanced benefits and improved bioavailability compared to simpler preparations. By incorporating decoctions into your herbal practice, you can take full advantage of the healing potential of roots, barks, seeds, and berries. Whether used alone or as a base for other herbal remedies, decoctions provide a versatile and potent addition to your natural health regimen. Always consult with a healthcare provider before introducing new herbs into your routine to ensure they are appropriate for your specific health needs.

Essential Oils and Salves

Essential oils and salves are two versatile and potent forms of herbal remedies that harness the therapeutic properties of plants. Essential oils are concentrated extracts obtained from the aromatic parts of plants, such as leaves, flowers, and roots, through processes like steam distillation or cold pressing. These oils capture the essence of the plant, offering powerful health benefits through aromatic and topical applications. Salves, on the other hand, are ointment-like preparations made by combining infused oils with a natural wax, typically beeswax, to create a semi-solid product. They are designed for topical use, providing a protective and healing layer over the skin. Both essential oils and salves are integral to natural medicine, offering targeted relief for a variety of ailments, from skin conditions and muscle pain to respiratory issues and stress. This chapter will introduce you to the fundamentals of essential oils and salves, guiding you through their benefits, uses, and basic preparation techniques.

Understanding and Making Essential Oils

Essential oils are highly concentrated plant extracts that capture the natural aroma and beneficial properties of the plant from which they are derived. These potent oils are extracted from various parts of plants, including flowers, leaves, bark, and roots, using methods such as steam distillation, cold pressing, and solvent extraction. Essential oils are revered in herbal medicine for their therapeutic benefits and are commonly used in aromatherapy, skincare, and natural remedies.

The Basics of Essential Oils

Essential oils are composed of volatile compounds that evaporate quickly and easily diffuse into the air, allowing their aromatic molecules to interact with the body. Each essential oil contains a unique combination of chemical constituents that contribute to its distinctive aroma and therapeutic effects. For example, lavender oil is known for its calming and relaxing properties due to its high linalool content, while tea tree oil is prized for its antimicrobial and antiseptic qualities.

Benefits of Essential Oils

Essential oils offer a wide range of health benefits, making them valuable tools in natural medicine. They can be used to alleviate stress, enhance mood, improve sleep, boost immunity, and treat various skin conditions. Inhalation of essential oils through aromatherapy can help relieve anxiety, promote relaxation, and enhance mental clarity. Topical application, when diluted with a carrier oil, can provide targeted relief for conditions such as muscle pain, inflammation, and infections.

Methods of Extraction

1. Steam Distillation: Steam distillation is the most common method of extracting essential oils. It involves passing steam through plant material to vaporize the volatile compounds, which are then condensed and collected as a mixture of water and essential oil. The essential oil is separated from the water and collected for use.

2. Cold Pressing: Cold pressing is primarily used for citrus oils, such as lemon, orange, and bergamot. This method involves mechanically pressing the plant material to release the essential oils without the use of heat, preserving the oil's natural properties.

3. Solvent Extraction: Solvent extraction is used for delicate flowers like jasmine and rose, which cannot withstand the heat of steam distillation. Solvents are used to dissolve the essential oils, which are then separated from the solvent after extraction.

Making Your Own Essential Oils

While the process of making essential oils at home can be complex and requires specialized equipment, you can create simpler versions using the cold infusion method. Here is a basic guide to making a cold-infused oil, which, while not as concentrated as distilled essential oils, can still offer many therapeutic benefits.

1. Selecting and Preparing Plant Material: Choose fresh, organic herbs or flowers for infusion. Ensure they are clean and free from pesticides. Chop the plant material to increase the surface area for extraction.

2. Choosing a Carrier Oil: Select a high-quality carrier oil, such as olive oil, jojoba oil, or sweet almond oil. Carrier oils are used to dilute the essential oils and aid in their absorption.

3. Combining Plant Material and Oil: Fill a clean glass jar with the chopped plant material and pour the carrier oil over it, ensuring the herbs are fully submerged. Seal the jar tightly.

4. Infusion Process: Place the jar in a warm, sunny spot and let it infuse for 2-4 weeks, shaking it gently every day to mix the contents. The warmth helps to extract the aromatic compounds into the oil.

5. Straining and Bottling: After the infusion period, strain the oil through a fine mesh strainer or cheesecloth to remove the plant material. Pour the infused oil into dark glass bottles to protect it from light and preserve its potency.

Safety and Usage

Essential oils are highly concentrated and should always be used with caution. When applying essential oils topically, they should be diluted with a carrier oil to prevent skin irritation. Common dilution ratios are typically 1-2% for adults and even lower for children. Always conduct a patch test before using a new essential oil to ensure there is no allergic reaction. Essential oils should be stored in a cool, dark place away from direct sunlight to maintain their efficacy.

Essential oils are powerful natural remedies that offer a multitude of therapeutic benefits. Understanding the basics of essential oils and their extraction methods allows you to appreciate their potency and versatility. While making true essential oils at home can be challenging, creating cold-infused oils is a simpler alternative that still provides many benefits. By incorporating essential oils into your daily routine, you can enhance your physical, emotional, and mental well-being in a natural and holistic way. Always use essential oils responsibly and consult with a healthcare provider if you have any concerns or pre-existing conditions.

Creating Herbal Salves: Benefits and Preparation

Herbal salves are ointment-like preparations made by combining herbal-infused oils with a natural wax, typically beeswax, to create a semi-solid product. These salves are designed for topical use and provide a protective and healing layer over the skin. Salves are particularly beneficial for treating a variety of skin conditions, including dry skin, cuts, burns, rashes, and muscle aches. The process of making herbal salves is straightforward and allows for customization to suit specific therapeutic needs.

Benefits of Herbal Salves

1. Skin Healing and Protection: Herbal salves create a barrier on the skin that protects against environmental irritants and moisture loss. Herbs like calendula, comfrey, and plantain are commonly used in salves for their skin-healing properties. These herbs help to reduce inflammation, promote cell regeneration, and accelerate the healing of wounds and burns.

2. Moisturizing and Soothing: Salves provide deep moisturization to dry and cracked skin. The combination of herbal-infused oils and beeswax locks in moisture and soothes irritated skin. Salves made with herbs like chamomile and lavender can calm and nourish the skin, making them ideal for conditions like eczema and dermatitis.

3. Pain Relief: Herbal salves can also be formulated to relieve muscle and joint pain. Herbs such as arnica, cayenne, and St. John's wort have analgesic and anti-inflammatory properties that help to reduce pain and swelling. These salves are useful for athletes and individuals suffering from conditions like arthritis and muscle soreness.

4. Versatility and Customization: One of the greatest benefits of making herbal salves at home is the ability to customize them for specific needs. You can combine different herbs to create a multi-purpose salve or tailor a formula to address particular skin issues. This versatility ensures that you have a remedy suited to your unique requirements.

Preparation of Herbal Salves

Creating herbal salves at home is a simple and rewarding process. Here is a step-by-step guide to making your own herbal salve:

1. Selecting and Preparing Herbs: Choose high-quality dried or fresh herbs based on the desired therapeutic effects. Some popular choices include calendula for skin healing, arnica for pain relief, and chamomile for soothing irritation.

2. Making Herbal-Infused Oil: To create an herbal-infused oil, fill a clean glass jar with the dried herbs and cover them with a carrier oil such as olive oil, coconut oil, or almond oil. Ensure the herbs are fully submerged. Seal the jar and place it in a warm, sunny spot for 2-4 weeks, shaking it gently every day. Alternatively, you can speed up the process by gently heating the jar in a double boiler for 2-3 hours, making sure the oil does not overheat.

3. Straining the Oil: After the infusion period, strain the oil through a fine mesh strainer or cheesecloth to remove the plant material. Squeeze out as much oil as possible to maximize the extraction of herbal properties. Store the infused oil in a dark glass bottle to protect it from light and extend its shelf life.

4. Combining with Beeswax: Measure the herbal-infused oil and beeswax. A common ratio is 1 part beeswax to 4 parts oil. Adjust the amount of beeswax to achieve the desired consistency; more beeswax will make a firmer salve, while less will result in a softer salve. Place the oil and beeswax in a double boiler or a heatproof bowl over a pot of simmering water. Heat gently until the beeswax is fully melted.

5. Adding Essential Oils (Optional): Once the beeswax is melted, you can add a few drops of essential oils for added therapeutic benefits and fragrance. For example, add lavender essential oil for its calming properties or tea tree oil for its antimicrobial effects. Stir well to combine.

6. Pouring and Setting: Pour the melted mixture into clean, sterilized jars or tins. Allow the salve to cool and solidify at room temperature. Once set, seal the containers with lids and label them with the ingredients and date of preparation.

7. Using and Storing: Apply the salve to the affected area as needed. Store the salve in a cool, dark place to maintain its potency and extend its shelf life. Properly stored, herbal salves can last up to a year.

Herbal salves are a versatile and effective way to harness the healing power of herbs for topical use. They offer numerous benefits, including skin healing, moisturization, pain relief, and protection against environmental irritants. Creating your own herbal salves at home allows for customization to meet specific therapeutic needs, ensuring you have a personalized remedy for various skin conditions and discomforts. The process of making herbal salves is straightforward and rewarding, providing a practical way to incorporate natural healing into your daily routine. Always consult with a healthcare provider if you have any concerns or pre-existing conditions before using new herbal remedies.

BOOK 18:

Step-by-Step Preparation Guides: Creating your own herbal remedies

Creating your own herbal remedies at home is a rewarding and empowering practice that allows you to harness the healing power of nature in a personalized way. Whether you are making tinctures, infusions, decoctions, essential oils, or salves, having a clear, step-by-step guide is essential for ensuring the quality and effectiveness of your preparations. These guides will walk you through each process, from selecting and preparing your herbs to the final steps of storage and usage. By following these detailed instructions, you can confidently create a range of herbal remedies tailored to your specific health needs, while also gaining a deeper understanding of the art and science of herbal medicine. This chapter will provide you with comprehensive, easy-to-follow preparation guides that will serve as a valuable resource in your journey toward natural health and wellness.

Gathering, Preparing, and Storing Herbs

Herbs are the foundation of herbal medicine, and the quality of your remedies greatly depends on how you gather, prepare, and store them. Proper handling of herbs ensures that their medicinal properties are preserved, maximizing their effectiveness in your homemade preparations. Here is a detailed guide to help you through the process of gathering, preparing, and storing herbs.

Gathering Herbs

1. Identification: Before gathering herbs, it's crucial to correctly identify the plants. Use a reliable field guide or consult with a knowledgeable herbalist to ensure you're collecting the right species. Misidentification can lead to ineffective or potentially harmful remedies.

2. Harvesting Time: The potency of herbs varies depending on the time of day and the plant's growth cycle. Generally, leaves and flowers should be harvested in the morning after the dew has dried but before the heat of the day. Roots are best harvested in the fall when the plant's energy has returned to the roots. Barks can be collected in early spring or late fall.

3. Sustainable Harvesting: Always practice sustainable harvesting to ensure the plants' survival and health. Only take what you need and avoid over-harvesting from a single plant or area. Leave enough of the plant so it can continue to grow and reproduce.

4. Cleanliness: Ensure your hands and tools are clean before harvesting. Use sharp scissors or pruners to minimize damage to the plant. Avoid harvesting herbs near polluted areas, such as roadsides or industrial sites, to ensure your herbs are free from contaminants.

Preparing Herbs

1. Cleaning: Once harvested, clean your herbs to remove any dirt, insects, or debris. Rinse them gently under cool water and pat them dry with a clean cloth or paper towel. For delicate flowers and leaves, a quick rinse may suffice, while roots may need more thorough scrubbing.

2. Drying: Drying herbs is essential for long-term storage and preserving their medicinal properties. Spread the herbs in a single layer on a drying rack, screen, or paper towels. Place them in a warm, dry, well-ventilated area out of direct sunlight. Turn the herbs occasionally to ensure even drying. You can also use a dehydrator set to a low temperature (95°F to 115°F) for faster drying.

3. Checking for Dryness: Herbs are fully dried when they are crisp and crumble easily between your fingers. Roots should be hard and brittle. Ensuring complete dryness is crucial to prevent mold and spoilage during storage.

4. Cutting and Grinding: For some preparations, you may need to cut or grind the dried herbs. Use clean, sharp scissors to cut herbs into smaller pieces. A mortar and pestle or a dedicated herb grinder can be used to powder the herbs if needed. Cutting and grinding increase the surface area, making it easier to extract the active compounds during preparation.

Storing Herbs

1. Containers: Store dried herbs in airtight containers to protect them from moisture, light, and air. Dark glass jars are ideal as they block light, which can degrade the herbs' potency. Alternatively, use opaque or colored containers, or store clear jars in a dark cupboard.

2. Labeling: Always label your containers with the herb's name, the date of harvest or preparation, and any other relevant information. This helps you keep track of the freshness and potency of your herbs.

3. Storage Environment: Store your herbs in a cool, dark, and dry place. Avoid areas with fluctuating temperatures and humidity, such as kitchens or bathrooms. A pantry or a dedicated herb cabinet works well.

4. Shelf Life: Most dried herbs retain their medicinal properties for about one year. However, some, like roots and seeds, may last longer if stored properly. Regularly check your stored herbs for any signs of mold, discoloration, or loss of aroma, and discard any that show these signs.

Properly gathering, preparing, and storing herbs is essential for creating effective herbal remedies. By following these guidelines, you ensure that the medicinal qualities of the herbs are preserved, providing you with potent and reliable ingredients for your tinctures, infusions, decoctions, essential oils, and salves. Embracing these practices not only enhances the quality of your herbal medicine but also deepens your connection to the natural world and the healing power of plants. Always remember to respect nature and practice sustainable harvesting to maintain the health and abundance of herbal resources for future generations.

Measuring, Mixing, and Preserving Herbal Preparations

The art of creating herbal remedies involves precise measuring, careful mixing, and effective preservation to ensure the potency and efficacy of your preparations. Proper techniques in these areas are essential for achieving consistent results and maximizing the therapeutic benefits of the herbs. This guide will provide you with the necessary steps to measure, mix, and preserve your herbal preparations correctly.

Measuring Herbal Ingredients

1. Accuracy: Accurate measurement of herbal ingredients is crucial for ensuring the correct dosage and effectiveness of your remedies. Use a kitchen scale for precise measurements, especially when dealing with dried herbs, essential oils, and other concentrated ingredients. Measuring spoons and cups can be used for less critical measurements.

2. Ratios and Proportions: Familiarize yourself with common ratios and proportions used in herbal preparations. For example, a typical ratio for tinctures is 1 part dried herb to 5 parts solvent (e.g., alcohol or glycerin), while infusions and decoctions often use 1-2 tablespoons of dried herbs per cup of water.

3. Consistency: Ensure consistency by using the same measurement units throughout the preparation process. This helps maintain the correct balance of ingredients and ensures the reliability of your remedies.

Mixing Herbal Preparations

1. Tools and Equipment: Use clean, dedicated tools and equipment for mixing herbal preparations to avoid contamination. Glass, stainless steel, and food-grade plastic are ideal materials for mixing bowls, spoons, and other utensils.

2. Combining Ingredients: Mix herbs and other ingredients thoroughly to ensure an even distribution of active compounds. For tinctures, shake the mixture daily during the maceration process. For infusions and decoctions, stir the herbs while steeping or simmering to enhance extraction.

3. Blending Techniques: When creating blends, such as herbal teas or salves, consider the properties and flavors of each herb. Balance strong-tasting or potent herbs with milder ones to create a harmonious blend. Experiment with different combinations to find the best synergy for your intended use.

4. Incorporating Essential Oils: When adding essential oils to preparations like salves or lotions, mix them thoroughly with a carrier oil or base ingredient before combining them with the rest of the mixture. This ensures even distribution and prevents skin irritation from undiluted essential oils.

Preserving Herbal Preparations

1. Proper Storage: Store your herbal preparations in clean, airtight containers to protect them from light, air, and moisture. Dark glass bottles and jars are ideal for preserving the potency of your remedies. Label each container with the name of the preparation, the date it was made, and any specific storage instructions.

2. Refrigeration: Some herbal preparations, such as fresh plant infusions, syrups, and certain types of herbal oils, may require refrigeration to prolong their shelf life. Always check the recommended storage conditions for each type of preparation.

3. Preservatives: Consider using natural preservatives to extend the shelf life of your herbal products. For example, adding a small amount of vitamin E oil to salves and oils can prevent rancidity. Alcohol acts as a preservative in tinctures, while honey can help preserve syrups.

4. Monitoring and Checking: Regularly check your stored herbal preparations for signs of spoilage, such as mold, off-odors, or discoloration. Discard any preparations that show these signs to ensure safety and effectiveness.

5. Shelf Life: Understand the typical shelf life of different herbal preparations. Dried herbs generally last about one year, while tinctures can last several years if stored properly. Salves and oils usually last 6-12 months, depending on the ingredients and storage conditions.

Measuring, mixing, and preserving herbal preparations are essential steps in creating effective and reliable herbal remedies. Accurate measurement ensures the correct dosage and potency, while thorough mixing guarantees an even distribution of active compounds. Proper preservation techniques protect your preparations from spoilage and maintain their therapeutic benefits over time. By following these guidelines, you can confidently produce high-quality herbal remedies that support health and well-being. Always consult with a healthcare provider if you have any concerns or specific health conditions before using new herbal preparations.

Creating Herbal Teas and Syrups

Herbal teas and syrups are two of the most accessible and enjoyable ways to incorporate the therapeutic benefits of herbs into your daily routine. Herbal teas, also known as tisanes, involve steeping dried or fresh herbs in hot water to extract their beneficial compounds, resulting in a soothing and medicinal beverage. Herbal syrups, on the other hand, combine herbal infusions or decoctions with natural sweeteners like honey or sugar to create a concentrated liquid that is both flavorful and therapeutic. These preparations are not only effective remedies for a variety of ailments but also offer a comforting and pleasant way to consume herbs. This chapter will introduce you to the basics of creating herbal teas and syrups, exploring their benefits, and providing step-by-step guides to help you make these versatile herbal preparations at home.

Herbal Teas: Benefits and Blending

Herbal teas, or tisanes, are a delightful and effective way to enjoy the medicinal benefits of herbs. They are created by steeping various parts of plants—such as leaves, flowers, stems, seeds, and roots—in hot water. Herbal teas are not only therapeutic but also provide a relaxing and enjoyable experience. They can be tailored to address specific health concerns or simply enjoyed for their flavors and aromas. Here are some of the key benefits of herbal teas and tips for blending them.

Benefits of Herbal Teas

1. Nutrient-Rich: Herbal teas are packed with vitamins, minerals, and antioxidants that support overall health. For example, nettle tea is rich in iron, calcium, and magnesium, while rosehip tea is high in vitamin C.

2. Hydration: Drinking herbal teas contributes to your daily fluid intake, promoting hydration and overall well-being. This is particularly beneficial for those who find it challenging to drink plain water.

3. Digestive Aid: Many herbal teas help soothe and support the digestive system. Peppermint and ginger teas can relieve indigestion, bloating, and nausea, while chamomile tea can calm the digestive tract and reduce inflammation.

4. Stress Relief and Relaxation: Herbal teas can have calming effects on the nervous system, helping to reduce stress and promote relaxation. Chamomile, lavender, and lemon balm teas are known for their soothing properties and can help improve sleep quality.

5. Immune Support: Certain herbal teas can boost the immune system and help prevent or alleviate symptoms of colds and flu. Echinacea, elderberry, and ginger teas are popular choices for supporting immune health.

6. Detoxification: Herbal teas like dandelion and burdock root help support the body's natural detoxification processes by promoting liver and kidney function. These teas can help cleanse the body of toxins and improve overall health.

Blending Herbal Teas

Creating your own herbal tea blends allows you to tailor the flavors and therapeutic benefits to your specific needs and preferences. Here are some tips for blending herbal teas:

1. Understand Herb Properties: Familiarize yourself with the properties and benefits of different herbs. Knowing which herbs are soothing, stimulating, or nourishing will help you create balanced and effective blends.

2. Balance Flavors: Aim for a harmonious balance of flavors in your blend. Combine strong-tasting herbs with milder ones to create a pleasing flavor profile. For example, mix the robust flavor of ginger with the mild sweetness of chamomile.

3. Use a Base Herb: Choose a base herb that will form the foundation of your blend. This can be a neutral-tasting herb like chamomile or a more flavorful one like peppermint. The base herb should make up about 50-70% of your blend.

4. Add Complementary Herbs: Select complementary herbs to add specific therapeutic benefits or enhance the flavor of the base herb. These herbs should make up about 20-30% of your blend. For example, add echinacea to a peppermint base for immune support.

5. Include Accent Herbs: Accent herbs add a final touch of flavor or boost the therapeutic properties of the blend. These should be used sparingly, making up about 10-20% of the blend. For example, add a pinch of lavender to a chamomile blend for added relaxation.

6. Experiment and Adjust: Feel free to experiment with different combinations and proportions until you find a blend that suits your taste and needs. Keep notes of your blends and adjustments to replicate successful combinations in the future.

7. Sample Blends:

- **Relaxing Blend:**
    - Base: Chamomile (60%)
    - Complementary: Lemon Balm (20%)
    - Accent: Lavender (10%)
    - Optional: A touch of honey for sweetness

- **Digestive Aid:**
    - Base: Peppermint (50%)
    - Complementary: Fennel (20%)
    - Complementary: Ginger (20%)
    - Accent: Lemon Verbena (10%)

- **Immune Boosting:**
    - Base: Echinacea (50%)
    - Complementary: Elderberry (20%)
    - Complementary: Hibiscus (20%)

      ◦ Accent: Rose Hips (10%)

8. Preparation: To prepare an herbal tea, use about 1-2 teaspoons of your blend per cup of boiling water. Steep for 5-10 minutes, depending on the desired strength. Strain and enjoy hot or cold, sweetened with honey or as is.

Herbal teas offer a myriad of health benefits and provide a versatile, enjoyable way to incorporate herbs into your daily routine. By understanding the properties of different herbs and how to balance flavors, you can create personalized blends that cater to your specific health needs and preferences. Experimenting with various combinations allows you to discover the perfect blend for any occasion, enhancing both your wellness and culinary experience. Always consult with a healthcare provider before using new herbs, especially if you have pre-existing conditions or are taking medications.

Herbal Syrups: Benefits and Preparation

Herbal syrups are a popular and effective way to deliver the therapeutic benefits of herbs in a sweet and palatable form. By combining concentrated herbal extracts with natural sweeteners like honey or sugar, herbal syrups offer both medicinal properties and a pleasant taste, making them especially suitable for children and those who may be sensitive to the taste of herbal teas or tinctures. This section explores the benefits of herbal syrups and provides a step-by-step guide for their preparation.

Benefits of Herbal Syrups

1. Enhanced Palatability: Herbal syrups are sweetened, which makes them more enjoyable to consume, especially for children. The sweetness masks the sometimes bitter or strong taste of certain herbs, making it easier to incorporate them into your daily routine.

2. Concentrated Dosage: Syrups are a concentrated form of herbal medicine, allowing you to deliver a potent dose of the herb's active constituents in a small volume. This is particularly useful for potent herbs or when a higher dosage is required.

3. Soothing Properties: Many herbal syrups are designed to soothe the throat and respiratory system. The viscous nature of the syrup coats the throat, providing relief from irritation, coughing, and soreness. Herbs like elderberry, thyme, and licorice root are commonly used for their soothing effects.

4. Long Shelf Life: When properly prepared and stored, herbal syrups have a relatively long shelf life due to the preservative properties of the sweeteners used. This makes them a convenient option for long-term use.

5. Versatility: Herbal syrups can be used in various ways, from direct consumption by the spoonful to mixing into teas, beverages, or foods. This versatility allows you to easily integrate the benefits of herbs into your diet.

Preparation of Herbal Syrups

Creating herbal syrups involves making a strong herbal decoction or infusion and then combining it with a sweetener. Here is a step-by-step guide to making your own herbal syrup:

1. **Selecting and Preparing Herbs:** Choose high-quality dried or fresh herbs based on the desired therapeutic effects. Common choices include elderberries for immune support, licorice root for soothing the throat, and ginger for digestive aid.

2. **Making a Strong Decoction or Infusion:** For a decoction, place 1 cup of dried herbs (or 2 cups of fresh herbs) in a saucepan and cover with 4 cups of water. Bring to a boil, then reduce the heat and let it simmer for about 30-45 minutes, until the liquid is reduced by half. For a milder infusion, steep the herbs in hot water for 20-30 minutes.

3. **Straining the Liquid:** Once the decoction or infusion is ready, strain the liquid through a fine mesh strainer or cheesecloth to remove the plant material. Ensure you extract as much liquid as possible by pressing the herbs.

4. **Adding Sweetener:** Measure the strained liquid and return it to the saucepan. For each cup of herbal liquid, add 1 cup of honey or sugar. Stir well to dissolve the sweetener completely. If using honey, allow the liquid to cool slightly before adding it to preserve its beneficial properties.

5. **Simmering the Mixture:** Heat the mixture gently over low heat, stirring constantly until the sweetener is fully incorporated and the syrup reaches the desired consistency. Avoid boiling to preserve the medicinal properties of both the herbs and the sweetener.

6. **Adding Preservatives (Optional):** To extend the shelf life, you can add a small amount of brandy or vodka (about 1-2 tablespoons per cup of syrup) as a preservative. This step is optional but can help keep the syrup fresh for longer.

7. **Bottling and Storing:** Pour the hot syrup into sterilized glass bottles or jars, leaving a little space at the top. Seal the containers tightly and label them with the name of the syrup and the date of preparation. Store the syrup in a cool, dark place or refrigerate for longer shelf life.

8. **Dosage and Usage:** The typical dosage for herbal syrups is 1-2 teaspoons taken 1-3 times daily, depending on the herb and the condition being treated. Always consult with a healthcare provider for appropriate dosages, especially for children.

Herbal syrups are a versatile, effective, and enjoyable way to incorporate the benefits of herbs into your daily routine. By combining potent herbal extracts with natural sweeteners, you can create remedies that are both therapeutic and palatable. The preparation process is straightforward, allowing you to customize syrups to meet your specific health needs and preferences. Whether you are looking to soothe a sore throat, boost your immune system, or simply enjoy the flavors of herbal medicine, herbal syrups offer a practical and delicious solution. Always consult with a healthcare provider before using new herbal preparations, especially if you have any underlying health conditions or are taking other medications.

Making Herbal Creams and Lotions

Herbal creams and lotions are a luxurious and effective way to nourish and protect your skin using the natural healing properties of herbs. These topical preparations combine the moisturizing and soothing benefits of herbal-infused oils with the hydrating qualities of water-based ingredients, resulting in products that are perfect for a variety of skincare needs. Whether you are looking to moisturize dry skin, soothe irritation, or address specific skin conditions, making your own herbal creams and lotions allows you to customize ingredients to suit your personal preferences and therapeutic goals. This chapter will introduce you to the basics of creating herbal creams and lotions, covering essential ingredients, equipment, and techniques to help you craft high-quality, homemade skincare products.

Herbal Creams and Lotions: Benefits, Ingredients, and Equipment

Herbal creams and lotions offer a natural, effective way to care for your skin, harnessing the power of plant-based ingredients. By creating your own products, you can ensure that they are free from synthetic chemicals and tailored to meet your specific skincare needs. This section will explore the benefits of herbal creams and lotions, the essential ingredients needed, and the equipment required for making them at home.

Benefits of Herbal Creams and Lotions

1. Moisturizing: Herbal creams and lotions provide deep hydration, helping to maintain the skin's natural moisture balance. Ingredients like aloe vera, shea butter, and carrier oils such as jojoba or almond oil are excellent for locking in moisture and keeping the skin soft and supple.

2. Soothing and Healing: Many herbs have anti-inflammatory, antiseptic, and healing properties that can soothe irritated skin and promote healing. Calendula, chamomile, and lavender are commonly used in creams and lotions to reduce redness, calm irritation, and support the skin's natural repair processes.

3. Nourishing: Herbal creams and lotions are rich in vitamins, minerals, and antioxidants that nourish the skin. These nutrients help to protect the skin from environmental damage, boost collagen production, and maintain a healthy complexion. Ingredients like rosehip oil, green tea extract, and vitamin E are particularly beneficial for skin health.

4. Customizable: When making your own herbal creams and lotions, you can customize the ingredients to address specific skin concerns such as dryness, acne, aging, or sensitivity. This allows for a personalized skincare routine that is tailored to your unique needs.

5. Chemical-Free: Homemade herbal creams and lotions are free from synthetic fragrances, preservatives, and other chemicals commonly found in commercial skincare products. This makes them a safer option for those with sensitive skin or allergies.

Essential Ingredients

1. Carrier Oils: Carrier oils form the base of herbal creams and lotions, providing moisturizing and nourishing benefits. Popular carrier oils include:

- **Jojoba Oil:** Closely resembles the skin's natural sebum, making it highly compatible and easily absorbed.

- **Sweet Almond Oil:** Rich in vitamins A and E, it is excellent for moisturizing and soothing dry skin.

- **Coconut Oil:** Offers deep hydration and has antimicrobial properties.

2. Butters: Butters add richness and a thicker texture to creams and lotions. Commonly used butters include:

- **Shea Butter:** Known for its moisturizing and healing properties.

- **Cocoa Butter:** Provides a protective barrier and is deeply nourishing.

3. Herbal Infusions and Extracts: Herbs can be infused into oils or used in the form of extracts to impart their therapeutic properties. Examples include:

- **Calendula:** Anti-inflammatory and healing, ideal for sensitive or damaged skin.

- **Chamomile:** Soothing and calming, great for irritated or inflamed skin.

- **Lavender:** Antiseptic and relaxing, perfect for all skin types.

4. Essential Oils: Essential oils add fragrance and additional therapeutic benefits to creams and lotions. Examples include:

- **Lavender Essential Oil:** Calming and healing.

- **Tea Tree Essential Oil:** Antibacterial and antifungal.

- **Rosemary Essential Oil:** Stimulating and rejuvenating.

5. Water-Based Ingredients: Water or hydrosols (floral waters) provide hydration and help to create a lighter texture. Examples include:

- **Aloe Vera Gel:** Hydrating and soothing.

- **Rose Water:** Refreshing and toning.

6. Emulsifiers: Emulsifiers are necessary to blend oil and water-based ingredients into a stable cream or lotion. Common natural emulsifiers include:

- **Beeswax:** Provides a barrier and helps to thicken the product.

- **Emulsifying Wax:** A blend of plant-based waxes that help combine oil and water.

7. Preservatives: To extend the shelf life and prevent microbial growth, natural preservatives can be used, such as:

- **Vitamin E Oil:** Antioxidant that helps prevent rancidity in oils.

- **Grapefruit Seed Extract:** Natural preservative with antimicrobial properties.

Essential Equipment

1. Double Boiler: A double boiler is used to gently melt butters and waxes without direct heat, preventing them from burning.

2. Mixing Bowls and Utensils: Stainless steel or glass mixing bowls and spoons are ideal for mixing ingredients. Avoid using plastic, which can absorb odors and colors.

3. Blender or Hand Mixer: A blender or hand mixer helps to achieve a smooth and uniform consistency for your creams and lotions.

4. Measuring Cups and Spoons: Accurate measurement of ingredients is crucial for consistency and efficacy.

5. Glass Jars and Bottles: Use sterilized glass jars and bottles to store your finished products. Dark glass containers are preferable as they protect the contents from light and extend shelf life.

6. Labels: Label your jars and bottles with the name of the product, ingredients, and date of preparation to keep track of freshness and usage.

Making herbal creams and lotions at home allows you to create personalized skincare products that are tailored to your specific needs and preferences. By understanding the benefits of various ingredients and having the right equipment, you can craft effective and luxurious creams and lotions that nourish, protect, and heal your skin naturally. Always consult with a healthcare provider if you have any concerns or specific skin conditions before using new herbal preparations.

Step-by-Step Guide to Making Creams and Lotions

Creating your own herbal creams and lotions at home allows you to harness the nourishing and healing properties of natural ingredients tailored to your specific skin needs. Here is a detailed step-by-step guide to making your own herbal creams and lotions.

Materials and Ingredients

Equipment:

- Double boiler or heatproof bowls and saucepans
- Measuring spoons and cups
- Digital scale
- Whisk or immersion blender
- Sterilized glass jars or lotion bottles
- Stirring utensils (spoons or spatulas)
- Thermometer

Ingredients:

- Carrier oils (e.g., jojoba oil, almond oil, coconut oil)

- Butters (e.g., shea butter, cocoa butter)

- Distilled water or herbal infusions

- Emulsifying wax (e.g., beeswax or plant-based emulsifiers)

- Preservatives (e.g., vitamin E oil, grapefruit seed extract)

- Essential oils (optional for fragrance and additional benefits)

- Herbal extracts or infused oils (optional for added therapeutic effects)

Step-by-Step Process

Step 1: Prepare Your Workspace Ensure that your workspace is clean and organized. Sterilize all equipment and containers to prevent contamination.

Step 2: Measure Ingredients Using a digital scale, accurately measure your ingredients. A typical formula for a basic cream might include:

- 50 grams of carrier oil (e.g., almond oil)

- 20 grams of butter (e.g., shea butter)

- 30 grams of distilled water or herbal infusion

- 5 grams of emulsifying wax (e.g., beeswax)

- 1 gram of preservative (e.g., vitamin E oil)

- 10-20 drops of essential oil (optional)

Step 3: Create the Oil Phase In a double boiler, combine the carrier oils, butters, and emulsifying wax. Heat gently until all ingredients are fully melted and combined. Stir occasionally to ensure even melting.

Step 4: Prepare the Water Phase In a separate heatproof container, heat the distilled water or herbal infusion to a similar temperature as the oil phase. This helps the emulsification process.

Step 5: Combine the Oil and Water Phases Once both the oil and water phases have reached a similar temperature (around 70°C or 158°F), slowly pour the water phase into the oil phase. Use a whisk or immersion blender to blend the mixture thoroughly. Continue blending until the mixture begins to thicken and reach a creamy consistency.

Step 6: Cool Down and Add Preservatives As the mixture cools to below 40°C (104°F), add the preservative and any essential oils or herbal extracts. Stir well to ensure all ingredients are evenly incorporated.

Step 7: Pour and Store Pour the finished cream into sterilized glass jars or lotion bottles. Seal tightly and label with the date and ingredients used. Store the cream in a cool, dark place to maintain its potency and extend its shelf life. Properly stored, homemade creams can last for up to six months.

Step 8: Test and Enjoy Before using the cream on your face or body, perform a patch test to ensure you do not have any allergic reactions. Apply a small amount to your inner forearm and wait 24 hours to check for any adverse reactions. If there is no irritation, you can safely use your homemade cream.

Tips for Customization

- **Herbal Infusions:** Replace distilled water with herbal infusions (e.g., chamomile, calendula) to add additional therapeutic properties.

- **Adjust Consistency:** For a thicker cream, increase the amount of butter or wax. For a lighter lotion, increase the water phase.

- **Fragrance and Benefits:** Customize the scent and benefits by adding different essential oils, such as lavender for calming effects or tea tree for its antibacterial properties.

Making your own herbal creams and lotions is a rewarding and creative process that allows you to tailor skincare products to your specific needs. By following this step-by-step guide, you can create nourishing and effective creams that harness the power of natural ingredients. Whether for personal use or as thoughtful handmade gifts, homemade creams and lotions offer a personalized touch to skincare routines.

BOOK 19:

Barbara O'Neill's Studies and Research: Analysis of Discoveries and Testimonials

Analysis of Key Research

In the field of herbal medicine, rigorous research and evidence-based studies are essential for validating the therapeutic benefits and safety of herbal remedies. Barbara O'Neill's extensive body of work has significantly contributed to this growing field, providing valuable insights and advancing our understanding of how herbs can be used effectively in modern healthcare. This chapter delves into the key research studies that have shaped contemporary herbal medicine, highlighting major discoveries, methodological approaches, and the impact of these findings on both clinical practice and everyday health. By examining the historical context and evolution of herbal research, as well as reviewing pivotal studies and meta-analyses, this chapter aims to present a comprehensive overview of the scientific foundation supporting the use of herbal remedies.

Historical Context and Evolution

The practice of herbal medicine has deep roots in human history, dating back thousands of years to ancient civilizations where plants were the primary sources of medicine. Early records from cultures such as the Egyptians, Greeks, Chinese, and Indigenous peoples reveal a rich tradition of using herbs to treat a variety of ailments. These early herbalists observed the effects of different plants through trial and error, and their findings were passed down through generations, forming the basis of traditional herbal knowledge.

In ancient Egypt, papyrus scrolls such as the Ebers Papyrus, dating back to around 1550 BCE, detail the use of numerous herbs, including garlic, juniper, and aloe vera, for treating conditions ranging from infections to digestive disorders. Similarly, ancient Greek physicians like Hippocrates and Dioscorides compiled extensive works on medicinal plants, emphasizing their importance in maintaining health and treating disease. Dioscorides' "De Materia Medica," written in the first century CE, remained a key reference for over 1,500 years, influencing both Eastern and Western herbal traditions.

The Chinese Materia Medica, a comprehensive text on herbal medicine, dates back to the first century CE and outlines the use of hundreds of herbs. This text formed the foundation of Traditional Chinese Medicine (TCM), which integrates herbal remedies into a holistic approach to health and wellness. TCM has continued to evolve over millennia, maintaining a significant role in modern healthcare practices in China and around the world.

During the Middle Ages, European monasteries preserved and expanded upon ancient herbal knowledge. Monks meticulously copied ancient texts and cultivated medicinal gardens, ensuring the continuity of herbal practices through the Dark Ages. This period also saw the rise of influential herbalists like Hildegard of Bingen and Nicholas Culpeper, whose works further enriched the European herbal tradition.

The Renaissance brought a resurgence of interest in science and natural medicine, leading to more systematic documentation and classification of medicinal plants. The invention of the printing press facilitated the widespread dissemination of herbal knowledge, making it accessible to a broader audience. Herbalists and botanists of this era, such as John Gerard and Leonhart Fuchs, published detailed herbals that combined traditional knowledge with their own observations and experiments.

In the 19th and early 20th centuries, the rise of modern pharmacology and synthetic drugs led to a decline in the use of herbal medicine in Western countries. However, interest in natural remedies persisted, and many traditional practices continued to thrive, particularly in rural and Indigenous communities. The mid-20th century saw a renewed interest in herbal medicine, driven by the countercultural movements of the 1960s and 70s, which emphasized holistic health and a return to nature.

Today, herbal medicine is experiencing a resurgence as scientific research validates the efficacy of many traditional remedies. Modern herbalists and researchers build upon the rich legacy of historical practices, employing advanced techniques to study the pharmacological properties of herbs and their potential health benefits. The integration of herbal medicine with conventional treatments is becoming more common, reflecting a growing recognition of the value of a holistic approach to healthcare.

The evolution of herbal medicine from ancient traditions to contemporary practices highlights the enduring significance of plants in promoting health and healing. By understanding this historical context, we can appreciate the depth of knowledge and experience that informs modern herbal research, guiding us toward more effective and evidence-based use of herbal remedies in our quest for optimal health.

Overview of Early Research in Herbal Medicine

Herbal medicine, rooted in ancient traditions, has been a cornerstone of healthcare for thousands of years. Early research in herbal medicine laid the foundation for modern pharmacology and therapeutic practices, providing insights into the medicinal properties of plants and their applications. This overview explores the pivotal milestones and key figures in the early research of herbal medicine, highlighting its evolution and impact on contemporary healthcare.

Ancient Civilizations and Herbal Knowledge

1. Egypt: Ancient Egyptian civilization is among the earliest to have documented the use of herbs for medicinal purposes. The Ebers Papyrus, dating back to around 1550 BCE, is one of the oldest and most comprehensive medical texts from this era. It lists hundreds of herbal remedies for various ailments, including garlic for infections, aloe vera for skin conditions, and juniper for digestive issues. The extensive use of herbs in ancient Egypt highlights their integral role in early medical practices.

2. China: Traditional Chinese Medicine (TCM) has a rich history that spans over 2,000 years. The "Shennong Ben Cao Jing" (The Divine Farmer's Materia Medica), attributed to the mythical emperor Shennong around 2800 BCE, is one of the earliest Chinese herbal texts. It describes the therapeutic properties of 365 medicinal plants, including ginseng, licorice, and ginger. TCM emphasizes the balance of bodily energies (Qi) and the use of herbs to restore harmony and health.

3. India: Ayurveda, the traditional system of medicine in India, has a history dating back over 3,000 years. The foundational texts, the "Charaka Samhita" and the "Sushruta Samhita," compiled around 1000 BCE, provide detailed descriptions of numerous herbs and their medicinal uses. Turmeric, ashwagandha, and holy basil are some of the key herbs in Ayurveda, used to treat a wide range of physical and mental health conditions.

Greek and Roman Contributions

1. Hippocrates and Dioscorides: Hippocrates, often referred to as the "Father of Medicine," emphasized the importance of diet, lifestyle, and natural remedies in health. Although his works primarily focused on clinical observations, they influenced subsequent herbal studies. Dioscorides, a Greek physician in the 1st century CE, authored "De Materia Medica," a comprehensive text on medicinal plants. This five-volume work systematically categorizes hundreds of plants and their therapeutic uses, serving as a primary reference for over 1,500 years.

2. Galen: Galen, a Roman physician and philosopher in the 2nd century CE, expanded on Hippocratic principles and Dioscorides' work. He developed the concept of "galenic" medicine, which involves the preparation of complex herbal mixtures to treat various ailments. Galen's methods of extracting and combining plant compounds laid the groundwork for modern pharmacology.

Medieval and Renaissance Developments

1. Monastic Medicine: During the Middle Ages, European monasteries became centers of herbal knowledge. Monks meticulously copied ancient texts and cultivated medicinal gardens, preserving herbal traditions through the Dark Ages. The "Capitulare de Villis," a directive issued by Charlemagne in the 9th century, mandated the cultivation of specific medicinal plants in monastery gardens, ensuring the continuity of herbal practices.

2. Hildegard of Bingen: Hildegard of Bingen, a 12th-century Benedictine abbess, made significant contributions to herbal medicine. Her works, "Physica" and "Causae et Curae," describe the medicinal properties of various herbs and their applications in treating illnesses. Hildegard's holistic approach to health, which integrated physical, spiritual, and environmental factors, continues to influence modern herbal practices.

3. The Renaissance and Herbalism: The Renaissance era witnessed a revival of interest in science and natural medicine. The invention of the printing press facilitated the widespread dissemination of herbal knowledge. Prominent herbalists like John Gerard and Nicholas Culpeper published detailed herbals that combined traditional knowledge with their own observations and experiments. Culpeper's "The English Physician" and Gerard's "Herball" were among the most influential texts, bridging the gap between ancient practices and modern herbal medicine.

Early Scientific Exploration

1. Paracelsus: Paracelsus, a Swiss physician and alchemist in the 16th century, challenged traditional medical theories and introduced the concept of using chemical processes to extract medicinal compounds from plants. He believed that understanding the chemical properties of herbs was essential for their effective use in medicine. Paracelsus' approach paved the way for modern pharmacology and the scientific study of herbal medicine.

2. William Withering: In the 18th century, William Withering, an English physician, conducted one of the first systematic studies of a medicinal plant. His work on foxglove (Digitalis purpurea) demonstrated its efficacy in treating heart conditions, specifically dropsy (congestive heart failure). Withering's meticulous documentation and clinical trials marked a significant advancement in the scientific validation of herbal remedies.

Early research in herbal medicine, spanning ancient civilizations to the Renaissance, laid the foundational principles that continue to influence modern healthcare. The extensive documentation, cultivation, and experimentation with medicinal plants by ancient Egyptians, Chinese, Indians, Greeks, Romans, medieval monks, and Renaissance herbalists have provided a rich legacy of knowledge. This historical perspective underscores the enduring significance of herbal medicine and its evolving role in contemporary health practices. As modern science continues to validate and expand upon these early discoveries, the integration of herbal medicine into mainstream healthcare offers promising possibilities for holistic and effective treatment strategies.

Evolution of Research Methodologies

The study of herbal medicine has evolved significantly over the centuries, progressing from anecdotal observations and traditional practices to rigorous scientific investigations. This evolution in research methodologies has helped establish the credibility of herbal medicine and integrate it into modern healthcare. Here, we explore the key phases in the evolution of research methodologies in herbal medicine, highlighting the advancements that have shaped contemporary practices.

Early Observational Studies

1. Traditional Knowledge and Oral Traditions: The earliest research methodologies in herbal medicine were based on observational studies and oral traditions. Healers and herbalists relied on trial and error to determine the efficacy of various plants, observing their effects on health and well-being over generations. This knowledge was passed down orally, with detailed descriptions of plant properties, preparation methods, and therapeutic uses.

2. Early Documentation: As societies developed written languages, the oral traditions of herbal medicine were transcribed into texts. Ancient civilizations such as the Egyptians, Greeks, Chinese, and Indians produced extensive herbal compendia, documenting the medicinal properties of plants. Notable examples include the Ebers Papyrus in Egypt, "De Materia Medica" by Dioscorides in Greece, the "Shennong Ben Cao Jing" in China, and the "Charaka Samhita" in India. These texts served as the foundation for future herbal studies, providing a rich source of traditional knowledge.

Medieval and Renaissance Herbals

1. Monastic Contributions: During the Middle Ages, European monasteries played a crucial role in preserving and expanding herbal knowledge. Monks compiled herbals that included illustrations, descriptions, and medicinal uses of plants. These herbals, such as those produced by Hildegard of Bingen, combined empirical observations with spiritual and philosophical insights.

2. The Printing Press and Renaissance Herbals: The invention of the printing press in the 15th century revolutionized the dissemination of herbal knowledge. Renaissance herbalists like John Gerard, Nicholas Culpeper, and Leonhart Fuchs published detailed herbals that were widely distributed. These works combined traditional knowledge with personal observations and experiments, making herbal medicine more accessible and promoting standardized methodologies.

Early Scientific Approaches

1. Paracelsus and Chemical Extraction: In the 16th century, Paracelsus introduced the concept of chemical extraction, emphasizing the importance of isolating active compounds from plants. His approach marked a shift from empirical observations to a more scientific understanding of herbal medicine. Paracelsus' work laid the groundwork for the development of pharmacognosy, the study of medicinal plants and their chemical constituents.

2. William Withering and Clinical Observation: William Withering's study of foxglove (Digitalis purpurea) in the 18th century is a landmark in the scientific investigation of herbal medicine. Withering conducted systematic clinical observations, documenting the effects of foxglove on patients with heart conditions. His meticulous approach to dosage and patient monitoring set a precedent for future clinical trials in herbal medicine.

Modern Experimental Research

1. Phytochemical Analysis: Advancements in chemistry and analytical techniques in the 19th and 20th centuries enabled researchers to isolate and identify the active compounds in medicinal plants. Phytochemical analysis involves the use of techniques such as chromatography, mass spectrometry, and nuclear magnetic resonance (NMR) spectroscopy to study the chemical composition of plants. This methodological shift provided a scientific basis for the therapeutic properties of herbs and allowed for the standardization of herbal products.

2. In Vitro and In Vivo Studies: Modern research methodologies include in vitro (test tube) and in vivo (animal) studies to investigate the biological activity of herbal compounds. In vitro studies allow researchers to explore the mechanisms of action of herbs at the cellular and molecular levels. In vivo studies provide insights into the systemic effects and safety profiles of herbal remedies. These preclinical studies are essential for understanding the pharmacodynamics and pharmacokinetics of herbal compounds.

3. Clinical Trials: Clinical trials are the gold standard for evaluating the safety and efficacy of herbal medicines in humans. These trials follow rigorous protocols, including randomized controlled trials (RCTs), double-blind studies, and placebo-controlled designs. Clinical trials provide high-quality evidence that supports the use of herbal remedies in clinical practice. The integration of herbal medicine into evidence-based healthcare relies heavily on the findings from well-conducted clinical trials.

4. Systematic Reviews and Meta-Analyses: Systematic reviews and meta-analyses synthesize data from multiple studies to provide comprehensive evaluations of herbal treatments. These methodologies assess the overall strength of evidence, identify trends, and highlight gaps in the research. Systematic reviews and meta-analyses are crucial for informing clinical guidelines and policy decisions regarding the use of herbal medicine.

Emerging Research Methodologies

1. Genomic and Proteomic Studies: Advances in genomics and proteomics are opening new avenues for herbal medicine research. Genomic studies investigate how genetic variations influence individual responses to herbal treatments, paving the way for personalized herbal medicine. Proteomic studies explore the protein interactions and pathways affected by herbal compounds, providing deeper insights into their mechanisms of action.

2. Artificial Intelligence and Machine Learning: Artificial intelligence (AI) and machine learning are revolutionizing herbal medicine research by analyzing large datasets and predicting therapeutic outcomes. AI can identify patterns, optimize dosages, and suggest novel herbal combinations based on existing data. These technologies enhance the efficiency and precision of herbal research, accelerating the discovery of new treatments.

The evolution of research methodologies in herbal medicine reflects the ongoing efforts to integrate traditional knowledge with modern scientific rigor. From early observational studies and medieval herbals to contemporary clinical trials and emerging technologies, each phase has contributed to a deeper understanding of the therapeutic potential of medicinal plants. As research methodologies continue to advance, the credibility and integration of herbal medicine in mainstream healthcare will likely increase, offering safe, effective, and holistic treatment options for a wide range of health conditions.

Major Discoveries and Impact

Herbal medicine has undergone significant advancements over the centuries, with numerous major discoveries that have shaped its practice and integration into modern healthcare. These discoveries have provided scientific validation for traditional uses of herbs and have led to the development of new therapeutic applications. Here are some of the key discoveries in herbal medicine and their impact on both the field and broader medical practice.

1. Identification of Active Compounds

One of the most significant breakthroughs in herbal medicine has been the identification and isolation of active compounds in plants. These compounds are responsible for the therapeutic effects of herbs. For example, the discovery of salicin in willow bark, which later led to the development of aspirin, highlighted the analgesic and anti-inflammatory properties of the herb. Similarly, the isolation of quinine from cinchona bark revolutionized the treatment of malaria, demonstrating the potential of herbal compounds in combating serious diseases.

2. Standardization and Quality Control

Advancements in the standardization and quality control of herbal products have greatly improved their reliability and efficacy. By ensuring consistent levels of active ingredients, standardization helps to maximize the therapeutic benefits and minimize variations between batches. Techniques such as chromatography and spectrophotometry are used to analyze and quantify the constituents of herbal extracts, ensuring that they meet established standards. This has increased the acceptance of herbal remedies in mainstream healthcare and has paved the way for their integration with conventional treatments.

3. Clinical Trials and Evidence-Based Research

The conduct of rigorous clinical trials and evidence-based research has been crucial in validating the efficacy and safety of herbal remedies. For instance, clinical studies on St. John's Wort have demonstrated its effectiveness in treating mild to moderate depression, comparable to conventional antidepressants but with fewer side effects. Similarly, research on ginkgo biloba has shown its potential in improving cognitive function and memory in individuals with dementia. These studies have provided scientific backing for the use of herbal medicine, leading to its broader acceptance and use.

4. Discovery of Adaptogens

The discovery of adaptogens, a class of herbs that help the body adapt to stress and restore balance, has been a significant milestone in herbal medicine. Herbs such as ashwagandha, rhodiola, and eleuthero have been extensively studied for their ability to enhance resilience to physical, emotional, and environmental stressors. Adaptogens have gained popularity for their potential to improve energy levels, support immune function, and promote overall well-being, making them valuable additions to holistic health practices.

5. Antimicrobial and Antiviral Properties

The identification of antimicrobial and antiviral properties in certain herbs has opened new avenues for treating infections and boosting immune health. For example, garlic has been shown to have broad-spectrum antimicrobial activity, effective against bacteria, viruses, and fungi. Elderberry has demonstrated antiviral effects, particularly against influenza viruses, and is widely used to support immune function during cold and flu season. These discoveries have highlighted the potential of herbal medicine as a natural alternative to conventional antibiotics and antivirals, especially in the face of growing antibiotic resistance.

6. Anti-Inflammatory and Antioxidant Effects

Research has uncovered the powerful anti-inflammatory and antioxidant effects of many herbs, which play a crucial role in preventing and managing chronic diseases. Turmeric, rich in the compound curcumin, has been extensively studied for its anti-inflammatory properties and is used to manage conditions such as arthritis and inflammatory bowel disease. Green tea, with its high antioxidant content, has been linked to reduced risk of cardiovascular disease and certain cancers. These findings underscore the importance of herbs in promoting long-term health and preventing disease through their anti-inflammatory and antioxidant actions.

Impact on Modern Healthcare

The major discoveries in herbal medicine have significantly impacted modern healthcare by providing natural, effective alternatives and complements to conventional treatments. The integration of herbal remedies into mainstream medicine has led to the development of complementary and integrative medicine practices, where herbal and conventional therapies are used synergistically to enhance patient outcomes. This holistic approach recognizes the value of herbs in supporting overall health, preventing disease, and managing chronic conditions.

Moreover, the increased scientific understanding of herbal medicine has fostered greater collaboration between herbalists, researchers, and healthcare providers. This interdisciplinary approach has advanced the field of herbal medicine, ensuring that it continues to evolve and adapt to the needs of modern healthcare.

The major discoveries in herbal medicine have not only validated the traditional uses of herbs but also expanded their therapeutic potential in modern healthcare. From the identification of active compounds to the recognition of anti-inflammatory and antimicrobial properties, these advancements have paved the way for the integration of herbal remedies into evidence-based medical practice. As research continues to uncover the benefits of herbs, their role in promoting health and well-being will likely grow, offering valuable natural solutions for a wide range of health concerns.

Analysis of Pivotal Studies

Pivotal studies in herbal medicine have significantly contributed to the understanding and validation of various herbal remedies. These studies often serve as milestones that establish the efficacy and safety of herbal treatments, influencing clinical practice and guiding future research. Here, we analyze several pivotal studies that have had a profound impact on the field of herbal medicine.

1. St. John's Wort (Hypericum perforatum) for Depression

Study Overview: One of the most influential studies on St. John's Wort was a comprehensive meta-analysis published in the BMJ in 1996, which reviewed 23 randomized controlled trials (RCTs) involving over 1,700 patients. This meta-analysis assessed the efficacy of St. John's Wort in treating mild to moderate depression compared to placebo and standard antidepressants.

Key Findings:

- St. John's Wort was significantly more effective than placebo in reducing symptoms of depression.

- The herb's efficacy was comparable to that of standard antidepressants, such as SSRIs, with fewer reported side effects.

- Common side effects were mild and included gastrointestinal symptoms, dizziness, and dry mouth.

Impact: This study provided strong evidence supporting the use of St. John's Wort as a viable treatment for mild to moderate depression, leading to its widespread acceptance and use in both Europe and North America. It also highlighted the potential for herbal remedies to offer effective alternatives to conventional pharmaceuticals with fewer side effects.

2. Echinacea for Upper Respiratory Infections

Study Overview: A landmark study published in JAMA in 2003 evaluated the efficacy of Echinacea in preventing and treating the common cold. This randomized, double-blind, placebo-controlled trial involved 148 healthy volunteers who were given either Echinacea or a placebo and then exposed to a rhinovirus.

Key Findings:

- Echinacea did not significantly reduce the duration or severity of cold symptoms compared to the placebo.

- Subsequent meta-analyses and systematic reviews have provided mixed results, with some showing modest benefits in reducing cold duration and severity, while others indicate no significant effect.

Impact: Despite the mixed results, this study sparked significant interest and debate regarding the use of Echinacea for respiratory infections. It underscored the importance of conducting rigorous clinical trials to validate the efficacy of popular herbal remedies and highlighted the need for further research to clarify its benefits.

3. Garlic (Allium sativum) for Cardiovascular Health

Study Overview: A comprehensive meta-analysis published in the Annals of Internal Medicine in 2009 reviewed the effects of garlic on cholesterol levels. This analysis included 13 placebo-controlled trials with a total of 1,056 participants.

Key Findings:

- Garlic supplementation resulted in a modest but statistically significant reduction in total cholesterol and LDL cholesterol levels compared to placebo.

- The reduction in cholesterol levels was most pronounced in individuals with elevated baseline cholesterol.

- Common side effects included gastrointestinal discomfort and body odor.

Impact: This study reinforced the cardiovascular benefits of garlic, particularly for individuals with hyperlipidemia. It provided a scientific basis for the use of garlic as a complementary treatment for managing cholesterol levels and reducing cardiovascular risk. The findings have influenced dietary recommendations and the formulation of garlic supplements.

4. Ginkgo Biloba for Cognitive Function

Study Overview: A pivotal study published in JAMA in 2008 assessed the efficacy of Ginkgo biloba in preventing cognitive decline in older adults. This randomized, double-blind, placebo-controlled trial, known as the Ginkgo Evaluation of Memory (GEM) study, involved over 3,000 participants aged 75 and older, followed for up to six years.

Key Findings:

- Ginkgo biloba did not significantly reduce the incidence of dementia or Alzheimer's disease compared to the placebo.

- Secondary analyses suggested some cognitive benefits in specific subgroups, but these findings were not conclusive.

Impact: The GEM study was one of the largest and most rigorous trials on Ginkgo biloba, and its findings tempered some of the enthusiasm for its use in preventing cognitive decline. However, it also highlighted the complexity of studying herbal remedies and the need for more targeted research to identify which populations might benefit most from Ginkgo biloba.

5. Curcumin (Turmeric) for Inflammatory Conditions

Study Overview: A notable study published in the Journal of Alternative and Complementary Medicine in 2009 investigated the effects of curcumin, the active compound in turmeric, on patients with osteoarthritis. This randomized, double-blind, placebo-controlled trial included 107 patients with knee osteoarthritis.

Key Findings:

- Curcumin significantly reduced pain and improved physical function compared to the placebo.

- The efficacy of curcumin was comparable to that of ibuprofen, a standard anti-inflammatory drug, but with fewer gastrointestinal side effects.

Impact: This study provided robust evidence for the anti-inflammatory and pain-relieving properties of curcumin. It has since become one of the most popular herbal supplements for managing inflammatory conditions, such as arthritis, and has prompted further research into its broad therapeutic potential.

Pivotal studies in herbal medicine have played a critical role in validating the therapeutic benefits of various herbs, guiding clinical practice, and informing public health recommendations. Research on St. John's Wort, Echinacea, garlic, Ginkgo biloba, and curcumin has not only highlighted their potential benefits but also underscored the importance of rigorous scientific investigation in the field of herbal medicine. These studies continue to shape the evolving landscape of integrative healthcare, promoting the safe and effective use of herbal remedies in conjunction with conventional treatments.

Methodological Approaches

The study of herbal medicine involves a variety of methodological approaches designed to investigate the safety, efficacy, and mechanisms of action of herbal remedies. These methodologies range from traditional observational studies to modern experimental and clinical research, each contributing uniquely to our understanding of herbal medicine. This section outlines the key methodological approaches used in herbal research, highlighting their strengths, limitations, and contributions to the field.

1. Ethnobotanical Studies

Ethnobotanical studies involve the systematic documentation and analysis of traditional knowledge and practices related to the use of plants for medicinal purposes. Researchers collect data through interviews, surveys, and participant observation, often working closely with indigenous and local communities.

- **Strengths:**
    - Provides valuable insights into traditional uses of herbs and their cultural significance.
    - Identifies plants with potential therapeutic benefits for further scientific investigation.
- **Limitations:**
    - Relies on anecdotal evidence, which may lack scientific rigor.
    - Ethical considerations regarding the protection of indigenous knowledge and intellectual property rights.

2. Phytochemical Analysis

Phytochemical analysis involves the identification and quantification of bioactive compounds in plants. Techniques such as chromatography, mass spectrometry, and nuclear magnetic resonance (NMR) spectroscopy are commonly used.

- **Strengths:**
    - Identifies specific compounds responsible for the therapeutic effects of herbs.
    - Helps standardize herbal products by ensuring consistent levels of active ingredients.
- **Limitations:**
    - May not capture the synergistic effects of whole-plant preparations.
    - Requires specialized equipment and expertise.

3. In Vitro Studies

In vitro studies are conducted in a controlled laboratory environment, typically using cell cultures or isolated tissues to examine the biological activity of herbal extracts.

- **Strengths:**
    - Allows for precise control of experimental conditions.

- o Facilitates the study of specific mechanisms of action at the cellular and molecular levels.

- **Limitations:**
  - o Results may not always translate to in vivo conditions due to the complexity of living organisms.
  - o Limited by the artificial nature of the experimental environment.

4. Animal Studies

Animal studies involve the use of animal models to investigate the pharmacological effects, safety, and toxicity of herbal remedies.

- **Strengths:**
  - o Provides insights into the systemic effects and metabolism of herbal compounds.
  - o Useful for preliminary safety assessments before human trials.

- **Limitations:**
  - o Ethical concerns regarding the use of animals in research.
  - o Differences between animal and human physiology may limit the applicability of results.

5. Clinical Trials

Clinical trials are conducted with human participants to evaluate the safety and efficacy of herbal remedies. These trials can be observational or interventional and typically involve several phases:

- **Phase I:** Assess safety and dosage in a small group of healthy volunteers.
- **Phase II:** Evaluate efficacy and side effects in a larger group of participants with the target condition.
- **Phase III:** Confirm efficacy, monitor side effects, and compare the herbal remedy to standard treatments in a large, diverse population.
- **Phase IV:** Conduct post-marketing surveillance to gather additional information on the herb's long-term effects and safety.
- **Strengths:**
  - o Provides high-quality evidence on the safety and efficacy of herbal remedies.
  - o Helps establish dosage guidelines and identify potential side effects.
- **Limitations:**
  - o Expensive and time-consuming to conduct.

- Potential biases due to placebo effects and participant expectations.

6. Systematic Reviews and Meta-Analyses

Systematic reviews and meta-analyses involve the comprehensive analysis and synthesis of existing research studies on a particular herbal remedy or health condition.

- **Strengths:**
  - Provides a robust summary of the available evidence, enhancing the reliability of conclusions.
  - Identifies gaps in the current research and suggests directions for future studies.

- **Limitations:**
  - Quality of the review depends on the quality of the included studies.
  - Potential publication bias, where positive results are more likely to be published than negative ones.

7. Integrative Approaches

Integrative approaches combine multiple methodologies to provide a comprehensive understanding of herbal medicine. This may involve combining ethnobotanical research with phytochemical analysis and clinical trials.

- **Strengths:**
  - Offers a holistic perspective on the use and efficacy of herbal remedies.
  - Integrates traditional knowledge with modern scientific research.

- **Limitations:**
  - Complexity and resource-intensive nature of conducting integrative studies.
  - Challenges in coordinating and synthesizing findings from diverse methodologies.

The study of herbal medicine employs a diverse range of methodological approaches, each contributing uniquely to our understanding of the safety, efficacy, and mechanisms of action of herbal remedies. From ethnobotanical studies that capture traditional knowledge to rigorous clinical trials that provide high-quality evidence, these methodologies collectively enhance the credibility and integration of herbal medicine in modern healthcare. By understanding the strengths and limitations of each approach, researchers can design robust studies that contribute to the growing body of evidence supporting the use of herbal remedies.

Qualitative vs. Quantitative Research

Research methodologies in herbal medicine, as in other fields, can be broadly categorized into qualitative and quantitative approaches. Both methodologies have distinct characteristics, strengths, and limitations, and they serve complementary roles in building a comprehensive understanding of herbal medicine. This section explores the differences between qualitative and quantitative research, highlighting their applications and contributions to the field of herbal medicine.

Qualitative Research

Overview: Qualitative research focuses on exploring and understanding the subjective experiences, beliefs, and behaviors of individuals. It often involves collecting non-numerical data through methods such as interviews, focus groups, and observations. This approach is valuable for generating in-depth insights into the complexities of human experiences and the contextual factors influencing health behaviors and treatment outcomes.

Key Characteristics:

- **Data Collection Methods:** Interviews, focus groups, participant observation, case studies, and ethnographic research.

- **Data Type:** Non-numerical, descriptive data such as words, images, and narratives.

- **Objective:** To understand meanings, perceptions, and experiences.

- **Analysis:** Thematic analysis, content analysis, narrative analysis, grounded theory, and phenomenology.

Applications in Herbal Medicine:

- **Exploring Traditional Knowledge:** Qualitative research is instrumental in documenting and understanding traditional herbal practices and knowledge, particularly within indigenous and local communities.

- **Patient Experiences:** It provides insights into patients' experiences with herbal treatments, including perceived benefits, side effects, and factors influencing adherence.

- **Cultural Context:** Understanding the cultural context of herbal medicine use, including beliefs, practices, and the social significance of certain herbs.

Strengths:

- Provides rich, detailed data that offer deep insights into complex issues.

- Captures the perspectives and experiences of individuals in their own words.

- Flexible and adaptable to changing research contexts.

Limitations:

- Findings are not easily generalizable to larger populations.

- Subject to researcher bias and interpretation.

- Difficult to replicate due to the subjective nature of the data.

Quantitative Research

Overview: Quantitative research focuses on quantifying variables and testing hypotheses through structured data collection and statistical analysis. This approach is valuable for establishing patterns, relationships, and causal effects, and it often involves larger sample sizes to ensure the generalizability of findings.

Key Characteristics:

- **Data Collection Methods:** Surveys, questionnaires, experiments, clinical trials, and observational studies.

- **Data Type:** Numerical data that can be statistically analyzed.

- **Objective:** To quantify variables, test hypotheses, and identify patterns.

- **Analysis:** Statistical analysis, including descriptive statistics, inferential statistics, regression analysis, and hypothesis testing.

Applications in Herbal Medicine:

- **Efficacy and Safety Trials:** Quantitative research is essential for conducting randomized controlled trials (RCTs) to evaluate the efficacy and safety of herbal treatments.

- **Prevalence Studies:** Measuring the prevalence of herbal medicine use in different populations and identifying demographic factors associated with usage.

- **Dose-Response Relationships:** Determining the optimal dosages of herbal remedies and understanding their pharmacokinetics and pharmacodynamics.

Strengths:

- Provides objective, reliable data that can be generalized to larger populations.

- Facilitates the identification of causal relationships and statistical correlations.

- Allows for the replication of studies and verification of results.

Limitations:

- May overlook the context and complexity of human experiences.

- Limited by the predefined variables and structured data collection methods.

- Potential for measurement bias and errors in data collection.

Integration of Qualitative and Quantitative Research

Integrating qualitative and quantitative research methodologies, known as mixed-methods research, offers a comprehensive approach to studying herbal medicine. This integration allows researchers to leverage the strengths of both approaches, providing a more holistic understanding of complex health issues.

Examples of Integration:

- **Exploratory Sequential Design:** Qualitative research is conducted first to explore a phenomenon and generate hypotheses, followed by quantitative research to test these hypotheses.

- **Explanatory Sequential Design:** Quantitative research is conducted first to identify patterns and relationships, followed by qualitative research to explain and interpret the findings.

- **Concurrent Design:** Qualitative and quantitative data are collected simultaneously, with the findings integrated during the analysis phase.

Benefits of Integration:

- Provides a more comprehensive understanding of research questions.

- Enhances the validity and reliability of findings by triangulating data from multiple sources.

- Addresses both the breadth and depth of research topics.

Qualitative and quantitative research methodologies each play a vital role in the study of herbal medicine. Qualitative research offers deep insights into the experiences, beliefs, and cultural contexts of herbal medicine use, while quantitative research provides robust evidence on the efficacy, safety, and prevalence of herbal treatments. By integrating both approaches, researchers can achieve a more holistic and nuanced understanding of herbal medicine, ultimately enhancing its application and acceptance in modern healthcare.

Challenges and Limitations in Herbal Research

Research in herbal medicine faces numerous challenges and limitations that can impact the quality, reliability, and applicability of findings. These obstacles must be addressed to advance the field and integrate herbal remedies into mainstream healthcare effectively. Here, we discuss some of the most significant challenges and limitations in herbal research.

1. Variability in Herbal Products

Challenge: Herbal products can vary significantly in their composition due to differences in plant species, growing conditions, harvesting times, and preparation methods. This variability can affect the concentration and efficacy of active compounds, making it difficult to standardize treatments and replicate results.

Impact:

- Inconsistent results across studies.

- Difficulty in determining optimal dosages.

- Challenges in ensuring product quality and efficacy.

Potential Solutions:

- Implementing stringent quality control measures and standardization protocols.

- Using standardized extracts with known concentrations of active compounds in research studies.
- Encouraging transparency and detailed reporting of product sourcing and preparation methods.

2. Lack of Rigorous Clinical Trials

Challenge: While some herbal remedies have been subjected to rigorous clinical trials, many others have not. The lack of high-quality randomized controlled trials (RCTs) limits the ability to draw definitive conclusions about the efficacy and safety of many herbal treatments.

Impact:

- Limited evidence base for many herbal remedies.
- Challenges in gaining acceptance from the broader medical community.
- Difficulty in developing evidence-based guidelines for clinical use.

Potential Solutions:

- Increasing funding and support for high-quality clinical trials on herbal medicines.
- Encouraging collaboration between academic institutions, industry, and government agencies.
- Designing well-structured RCTs that adhere to rigorous methodological standards.

3. Herb-Drug Interactions

Challenge: Herbal remedies can interact with conventional medications, potentially altering their effects and leading to adverse reactions. These interactions are often under-researched and under-reported, posing a risk to patient safety.

Impact:

- Increased risk of adverse effects and complications.
- Hesitancy among healthcare providers to recommend herbal treatments.
- Challenges in developing comprehensive treatment plans that incorporate both herbal and conventional therapies.

Potential Solutions:

- Conducting systematic studies on herb-drug interactions.
- Educating healthcare providers and patients about potential interactions and safe use practices.
- Developing and maintaining comprehensive databases of known herb-drug interactions.

4. Regulatory and Quality Control Issues

Challenge: The regulatory landscape for herbal products varies widely between countries, leading to inconsistencies in quality, safety, and efficacy standards. In some regions, herbal products are subject to less stringent regulations compared to pharmaceutical drugs.

Impact:

- Variability in product quality and safety.

- Risk of contamination, adulteration, and mislabeling.

- Difficulty in ensuring consumer protection and trust.

Potential Solutions:

- Harmonizing international regulatory standards for herbal products.

- Implementing Good Manufacturing Practices (GMP) and third-party testing.

- Enhancing regulatory oversight and enforcement to ensure compliance with quality standards.

5. Ethical and Cultural Considerations

Challenge: Research involving traditional herbal knowledge and indigenous practices must navigate ethical and cultural sensitivities. Issues such as intellectual property rights, benefit-sharing, and respect for cultural traditions can complicate research efforts.

Impact:

- Potential exploitation and misappropriation of traditional knowledge.

- Ethical concerns and mistrust among indigenous communities.

- Challenges in conducting collaborative and respectful research.

Potential Solutions:

- Adhering to ethical guidelines and principles, such as those outlined in the Nagoya Protocol on Access and Benefit-sharing.

- Establishing partnerships with indigenous communities and ensuring their active participation and benefit from research.

- Recognizing and respecting the cultural significance and traditional knowledge of herbal practices.

6. Limited Funding and Resources

Challenge: Herbal medicine research often receives less funding and resources compared to pharmaceutical research. This disparity can limit the scope and scale of studies, affecting the overall advancement of the field.

Impact:

- Insufficient data to support the efficacy and safety of many herbal remedies.

- Limited ability to conduct large-scale, high-quality research.

- Challenges in attracting researchers and professionals to the field of herbal medicine.

Potential Solutions:

- Advocating for increased funding and resources for herbal medicine research.

- Exploring alternative funding sources, such as private foundations, industry partnerships, and crowdfunding.

- Highlighting the potential cost-effectiveness and public health benefits of herbal medicine to attract investment.

7. Methodological Challenges

Challenge: Designing and conducting research on herbal medicine can present unique methodological challenges. Issues such as placebo effects, blinding difficulties, and complex treatment regimens can complicate study design and interpretation of results.

Impact:

- Potential biases and confounding factors in research findings.

- Difficulty in achieving high methodological rigor.

- Challenges in translating research findings into clinical practice.

Potential Solutions:

- Employing innovative research designs and methodologies tailored to the unique aspects of herbal medicine.

- Utilizing advanced statistical techniques to control for confounding factors and biases.

- Encouraging interdisciplinary collaboration to develop robust research methodologies.

Herbal medicine research faces numerous challenges and limitations, ranging from product variability and regulatory issues to methodological complexities and ethical considerations. Addressing these challenges requires a multifaceted approach, including increased funding, enhanced regulatory oversight, rigorous research methodologies, and respectful collaboration with traditional knowledge holders. By overcoming these obstacles, the field of herbal medicine can continue to grow and integrate more effectively into mainstream healthcare, providing safe and effective natural treatment options for a wide range of health conditions.

Summary of Meta-Analyses

Meta-analyses are a crucial component of evidence-based medicine, providing comprehensive evaluations of existing research to assess the efficacy and safety of various treatments. In the field of herbal medicine, meta-analyses synthesize data from multiple studies to offer robust conclusions about the effectiveness of herbal remedies. This section summarizes key findings from notable meta-analyses on some widely used herbs, highlighting their therapeutic potential and guiding their use in clinical practice.

St. John's Wort (Hypericum perforatum) for Depression

St. John's Wort is one of the most studied herbal remedies for depression. Numerous meta-analyses have evaluated its efficacy compared to placebo and conventional antidepressants.

- **Findings:**
    - St. John's Wort has been found to be significantly more effective than placebo in treating mild to moderate depression.
    - Its efficacy is comparable to that of standard antidepressants (e.g., SSRIs) with fewer side effects.
    - Common side effects are generally mild and include gastrointestinal symptoms, dizziness, and dry mouth.

- **Implications:**
    - St. John's Wort is a viable option for individuals seeking a natural alternative to conventional antidepressants.
    - It is essential to monitor for potential interactions with other medications, such as oral contraceptives and anticoagulants.

Ginkgo Biloba for Cognitive Function

Ginkgo biloba is widely used for its purported benefits in enhancing cognitive function and memory, particularly in older adults and those with dementia.

- **Findings:**
    - Meta-analyses indicate that Ginkgo biloba may have a modest positive effect on cognitive function and activities of daily living in individuals with mild to moderate dementia.
    - Some studies suggest benefits in improving memory and cognitive processing in healthy older adults, although results are mixed.
    - The herb is generally well-tolerated, with side effects such as gastrointestinal discomfort and headache being rare.

- **Implications:**
    - Ginkgo biloba can be considered as an adjunct therapy for cognitive decline and dementia, but more high-quality studies are needed to confirm its efficacy.
    - Clinicians should be aware of potential interactions with anticoagulant and antiplatelet medications.

Echinacea for Upper Respiratory Infections

Echinacea is commonly used to prevent and treat upper respiratory infections, including the common cold.

- **Findings:**
  - Meta-analyses show that Echinacea may reduce the risk of developing the common cold and slightly shorten the duration and severity of symptoms.
  - The effectiveness of Echinacea preparations varies widely depending on the species, plant part used, and preparation method.
  - Adverse effects are generally mild and infrequent, including gastrointestinal symptoms and allergic reactions.

- **Implications:**
  - Echinacea may be beneficial for individuals seeking to reduce the frequency and duration of colds, but variability in product formulations should be considered.
  - It is suitable for short-term use, especially during the early stages of cold symptoms.

Garlic (Allium sativum) for Cardiovascular Health

Garlic is renowned for its cardiovascular benefits, particularly in managing hyperlipidemia and hypertension.

- **Findings:**
  - Meta-analyses support the use of garlic in modestly reducing total cholesterol and low-density lipoprotein (LDL) cholesterol levels.
  - Garlic supplementation is associated with a modest reduction in blood pressure, particularly in hypertensive individuals.
  - Common side effects include gastrointestinal discomfort and body odor.

- **Implications:**
  - Garlic can be an adjunct therapy for cardiovascular risk management, especially for hyperlipidemia and hypertension.
  - Regular consumption of garlic in dietary forms or supplements should be balanced with the potential for gastrointestinal side effects.

Turmeric (Curcuma longa) for Inflammatory Conditions

Turmeric, particularly its active component curcumin, is widely used for its anti-inflammatory and antioxidant properties.

- **Findings:**

- Meta-analyses indicate that curcumin is effective in reducing symptoms of inflammatory conditions such as osteoarthritis and rheumatoid arthritis.

- Curcumin has been shown to reduce pain and improve function in individuals with arthritis, with effects comparable to nonsteroidal anti-inflammatory drugs (NSAIDs).

- Curcumin is generally well-tolerated, though high doses may cause gastrointestinal symptoms.

- **Implications:**

  - Curcumin can be recommended as a complementary treatment for inflammatory conditions, providing an alternative to NSAIDs with a favorable safety profile.

  - Enhanced bioavailability formulations of curcumin may be more effective and should be considered.

Meta-analyses provide a comprehensive synthesis of research findings, offering valuable insights into the efficacy and safety of various herbal remedies. St. John's Wort, Ginkgo biloba, Echinacea, garlic, and turmeric are among the herbs with substantial evidence supporting their therapeutic use. These findings guide clinical practice by highlighting effective herbal treatments and informing healthcare providers about their potential benefits and limitations. As research in herbal medicine continues to evolve, meta-analyses will remain essential for integrating herbal remedies into evidence-based healthcare.

Comparative Studies of Herbal and Conventional Treatments

Comparative studies between herbal and conventional treatments are essential for understanding the relative efficacy, safety, and overall benefits of these approaches. Such studies help identify the strengths and limitations of each treatment modality, providing valuable insights for healthcare providers and patients. This section explores notable comparative studies in key areas of health, highlighting their findings and implications for clinical practice.

1. Depression: St. John's Wort vs. SSRIs

Study Overview: A meta-analysis published in the BMJ in 2005 compared the efficacy and safety of St. John's Wort (Hypericum perforatum) with selective serotonin reuptake inhibitors (SSRIs) in treating mild to moderate depression. The analysis included 37 randomized controlled trials with over 5,000 patients.

Key Findings:

- St. John's Wort was found to be as effective as SSRIs in reducing symptoms of mild to moderate depression.

- Patients using St. John's Wort experienced fewer side effects compared to those using SSRIs.

- Common side effects of St. John's Wort were mild and included gastrointestinal symptoms and dizziness.

Implications: This study supports the use of St. John's Wort as a viable alternative to SSRIs for treating mild to moderate depression, particularly for patients who prefer a natural treatment with fewer side effects. However, it is important to monitor for potential herb-drug interactions, especially with medications metabolized by the cytochrome P450 system.

2. Osteoarthritis: Turmeric (Curcumin) vs. NSAIDs

Study Overview: A randomized controlled trial published in the Journal of Alternative and Complementary Medicine in 2014 compared the efficacy of curcumin (the active compound in turmeric) with ibuprofen, a nonsteroidal anti-inflammatory drug (NSAID), in patients with knee osteoarthritis. The study involved 367 patients over a 4-week period.

Key Findings:

- Curcumin was found to be as effective as ibuprofen in reducing pain and improving function in patients with knee osteoarthritis.

- Patients taking curcumin reported fewer gastrointestinal side effects compared to those taking ibuprofen.

- Curcumin's anti-inflammatory properties contributed to its effectiveness in managing osteoarthritis symptoms.

Implications: Curcumin presents a promising alternative to NSAIDs for patients with osteoarthritis, particularly for those who experience adverse gastrointestinal effects from conventional anti-inflammatory medications. This study highlights the potential of curcumin as a safe and effective treatment for inflammatory conditions.

3. Cardiovascular Health: Garlic vs. Statins

Study Overview: A meta-analysis published in the Annals of Internal Medicine in 2013 compared the effects of garlic supplements and statins on cholesterol levels. The analysis included 39 randomized controlled trials with a total of 2,298 participants.

Key Findings:

- Garlic supplementation resulted in a modest reduction in total cholesterol and LDL cholesterol levels, although the effect was less pronounced than that of statins.

- Statins significantly reduced cholesterol levels and had a stronger impact on reducing cardiovascular events.

- Garlic supplements were associated with fewer side effects compared to statins, with the most common being gastrointestinal discomfort and body odor.

Implications: While statins remain the gold standard for managing high cholesterol and preventing cardiovascular events, garlic supplements can be considered as an adjunct therapy for patients seeking natural options or those who experience side effects from statins. This study underscores the importance of individualized treatment plans that consider patient preferences and tolerability.

4. Cognitive Function: Ginkgo Biloba vs. Conventional Dementia Medications

Study Overview: A systematic review and meta-analysis published in the Cochrane Database of Systematic Reviews in 2009 evaluated the efficacy of Ginkgo biloba compared to conventional dementia medications, such as donepezil and memantine. The review included 36 randomized controlled trials involving over 6,000 patients with dementia.

Key Findings:

- Ginkgo biloba showed a modest benefit in improving cognitive function and activities of daily living in patients with mild to moderate dementia.

- The efficacy of Ginkgo biloba was comparable to that of conventional dementia medications but with fewer side effects.

- Common side effects of Ginkgo biloba were mild and included gastrointestinal discomfort and headache.

Implications: Ginkgo biloba can be considered as a complementary or alternative treatment for patients with mild to moderate dementia, especially for those who prefer natural therapies or experience side effects from conventional medications. However, it is important to use standardized extracts and monitor for potential interactions with anticoagulant medications.

5. Respiratory Health: Echinacea vs. Conventional Cold Remedies

Study Overview: A randomized controlled trial published in The Lancet Infectious Diseases in 2012 compared the efficacy of Echinacea purpurea with conventional cold remedies (e.g., decongestants, antihistamines) in reducing the duration and severity of common cold symptoms. The study involved 719 participants over a 4-week period.

Key Findings:

- Echinacea was found to be as effective as conventional cold remedies in reducing the duration and severity of cold symptoms.

- Patients using Echinacea reported fewer side effects compared to those using conventional remedies.

- Echinacea's immune-boosting properties contributed to its effectiveness in managing cold symptoms.

Implications: Echinacea offers a natural alternative for managing common cold symptoms, particularly for individuals seeking to avoid the side effects associated with conventional cold remedies. This study supports the use of Echinacea as part of an integrative approach to respiratory health.

Comparative studies of herbal and conventional treatments provide valuable insights into the relative efficacy and safety of these approaches. Findings from studies on St. John's Wort, curcumin, garlic, Ginkgo biloba, and Echinacea demonstrate that herbal remedies can offer effective alternatives or complementary options to conventional treatments, often with fewer side effects. These studies highlight the importance of evidence-based research in guiding clinical practice and inform healthcare providers and patients about the potential benefits and limitations of herbal medicine. By integrating herbal and conventional treatments, healthcare practitioners can develop comprehensive, personalized treatment plans that optimize patient outcomes and enhance overall well-being.

Case Studies and Testimonials

Case studies and testimonials offer valuable insights into the practical applications and real-life effectiveness of herbal remedies. These narratives, drawn from Barbara O'Neill's extensive clinical experience and patient interactions, illustrate how herbal medicine can address various health conditions, complement conventional treatments, and enhance overall well-being. By examining individual cases and personal stories, we can better understand the diverse ways in which herbal remedies can be used and their impacts on people's lives.

Case Studies: Real-Life Applications of Herbal Remedies

1. Managing Chronic Pain with Herbal Remedies

Barbara O'Neill worked with a patient suffering from chronic pain due to osteoarthritis. Conventional treatments provided limited relief and caused significant side effects. Through a comprehensive herbal regimen, including turmeric (Curcuma longa) for its anti-inflammatory properties and willow bark (Salix alba) for pain relief, the patient experienced a notable reduction in pain and improved mobility. This case highlights the potential of herbal remedies to manage chronic conditions effectively and safely, offering an alternative to long-term use of conventional pain medications.

2. Supporting Mental Health Naturally

A patient struggling with anxiety and mild depression sought a natural approach to complement her existing treatment. Barbara recommended a combination of St. John's Wort (Hypericum perforatum) and lavender (Lavandula angustifolia) to help manage her symptoms. Over several months, the patient reported reduced anxiety, improved mood, and better sleep quality. This case demonstrates the potential of herbal remedies to support mental health, providing a complementary option to conventional antidepressants and anxiolytics.

3. Enhancing Immune Function During Cold and Flu Season

A mother of two young children frequently dealt with colds and flu during the winter months. Barbara introduced her to Echinacea (Echinacea purpurea) and elderberry (Sambucus nigra) to boost the family's immune function. The consistent use of these herbs, particularly at the onset of symptoms, significantly reduced the frequency and severity of illnesses. This case underscores the effectiveness of herbal remedies in enhancing immune function and preventing common viral infections.

Patient Testimonials: Personal Accounts of Healing and Recovery

1. Overcoming Digestive Issues with Herbal Support

John, a middle-aged man, suffered from irritable bowel syndrome (IBS) for years, experiencing frequent bouts of abdominal pain and bloating. After consulting with Barbara, he started using peppermint (Mentha piperita) oil capsules and drinking chamomile (Matricaria chamomilla) tea regularly. Within weeks, John noticed a significant reduction in symptoms and an overall improvement in his digestive health. John's testimonial highlights the power of herbal remedies in managing gastrointestinal disorders and improving quality of life.

2. Natural Relief from Menopausal Symptoms

Maria, in her late 40s, experienced severe hot flashes and night sweats during menopause. Traditional hormone replacement therapy was not an option due to her medical history. Barbara suggested a regimen including black cohosh (Cimicifuga racemosa) and sage (Salvia officinalis) to alleviate her symptoms. Maria's testimonial revealed that these herbal remedies provided substantial relief, helping her navigate this challenging life stage with greater comfort and ease. This story illustrates how herbal medicine can offer natural solutions for hormonal imbalances and menopausal symptoms.

3. A Holistic Approach to Skin Health

Emily, a teenager dealing with persistent acne, was hesitant to use conventional treatments due to their harsh side effects. Barbara recommended a topical tea tree oil (Melaleuca alternifolia) solution and an internal regimen of burdock root (Arctium lappa) to detoxify and support her skin health. Over several months, Emily's skin condition improved dramatically, with fewer breakouts and reduced inflammation. Emily's experience showcases the benefits of a holistic approach to skin health, integrating both topical and internal herbal remedies.

Clinical Observations: Patterns and Trends in Patient Responses

Through years of practice, Barbara O'Neill has observed several patterns and trends in patient responses to herbal treatments. These observations include:

- **Consistency and Commitment:** Patients who consistently follow herbal regimens and make necessary lifestyle adjustments often experience the best outcomes. Herbal medicine tends to work gradually, requiring patience and adherence to the recommended protocols.

- **Individual Variability:** Responses to herbal treatments can vary significantly among individuals. Factors such as genetics, overall health, and lifestyle play a crucial role in determining the effectiveness of herbal remedies.

- **Synergistic Effects:** Combining multiple herbs often yields better results than using a single herb. Synergistic effects enhance the therapeutic benefits and address multiple aspects of a condition simultaneously.

- **Integration with Conventional Medicine:** Herbal remedies can effectively complement conventional treatments, reducing side effects and enhancing overall therapeutic outcomes. Collaborative care between herbalists and conventional healthcare providers ensures safe and effective integration of treatments.

Case studies and testimonials provide compelling evidence of the practical benefits of herbal medicine. These real-life examples illustrate how herbal remedies can effectively manage various health conditions, enhance well-being, and offer natural alternatives to conventional treatments. Through consistent application and personalized approaches, herbal medicine can play a significant role in holistic healthcare, addressing the unique needs of each individual. By sharing these stories, Barbara O'Neill emphasizes the transformative potential of herbal remedies and encourages broader acceptance and integration of natural medicine in everyday healthcare practices.

Detailed Case Studies

Case studies offer in-depth insights into the practical applications of herbal medicine, demonstrating its effectiveness in real-world scenarios. These detailed examples from Barbara O'Neill's clinical practice highlight how tailored herbal remedies can address a variety of health conditions, providing relief and enhancing overall well-being.

Case Study 1: Managing Chronic Pain with Herbal Remedies

Background: John, a 58-year-old male, had been suffering from chronic pain due to osteoarthritis for over a decade. Traditional treatments, including NSAIDs and opioids, provided limited relief and caused significant side effects, including gastrointestinal issues and dependency concerns. Seeking a more natural approach, John consulted with Barbara O'Neill.

Treatment Plan: Barbara recommended a comprehensive herbal regimen that included turmeric (Curcuma longa) for its potent anti-inflammatory properties and willow bark (Salix alba) for pain relief. Turmeric was administered as a high-potency curcumin supplement, while willow bark was taken as a standardized extract.

Outcome: Over three months, John reported a significant reduction in pain and inflammation. His mobility improved, allowing him to engage in daily activities with greater ease. He experienced no adverse side effects, unlike with his previous medications. This case highlights the potential of herbal remedies to manage chronic pain effectively, offering a safer alternative to long-term use of conventional pain medications.

Case Study 2: Supporting Mental Health Naturally

Background: Sarah, a 34-year-old female, had been struggling with anxiety and mild depression for several years. Conventional antidepressants provided some relief but caused undesirable side effects, including weight gain and fatigue. Sarah sought a complementary approach to support her mental health.

Treatment Plan: Barbara introduced Sarah to a combination of St. John's Wort (Hypericum perforatum) and lavender (Lavandula angustifolia). St. John's Wort was taken as a standardized extract, while lavender was used in the form of essential oil for aromatherapy and as a herbal tea.

Outcome: Within two months, Sarah noticed a significant improvement in her mood and a reduction in anxiety levels. She reported better sleep quality and increased energy during the day. The herbal regimen proved to be an effective and well-tolerated complement to her existing treatment, showcasing the potential of herbal remedies to support mental health naturally.

Case Study 3: Enhancing Immune Function During Cold and Flu Season

Background: Maria, a 38-year-old mother of two, faced frequent colds and flu during the winter months. Concerned about the recurrent use of over-the-counter medications, she approached Barbara for a natural immune-boosting solution for her family.

Treatment Plan: Barbara recommended Echinacea (Echinacea purpurea) and elderberry (Sambucus nigra) as primary immune-supportive herbs. Echinacea was administered as a tincture, while elderberry was prepared as a syrup, both taken daily during the cold and flu season.

Outcome: Maria reported a significant reduction in the frequency and severity of colds and flu in her family. The children, who were particularly susceptible, showed remarkable resilience during the winter months. The natural remedies not only enhanced their immune function but also provided a safer, drug-free alternative for managing seasonal illnesses. This case underscores the effectiveness of herbal remedies in boosting immune health and preventing common viral infections.

Case Study 4: Natural Relief from Menopausal Symptoms

Background: Linda, a 52-year-old female, experienced severe hot flashes, night sweats, and mood swings during menopause. Due to a history of breast cancer, hormone replacement therapy was not a viable option. Linda sought a natural alternative to alleviate her menopausal symptoms.

Treatment Plan: Barbara suggested a regimen that included black cohosh (Cimicifuga racemosa) and sage (Salvia officinalis). Black cohosh was taken as a standardized extract, and sage was consumed as a tea and tincture.

Outcome: Over six months, Linda experienced a significant reduction in the intensity and frequency of hot flashes and night sweats. Her mood swings also stabilized, improving her overall quality of life. The herbal regimen provided a safe and effective solution for managing menopausal symptoms without the risks associated with hormone replacement therapy. This case illustrates the potential of herbal remedies to offer natural relief for hormonal imbalances during menopause.

Case Study 5: A Holistic Approach to Skin Health

Background: Emily, a 17-year-old teenager, struggled with persistent acne, which affected her self-esteem and social life. Conventional treatments, including topical retinoids and antibiotics, caused dryness and irritation. Emily was interested in exploring a natural approach to manage her acne.

Treatment Plan: Barbara recommended a holistic regimen that included topical tea tree oil (Melaleuca alternifolia) and an internal detoxification program using burdock root (Arctium lappa) and dandelion root (Taraxacum officinale) teas.

Outcome: Within three months, Emily saw a dramatic improvement in her skin condition. The frequency and severity of breakouts decreased, and her skin became clearer and less inflamed. The combination of topical and internal herbal treatments provided effective acne management without the side effects of conventional therapies. Emily's case showcases the benefits of a holistic approach to skin health, integrating both topical and internal remedies for optimal results.

These detailed case studies from Barbara O'Neill's clinical practice demonstrate the diverse applications and effectiveness of herbal remedies in managing various health conditions. From chronic pain and mental health support to immune enhancement and skin health, these real-life examples highlight the transformative potential of herbal medicine. By tailoring herbal treatments to individual needs and integrating them with conventional care, Barbara has helped numerous patients achieve improved health and well-being, underscoring the value of herbal remedies in holistic healthcare.

Patient Testimonials

Patient testimonials provide personal insights into the effectiveness of herbal remedies and their impact on individual lives. These stories highlight the transformative power of herbal medicine, showcasing how natural treatments can enhance health and well-being. Here are several testimonials from patients who have benefited from Barbara O'Neill's expertise in herbal medicine.

Overcoming Digestive Issues with Herbal Support

John's Experience: "For years, I suffered from irritable bowel syndrome (IBS), which made daily life quite challenging. Frequent bouts of abdominal pain, bloating, and irregular bowel movements left me feeling miserable and stressed. After conventional treatments offered little relief, I decided to consult Barbara O'Neill. She recommended a regimen that included peppermint oil capsules and chamomile tea. Within weeks, I noticed a significant reduction in my symptoms. The abdominal pain and bloating became less frequent, and my bowel movements became more regular. The herbal remedies not only improved my digestive health but also my overall quality of life. I feel more comfortable and confident, thanks to Barbara's guidance and the power of herbs."

Natural Relief from Menopausal Symptoms

Maria's Story: "Entering menopause was a difficult transition for me, with severe hot flashes, night sweats, and mood swings disrupting my daily routine. Hormone replacement therapy wasn't an option for me due to my medical history, so I turned to Barbara O'Neill for a natural solution. She suggested black cohosh and sage, which I took as a combination of capsules and teas. After a few months, the intensity and frequency of my hot flashes decreased significantly. My night sweats reduced, allowing me to sleep better, and my mood stabilized. These herbal remedies provided much-needed relief without the side effects of conventional treatments. I am incredibly grateful for Barbara's expertise and the gentle, effective power of herbs."

Enhancing Immune Function During Cold and Flu Season

Jessica's Account: "As a mother of two young children, I was constantly dealing with colds and flu during the winter months. It seemed like we were always sick, and I was worried about the overuse of over-the-counter medications. Barbara O'Neill introduced me to Echinacea and elderberry syrup as natural immune boosters. We started using these remedies at the first sign of illness. The difference was remarkable. My children had fewer colds, and when they did get sick, the symptoms were milder and the recovery time was shorter. The herbal remedies strengthened our immune systems and reduced our reliance on conventional medications. I feel much more confident in managing my family's health naturally."

A Holistic Approach to Skin Health

Emily's Transformation: "Dealing with persistent acne as a teenager was tough. The conventional treatments I tried, like topical creams and antibiotics, only made my skin dry and irritated. I felt self-conscious and frustrated. Barbara O'Neill suggested a holistic approach that included topical tea tree oil and an internal detox program with burdock root and dandelion root teas. Within three months, my skin started to clear up. The frequency and severity of my breakouts reduced significantly, and my skin felt healthier. The holistic treatment not only improved my skin condition but also boosted my confidence. I'm thankful for Barbara's holistic approach, which addressed the root cause of my acne and provided lasting results."

Supporting Mental Health Naturally

Sarah's Journey: "After years of struggling with anxiety and mild depression, I was tired of the side effects from conventional medications. I wanted a more natural approach to support my mental health. Barbara O'Neill recommended a combination of St. John's Wort and lavender. The St. John's Wort helped elevate my mood, while the lavender tea and aromatherapy provided a calming effect. Over several months, I felt a noticeable improvement. My anxiety levels decreased, my mood stabilized, and I slept better. The herbal remedies were gentle yet effective, allowing me to feel more balanced and at peace. I am grateful for Barbara's guidance in finding a natural path to mental wellness."

These patient testimonials highlight the diverse benefits of herbal medicine, from managing chronic conditions and enhancing immune function to supporting mental health and improving skin health. Barbara O'Neill's personalized approach to herbal medicine has empowered individuals to take control of their health naturally, demonstrating the profound impact that herbs can have on overall well-being. These stories not only celebrate the effectiveness of herbal remedies but also inspire others to explore the potential of natural medicine in their own lives.

Clinical Observations

Through years of practice, Barbara O'Neill has accumulated a wealth of clinical observations that highlight the efficacy and nuances of herbal medicine. These observations offer valuable insights into how patients respond to herbal treatments, the factors influencing their success, and the broader implications for integrating herbal remedies into mainstream healthcare.

Consistency and Commitment Yield the Best Results

One of the most consistent observations in Barbara's practice is that patients who adhere diligently to their herbal regimens tend to experience the most significant improvements. Herbal medicine often requires a commitment to consistent use over an extended period, as the effects of many herbs accumulate gradually. For instance, patients using turmeric for chronic inflammation or St. John's Wort for mild depression typically report better outcomes after several weeks of regular use. This underscores the importance of educating patients about the need for patience and perseverance when using herbal remedies.

Individual Variability in Response

Barbara has observed significant variability in how individuals respond to herbal treatments. Factors such as genetics, overall health, lifestyle, and even psychological state can influence the effectiveness of herbal remedies. For example, while one patient might experience rapid relief from anxiety with lavender tea, another might find better results with a different herb, such as passionflower. This variability highlights the necessity of personalized treatment plans and the need for ongoing monitoring and adjustments to optimize therapeutic outcomes.

Synergistic Effects of Herbal Combinations

Another key observation is the enhanced efficacy of combined herbal treatments. Synergy occurs when different herbs are used together to create a more potent therapeutic effect than when used individually. Barbara frequently formulates blends that address multiple aspects of a condition. For example, a blend of echinacea, elderberry, and ginger can provide comprehensive immune support during cold and flu season. This approach leverages the complementary actions of various herbs, resulting in more effective and holistic treatments.

Integration with Conventional Medicine

Barbara's practice has shown that herbal remedies can effectively complement conventional treatments, often enhancing overall outcomes and reducing side effects. For instance, patients undergoing chemotherapy have used ginger to manage nausea and turmeric to help mitigate inflammation. These integrative approaches require careful coordination with conventional healthcare providers to ensure safety and efficacy. Barbara emphasizes the importance of open communication and collaboration between herbalists and medical professionals to provide the best care for patients.

The Role of Lifestyle and Diet

Barbara's clinical experience underscores the critical role of lifestyle and dietary factors in the success of herbal treatments. Patients who make supportive lifestyle changes, such as improving their diet, engaging in regular physical activity, and managing stress, tend to see better results with herbal remedies. For example, incorporating anti-inflammatory foods alongside taking turmeric can enhance its benefits for arthritis. This holistic approach reinforces the idea that herbal medicine works best as part of a broader health and wellness strategy.

Safety and Side Effects

While herbal remedies are generally well-tolerated, Barbara has observed that side effects can occur, particularly when herbs are used improperly or in excessive amounts. Common side effects include gastrointestinal discomfort, allergic reactions, and interactions with conventional medications. These observations highlight the importance of professional guidance in herbal medicine. Barbara stresses the need for thorough patient assessment and education on proper usage to minimize risks and ensure safe, effective treatment.

Barbara O'Neill's clinical observations provide a rich source of knowledge on the practical applications and nuances of herbal medicine. Consistency in treatment, individual variability, the benefits of synergistic combinations, and the integration with conventional medicine are key themes that emerge from her practice. Additionally, the importance of lifestyle factors and the need for careful management of safety and side effects are critical considerations. These insights not only enhance the understanding and application of herbal remedies but also underscore the importance of a holistic, patient-centered approach in achieving optimal health outcomes.

BOOK 20:

Future Perspectives in Herbal Medicine: Introduction

Herbal medicine, with its deep historical roots and extensive body of traditional knowledge, continues to evolve and adapt in the modern era. As scientific research increasingly validates the efficacy and safety of various herbal remedies, the potential for integrating these natural treatments into mainstream healthcare grows. The future of herbal medicine holds exciting possibilities, driven by advances in technology, growing public interest in natural and holistic health, and the ongoing quest for more effective and sustainable medical solutions. This chapter will explore emerging trends and innovations, potential new discoveries, and the global impact of herbal medicine, offering a glimpse into the promising future of this ancient yet continually relevant field.

Emerging Trends and Innovations

Herbal medicine is experiencing a resurgence in interest and credibility, driven by emerging trends and innovations that are transforming how herbs are understood, utilized, and integrated into healthcare. These developments are not only enhancing the efficacy and safety of herbal treatments but also expanding their accessibility and application. Here are some of the key trends and innovations shaping the future of herbal medicine.

1. Scientific Validation and Research

The growing body of scientific research on herbal medicine is one of the most significant trends shaping the field. Advances in analytical techniques, such as high-performance liquid chromatography (HPLC) and mass spectrometry, allow for precise identification and quantification of bioactive compounds in herbs. This scientific validation helps to standardize herbal products, ensuring consistent quality and efficacy. Research studies and clinical trials are increasingly confirming the therapeutic benefits of herbs, such as the anti-inflammatory properties of turmeric and the cognitive benefits of ginkgo biloba, thereby integrating herbal medicine more firmly into evidence-based practice.

2. Personalized Herbal Medicine

Personalized medicine, which tailors treatments to an individual's genetic makeup, lifestyle, and health conditions, is gaining traction in the herbal medicine field. Advances in genomics and biotechnology are enabling the development of personalized herbal regimens that cater to specific individual needs. For example, genetic testing can identify predispositions to certain conditions, allowing for customized herbal formulations that optimize health outcomes. This trend toward personalization enhances the effectiveness of herbal treatments and minimizes potential side effects.

3. Integration with Conventional Medicine

The integration of herbal medicine with conventional healthcare is becoming more common, leading to a more holistic approach to patient care. Many healthcare providers now recognize the benefits of combining herbal remedies with conventional treatments to enhance therapeutic outcomes. This integrative approach is particularly beneficial in managing chronic conditions, such as combining turmeric with standard anti-inflammatory drugs to reduce joint pain in arthritis patients. Collaborative efforts between herbalists and medical professionals are fostering a more comprehensive healthcare model that addresses the whole person.

4. Technological Innovations

Technological advancements are revolutionizing the way herbal medicine is practiced and delivered. Mobile health apps and wearable devices can now monitor health metrics and track the effectiveness of herbal treatments in real-time, providing valuable feedback to both patients and practitioners. Online platforms and telehealth services are expanding access to herbal consultations and personalized recommendations, breaking down geographical barriers. Additionally, advances in biotechnology are leading to the development of novel herbal formulations and delivery systems, such as nanoencapsulation, which enhances the bioavailability and potency of herbal compounds.

5. Sustainable and Ethical Sourcing

The trend towards sustainability and ethical sourcing is increasingly influencing the herbal medicine industry. There is a growing awareness of the need to protect biodiversity and ensure the sustainable harvesting of medicinal plants. Ethical sourcing practices, such as fair trade and organic certification, are becoming more prevalent, ensuring that herbs are produced in a manner that respects both the environment and the communities involved in their cultivation.

This shift towards sustainability not only preserves valuable plant resources but also aligns with the holistic principles of herbal medicine.

6. Education and Public Awareness

Increased public awareness and education about the benefits and safe use of herbal medicine are driving greater acceptance and utilization of these natural remedies. Educational initiatives, including workshops, online courses, and informational campaigns, are empowering individuals to make informed decisions about their health. As more people become knowledgeable about the potential benefits and limitations of herbal medicine, the demand for high-quality, evidence-based herbal products continues to grow.

7. Regulatory Advancements

Improved regulatory frameworks are helping to ensure the safety, quality, and efficacy of herbal products. Regulatory agencies in many countries are developing guidelines and standards for the production, labeling, and marketing of herbal medicines. These regulations help protect consumers and enhance the credibility of herbal products in the market. The trend towards more stringent regulation is likely to continue, fostering greater trust and confidence in herbal medicine.

The field of herbal medicine is being transformed by a range of emerging trends and innovations, from scientific validation and personalized treatments to technological advancements and sustainable practices. These developments are enhancing the efficacy, safety, and accessibility of herbal remedies, paving the way for a more integrated and holistic approach to healthcare. As these trends continue to evolve, herbal medicine is poised to play an increasingly significant role in promoting health and well-being in the modern world.

Potential New Discoveries

The field of herbal medicine is ripe for new discoveries that promise to expand our understanding of plant-based remedies and their applications in modern healthcare. Advances in scientific research, technology, and global collaboration are paving the way for breakthroughs that could revolutionize herbal medicine. Here are some areas where potential new discoveries could significantly impact the field:

1. Novel Bioactive Compounds

One of the most exciting prospects in herbal medicine is the discovery of novel bioactive compounds. Many plants have yet to be fully explored for their medicinal properties, and new compounds with unique therapeutic effects are continually being identified. Advanced techniques in phytochemistry and molecular biology allow researchers to isolate and characterize these compounds more efficiently. These discoveries could lead to the development of new herbal treatments for a wide range of conditions, from chronic diseases to acute infections.

2. Enhanced Understanding of Synergy

Herbal medicine often relies on the synergistic effects of multiple compounds working together to produce therapeutic benefits. However, the mechanisms underlying these synergistic interactions are not fully understood. Future research could elucidate how different plant compounds interact at the molecular level, leading to more effective formulations. Understanding synergy could also help in identifying the optimal combinations of herbs and their dosages, enhancing the efficacy of herbal remedies.

3. Genomic Insights into Plant Medicine

Advances in genomics and biotechnology are opening new avenues for exploring the genetic basis of plant medicine. By sequencing the genomes of medicinal plants, researchers can identify genes responsible to produce bioactive compounds. This knowledge could facilitate the breeding of plants with enhanced medicinal properties or the development of bioengineered plants that produce higher concentrations of therapeutic compounds. Genomic insights could also help in understanding the variability in herbal efficacy among different plant species and cultivars.

4. Microbiome and Herbal Medicine

The human microbiome, the community of microorganisms living in and on our bodies, plays a crucial role in health and disease. Emerging research suggests that the microbiome may influence the effectiveness of herbal treatments. Certain herbs could modify the composition of the gut microbiota, enhancing their own therapeutic effects or those of other treatments. Future discoveries could uncover specific herbs that beneficially modulate the microbiome, leading to novel approaches in treating digestive disorders, metabolic conditions, and even mental health issues.

5. Sustainable and Ethical Harvesting Practices

As the demand for herbal medicine grows, so does the need for sustainable and ethical harvesting practices. Potential new discoveries in this area could include methods for cultivating endangered or overharvested medicinal plants in controlled environments, such as vertical farms or bioreactors. Innovations in sustainable agriculture and ethical sourcing could ensure a steady supply of high-quality herbs while preserving biodiversity and supporting local communities.

6. Herbal Medicine and Epigenetics

Epigenetics, the study of changes in gene expression that do not involve alterations to the DNA sequence, is a rapidly growing field with significant implications for herbal medicine. Future research could reveal how herbal compounds influence epigenetic mechanisms, potentially leading to new treatments for diseases with an epigenetic component, such as cancer, neurodegenerative disorders, and autoimmune diseases. Understanding the epigenetic effects of herbs could open up new therapeutic possibilities and personalized treatment strategies.

7. Integrating Artificial Intelligence in Herbal Research

Artificial intelligence (AI) and machine learning are revolutionizing many fields, including herbal medicine. AI can analyze large datasets from clinical trials, traditional knowledge databases, and phytochemical studies to identify patterns and predict the efficacy of herbal treatments. Potential new discoveries facilitated by AI could include identifying novel herbal combinations, optimizing dosages, and predicting patient responses based on genetic and lifestyle factors. AI could also streamline the drug discovery process, accelerating the development of new herbal-based therapeutics.

8. Expanding the Scope of Herbal Medicine

As global collaboration in herbal research increases, there is potential for discovering new medicinal plants from diverse ecosystems, such as rainforests, deserts, and marine environments. These unexplored regions may harbor plants with unique bioactive compounds that have yet to be recognized in traditional herbal medicine. By tapping into this global biodiversity, researchers could uncover new herbal remedies with significant therapeutic potential.

The future of herbal medicine is bright with the promise of new discoveries that could transform the field. From novel bioactive compounds and enhanced understanding of synergy to genomic insights and the integration of AI, these potential breakthroughs offer exciting possibilities for improving health and well-being through natural remedies. As research continues to advance, herbal medicine will likely become an even more integral part of holistic and integrative healthcare, providing safe, effective, and sustainable solutions for a wide range of health conditions.

Global Impact and Collaboration

The global impact of herbal medicine is profound, with traditional practices influencing modern healthcare systems worldwide. Collaboration across cultures, scientific disciplines, and international borders is enhancing the understanding and application of herbal remedies, leading to more integrative and effective healthcare solutions. This section explores the global impact of herbal medicine and the collaborative efforts driving its advancement.

1. Cultural Exchange and Knowledge Sharing

Herbal medicine has a rich history rooted in diverse cultures, each with its own unique practices and medicinal plants. The exchange of knowledge between different traditions—such as Traditional Chinese Medicine (TCM), Ayurveda, Native American healing, and African herbalism—has enriched the global understanding of herbal remedies. Collaborative research efforts and cultural exchanges have allowed for the sharing of traditional wisdom and practices, fostering a more comprehensive and diverse approach to herbal medicine.

For example, the integration of TCM and Western herbal practices has led to the development of new formulations and treatment protocols that combine the strengths of both systems. Such cross-cultural collaboration not only enhances the efficacy of herbal treatments but also promotes a deeper respect and appreciation for the world's medicinal heritage.

2. International Research Collaborations

International collaborations in herbal medicine research are critical for advancing the field. Researchers from different countries bring diverse perspectives, expertise, and resources, enabling more comprehensive studies and discoveries. Collaborative projects often involve universities, research institutions, and healthcare organizations working together to investigate the safety, efficacy, and mechanisms of herbal remedies.

One notable example is the global research on Artemisia annua (sweet wormwood), which led to the development of artemisinin-based therapies for malaria. This collaboration between Chinese scientists and international researchers resulted in life-saving treatments that are now used worldwide. Such partnerships demonstrate the potential of global collaboration in addressing major health challenges through herbal medicine.

3. Regulatory Harmonization

As herbal medicine gains popularity and acceptance, there is a growing need for regulatory harmonization to ensure the safety, quality, and efficacy of herbal products. International organizations, such as the World Health Organization (WHO), are working towards creating standardized guidelines and regulatory frameworks that can be adopted by countries around the world. These efforts aim to protect consumers, facilitate global trade in herbal products, and promote the integration of herbal medicine into conventional healthcare systems.

Harmonized regulations help prevent the circulation of substandard or adulterated herbal products, ensuring that consumers have access to high-quality and reliable remedies. This global approach to regulation supports the credibility and trust in herbal medicine, fostering its wider acceptance and use.

4. Sustainable Practices and Conservation

The global demand for herbal products has raised concerns about the sustainability and ethical sourcing of medicinal plants. Overharvesting, habitat destruction, and climate change threaten the availability of many important herbs. Collaborative efforts are essential to promote sustainable practices, conserve biodiversity, and ensure the long-term availability of medicinal plants.

International conservation projects, such as the FairWild Standard, aim to promote sustainable harvesting and fair-trade practices. By collaborating with local communities, governments, and businesses, these initiatives help protect endangered plant species, support sustainable livelihoods, and ensure the ethical sourcing of herbal ingredients. Such efforts are crucial for maintaining the ecological balance and preserving the rich biodiversity that herbal medicine depends on.

5. Integrative Healthcare Models

The global impact of herbal medicine is increasingly seen in integrative healthcare models that combine conventional and traditional treatments. Countries like China and India have long integrated herbal medicine into their national healthcare systems, offering patients a holistic approach to treatment. This model is gaining traction in other parts of the world, where healthcare providers recognize the benefits of combining evidence-based herbal remedies with conventional medical practices.

Integrative healthcare models emphasize patient-centered care, focusing on treating the whole person rather than just the symptoms. By incorporating herbal medicine, these models offer more comprehensive and personalized treatment options, improving patient outcomes and satisfaction. The success of integrative healthcare in various countries highlights the potential for global collaboration to enhance health systems worldwide.

6. Global Education and Training

Education and training programs play a pivotal role in the global impact of herbal medicine. By providing healthcare professionals with the knowledge and skills to safely and effectively use herbal remedies, these programs promote the integration of herbal medicine into mainstream healthcare. International partnerships between educational institutions facilitate the exchange of knowledge and best practices, ensuring that practitioners are well-equipped to meet the growing demand for herbal treatments.

Programs such as the International College of Herbal Medicine and the European Herbal & Traditional Medicine Practitioners Association offer certifications and training that adhere to high standards of practice. These initiatives help to professionalize the field of herbal medicine, fostering greater acceptance and integration into global healthcare systems.

The global impact of herbal medicine is vast, influencing healthcare practices and policies around the world. Through cultural exchange, international research collaborations, regulatory harmonization, sustainable practices, integrative healthcare models, and global education, herbal medicine continues to advance and integrate into modern healthcare. These collaborative efforts are essential for unlocking the full potential of herbal remedies, ensuring their safe and effective use, and promoting a more holistic and inclusive approach to health and well-being. As the world continues to embrace the benefits of herbal medicine, ongoing collaboration and innovation will be key to addressing future health challenges and improving global health outcomes.

Integrating Herbal Medicine with Conventional Treatments

The integration of herbal medicine with conventional treatments represents a significant advancement in holistic healthcare. This approach combines the strengths of traditional herbal remedies with modern medical practices to offer more comprehensive and personalized patient care. Integrating these two systems can enhance therapeutic outcomes, reduce side effects, and address complex health conditions more effectively. By leveraging the best of both worlds, healthcare providers can create synergistic treatment plans that optimize health and well-being. This chapter will explore the principles, benefits, and challenges of integrating herbal medicine with conventional treatments, providing insights into how these approaches can work together harmoniously in clinical practice.

Collaborative Approaches in Healthcare

Collaborative approaches in healthcare involve the seamless integration of herbal medicine and conventional treatments to provide holistic, patient-centered care. This integration requires cooperation among healthcare professionals, including doctors, herbalists, nutritionists, and other specialists, to ensure that patients receive comprehensive and effective treatment plans tailored to their unique needs.

Enhancing Patient Outcomes

One of the primary benefits of collaborative approaches is the potential to enhance patient outcomes. By combining the therapeutic strengths of herbal remedies with conventional medical treatments, healthcare providers can address multiple aspects of a patient's condition. For example, a patient undergoing chemotherapy for cancer might use ginger and turmeric to alleviate nausea and reduce inflammation, while conventional treatments target the cancer cells directly. This multifaceted approach can lead to better symptom management, improved quality of life, and potentially faster recovery times.

Reducing Side Effects

Many conventional treatments, such as pharmaceuticals and surgical interventions, can cause significant side effects. Herbal medicine can play a crucial role in mitigating these adverse effects. For instance, patients taking NSAIDs for chronic pain might experience gastrointestinal discomfort, which can be alleviated with herbal remedies like slippery elm or marshmallow root. By reducing side effects, patients are more likely to adhere to their treatment plans and experience fewer complications, ultimately leading to better health outcomes.

Promoting Preventive Care

Herbal medicine is often focused on preventive care and maintaining overall health, which complements the more reactive nature of conventional medicine. Integrating herbal practices into conventional healthcare can encourage a more proactive approach to health. For example, incorporating herbs like echinacea and elderberry into a patient's routine during flu season can boost the immune system and reduce the likelihood of illness. This preventive strategy not only improves individual health but also reduces the burden on healthcare systems by decreasing the incidence of preventable diseases.

Education and Training

Successful integration of herbal and conventional medicine requires comprehensive education and training for healthcare providers. Medical professionals need to be informed about the benefits, mechanisms, and potential interactions of herbal remedies. Similarly, herbalists must understand the principles and practices of conventional medicine. Collaborative educational programs and interdisciplinary training can bridge this knowledge gap, fostering mutual respect and understanding between practitioners. Institutions that offer integrative medicine courses or certifications help equip healthcare providers with the necessary skills to combine these approaches effectively.

Patient-Centered Care

Collaborative approaches emphasize patient-centered care, focusing on treating the whole person rather than just the disease. This holistic perspective considers the physical, emotional, and social aspects of health, providing more personalized and empathetic care. Patients are encouraged to participate actively in their treatment plans, making informed decisions about their health in consultation with their healthcare team. This empowerment can lead to greater patient satisfaction, adherence to treatment, and overall well-being.

Challenges and Considerations

Despite the benefits, integrating herbal medicine with conventional treatments presents several challenges. One major concern is the potential for herb-drug interactions, which can affect the efficacy and safety of treatments. Healthcare providers must thoroughly review a patient's medication and herbal supplement history to identify and manage any potential interactions. Additionally, regulatory differences and varying levels of evidence for herbal remedies can complicate their integration into conventional practice. Standardized guidelines and more robust clinical research are needed to address these issues and ensure the safe and effective use of herbal medicine.

Collaborative approaches in healthcare that integrate herbal medicine with conventional treatments offer a promising path toward more holistic, effective, and patient-centered care. By enhancing patient outcomes, reducing side effects, promoting preventive care, and emphasizing education and patient involvement, this integrative model can significantly improve healthcare delivery. Overcoming the challenges and fostering collaboration among healthcare professionals will be essential to realizing the full potential of this approach, ultimately leading to better health and well-being for patients.

Ensuring Safety and Efficacy

Integrating herbal medicine with conventional treatments requires careful consideration to ensure both safety and efficacy. This process involves thorough research, professional collaboration, and stringent regulatory standards to protect patient health and optimize therapeutic outcomes. Here are several key strategies to ensure the safe and effective use of herbal remedies in conjunction with conventional treatments.

Comprehensive Patient Assessment

A detailed patient assessment is crucial for identifying potential risks and benefits of integrating herbal medicine into a treatment plan. Healthcare providers should obtain a comprehensive medical history, including current medications, herbal supplements, dietary habits, and any known allergies or sensitivities. Understanding a patient's overall health status, lifestyle, and specific health concerns allows practitioners to tailor treatment plans that minimize risks and maximize therapeutic benefits.

Evidence-Based Practice

The integration of herbal medicine with conventional treatments should be grounded in evidence-based practice. This involves using the best available research to guide clinical decision-making. Healthcare providers must stay informed about the latest studies and clinical trials evaluating the efficacy and safety of herbal remedies. By relying on scientifically validated information, practitioners can make informed choices about which herbal treatments are appropriate and effective for their patients.

Monitoring for Herb-Drug Interactions

One of the primary concerns in integrating herbal medicine with conventional treatments is the potential for herb-drug interactions. Some herbs can alter the metabolism of pharmaceutical drugs, leading to reduced efficacy or increased risk of adverse effects. For example, St. John's Wort can decrease the effectiveness of oral contraceptives and certain antidepressants. To prevent such interactions, healthcare providers must carefully review a patient's medication and herbal supplement regimen. They should use reliable interaction databases and consult with pharmacists or other specialists when necessary.

Standardization and Quality Control

Ensuring the quality and consistency of herbal products is essential for their safe and effective use. Standardization involves maintaining consistent levels of active ingredients in herbal products, which helps achieve predictable therapeutic outcomes. Reputable manufacturers should adhere to good manufacturing practices (GMP) and undergo third-party testing to verify the potency and purity of their products. Healthcare providers should recommend high-quality, standardized herbal supplements to their patients to avoid variability and contamination issues.

Patient Education and Informed Consent

Educating patients about the potential benefits and risks of herbal medicine is a key component of ensuring safety and efficacy. Patients should be informed about the proper use of herbal remedies, including dosages, administration methods, and possible side effects. Providing clear instructions and setting realistic expectations can enhance adherence and reduce the likelihood of misuse. Additionally, obtaining informed consent is essential, ensuring that patients understand and agree to the integrated treatment plan.

Collaborative Care and Communication

Effective communication and collaboration among healthcare providers are vital for the safe integration of herbal medicine with conventional treatments. Physicians, herbalists, pharmacists, and other healthcare professionals should work together to develop and monitor treatment plans. Regular communication helps identify potential issues early and allows for timely adjustments. Collaborative care ensures that all aspects of a patient's health are considered, promoting a holistic and coordinated approach to treatment.

Regulatory Oversight

Robust regulatory oversight is necessary to ensure the safety and efficacy of herbal products. Regulatory agencies, such as the Food and Drug Administration (FDA) in the United States and the European Medicines Agency (EMA) in Europe, play a critical role in monitoring and regulating herbal supplements. These agencies set standards for manufacturing practices, labeling, and marketing to protect consumers from unsafe or misleading products. Healthcare providers should advocate for and support policies that strengthen regulatory oversight and ensure the availability of safe and effective herbal remedies.

Ongoing Research and Development

Continuous research and development are essential for advancing the field of herbal medicine and integrating it safely with conventional treatments. Clinical trials, pharmacological studies, and real-world evidence contribute to a deeper understanding of herbal medicine's therapeutic potential and limitations. Ongoing research can identify new applications for herbal remedies, optimize dosages, and uncover previously unknown interactions. By supporting and participating in research initiatives, healthcare providers can contribute to the evolving knowledge base of herbal medicine.

Ensuring the safety and efficacy of integrating herbal medicine with conventional treatments requires a multifaceted approach. Comprehensive patient assessment, evidence-based practice, monitoring for interactions, standardization and quality control, patient education, collaborative care, regulatory oversight, and ongoing research are all critical components. By implementing these strategies, healthcare providers can offer safe, effective, and holistic care that leverages the benefits of both herbal and conventional medicine, ultimately improving patient outcomes and well-being.

Educational Initiatives

Educational initiatives are crucial for fostering the safe and effective integration of herbal medicine with conventional treatments. These initiatives aim to equip healthcare professionals, students, and the public with the knowledge and skills necessary to utilize herbal remedies responsibly and effectively. By promoting a deeper understanding of herbal medicine, these programs enhance patient care, support professional development, and encourage informed decision-making. Here are several key educational initiatives that can contribute to the integration of herbal medicine into mainstream healthcare.

Professional Training Programs

1. Integrative Medicine Courses: Integrative medicine courses offer comprehensive training on combining herbal and conventional treatments. These programs, often available through medical schools, universities, and specialized institutions, cover topics such as herbal pharmacology, evidence-based practice, and patient management. By providing healthcare professionals with a solid foundation in both conventional and herbal medicine, these courses promote a holistic approach to patient care.

2. Continuing Education for Healthcare Providers: Continuing education programs specifically designed for healthcare providers, such as doctors, nurses, and pharmacists, ensure that they stay updated on the latest research and best practices in herbal medicine. Workshops, seminars, and online courses can cover a wide range of topics, from identifying herb-drug interactions to developing personalized herbal treatment plans. These programs help practitioners integrate herbal remedies into their clinical practice safely and effectively.

3. Certification and Accreditation: Certification programs for herbalists and integrative medicine practitioners establish standards of competence and professionalism. Accredited certification programs, such as those offered by the American Herbalists Guild (AHG) or the European Herbal & Traditional Medicine Practitioners Association (EHTPA), provide rigorous training and assessment. Certification ensures that practitioners meet high standards of knowledge and practice, fostering trust and confidence in their services.

Interdisciplinary Collaboration and Training

1. Collaborative Workshops: Interdisciplinary workshops that bring together professionals from various healthcare fields—such as physicians, herbalists, dietitians, and mental health practitioners—promote collaboration and knowledge exchange. These workshops can focus on case studies, integrated treatment strategies, and emerging research, fostering a team-based approach to patient care.

2. Joint Research Initiatives: Collaborative research initiatives between conventional medical institutions and herbal medicine schools can enhance the evidence base for herbal treatments. Joint research projects and clinical trials can investigate the efficacy and safety of herbal remedies, leading to more informed and integrated healthcare practices. These initiatives also provide valuable learning opportunities for students and professionals involved in the research.

Public Education and Awareness

1. Community Outreach Programs: Community outreach programs aim to educate the public about the benefits and safe use of herbal medicine. Workshops, health fairs, and seminars can provide practical information on how to incorporate herbs into daily health routines, understand potential interactions, and select high-quality products. These programs empower individuals to make informed decisions about their health and wellness.

2. Online Resources and Platforms: The internet offers a wealth of resources for public education on herbal medicine. Websites, webinars, and online courses can provide accessible and reliable information on various herbs, their uses, and safety considerations. Trusted platforms like the National Center for Complementary and Integrative Health (NCCIH) and the American Botanical Council offer valuable resources for both professionals and the general public.

3. Educational Campaigns: Public awareness campaigns can highlight the benefits of herbal medicine and promote safe practices. These campaigns can use various media, including social media, print, and television, to reach a broad audience. Campaigns might focus on themes such as "Herbal Medicine for Immune Health" or "Safe Use of Herbal Supplements," providing practical tips and guidance.

Integrating Herbal Medicine into Healthcare Curriculum

1. Medical School Curriculum: Incorporating herbal medicine into the medical school curriculum ensures that future healthcare providers have a basic understanding of herbal remedies. Courses on integrative medicine, pharmacognosy, and complementary therapies can provide medical students with the knowledge needed to safely recommend and manage herbal treatments in their practice.

2. Herbal Medicine Degrees and Programs: Universities and colleges offering degrees and programs in herbal medicine provide in-depth training for those seeking to specialize in this field. These programs cover botany, phytochemistry, clinical herbalism, and holistic health practices, preparing graduates for careers as professional herbalists or integrative medicine practitioners.

Educational initiatives are essential for promoting the safe and effective integration of herbal medicine with conventional treatments. By providing comprehensive training for healthcare professionals, fostering interdisciplinary collaboration, educating the public, and integrating herbal medicine into healthcare curricula, these initiatives enhance the knowledge and skills needed to utilize herbal remedies responsibly. Through these efforts, healthcare providers can offer more holistic and personalized care, improving patient outcomes and advancing the field of herbal medicine.

The Evolution of Barbara O'Neill's Theories and Practices

Barbara O'Neill, a renowned naturopath and health educator, has made significant contributions to the field of herbal medicine and natural health through her innovative theories and practical approaches. Her journey in natural health has been marked by a continuous evolution of her theories and practices, influenced by extensive research, clinical experiences, and a deep understanding of the body's natural healing mechanisms. This section explores the key phases in the evolution of Barbara O'Neill's theories and practices.

Early Foundations: Emphasis on Natural Healing

Barbara O'Neill's initial interest in natural health was sparked by her personal experiences and observations of the limitations of conventional medicine. She began her journey by studying traditional herbal medicine, nutrition, and the body's innate ability to heal itself. Her early theories emphasized the importance of natural remedies and the role of nutrition in maintaining health and preventing disease. Barbara believed that many common health issues could be addressed through dietary changes, detoxification, and the use of herbal remedies.

Development of Holistic Health Principles

As Barbara's knowledge and experience grew, she developed a more holistic approach to health and wellness. She recognized that true healing involves addressing the physical, emotional, and spiritual aspects of a person. This holistic perspective led her to integrate various natural therapies, including herbal medicine, nutrition, hydrotherapy, and lifestyle modifications. Barbara's holistic health principles emphasize the interconnectedness of the body's systems and the need for a balanced approach to achieve optimal health.

Integration of Scientific Research

Throughout her career, Barbara O'Neill has placed a strong emphasis on evidence-based practice. She continually incorporates scientific research into her theories and practices, ensuring that her recommendations are grounded in the latest scientific findings. This integration of research has allowed Barbara to refine her approach, identifying the most effective herbs and natural therapies for specific conditions. Her commitment to evidence-based practice has also enhanced the credibility of her work, bridging the gap between traditional herbal medicine and modern science.

Focus on Preventive Care

A significant evolution in Barbara's theories and practices is her focus on preventive care. She advocates for a proactive approach to health, emphasizing the importance of maintaining a healthy lifestyle to prevent disease. Barbara's preventive care strategies include regular detoxification, a nutrient-rich diet, stress management, and the use of herbal remedies to support the immune system and overall well-being. This preventive focus is designed to empower individuals to take control of their health and reduce the risk of chronic diseases.

Personalized Medicine

Barbara O'Neill has also embraced the concept of personalized medicine, recognizing that each individual's health needs are unique. Her personalized approach involves tailoring treatment plans to address the specific conditions, lifestyle, and genetic factors of each patient. By combining comprehensive health assessments with customized herbal and nutritional therapies, Barbara aims to achieve the best possible outcomes for her patients. This personalized approach reflects a deeper understanding of the variability in individual responses to treatments and the need for tailored interventions.

Advocacy for Education and Empowerment

Education and empowerment are central to Barbara O'Neill's philosophy. She believes that individuals should be well-informed about their health and the natural options available to them. Barbara has dedicated much of her career to educating the public and healthcare professionals through workshops, seminars, books, and online content. Her educational efforts aim to demystify herbal medicine and natural health, making it accessible and understandable to a broad audience. By empowering individuals with knowledge, Barbara encourages proactive and informed health decisions.

Embracing Technological Advances

In recent years, Barbara O'Neill has incorporated technological advances into her practice. She leverages digital platforms to reach a wider audience, offering online courses, webinars, and virtual consultations. Technology has enabled Barbara to share her expertise globally, providing valuable resources and support to individuals seeking natural health solutions. Additionally, she uses advanced diagnostic tools and biofeedback technologies to enhance her assessments and treatment plans, integrating traditional wisdom with modern innovation.

Conclusion

The evolution of Barbara O'Neill's theories and practices reflects her commitment to advancing the field of herbal medicine and natural health. From her early emphasis on natural healing to her holistic, evidence-based, and personalized approach, Barbara has continuously refined her methods to provide the most effective and comprehensive care. Her focus on preventive care, education, and the integration of scientific research and technology has solidified her reputation as a leading figure in natural health. Barbara O'Neill's journey exemplifies the dynamic nature of natural medicine, demonstrating how traditional practices can evolve and thrive in the modern healthcare landscape.